Handbook ...nce ...ics

Handbook of Sports Medicine and Science

Gymnastics

EDITED BY

Dennis J. Caine, PhD

Professor and Interim Dean
College of Education and Human Development
University of North Dakota
Grand Forks, ND, USA

Keith Russell, PhD

President
Scientific Commission
Federation Internationale de Gymnastique (FIG);
Professor, College of Kinesiology
University of Saskatchewan
Saskatoon, SK, Canada

Liesbeth Lim, MD

Former National Sports Physician of the Royal Dutch Gymnastics Federation, 1997–2012;
Sports Physician, Sports Medical Advice Center Aalsmeer
Aalsmeer;
Sports Medical Advice Center Annatommie (Centers for Orthopedics and Movement)
Amsterdam, The Netherlands

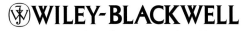

A John Wiley & Sons, Ltd., Publication

This edition first published 2013, © 2013 International Olympic Committee
Published by John Wiley & Sons, Ltd

Wiley-Blackwell is an imprint of John Wiley & Sons, formed by the merger of Wiley's global Scientific, Technical and Medical business with Blackwell Publishing.

Registered office:
John Wiley & Sons, Ltd, The Atrium, Southern Gate, Chichester, West Sussex, PO19 8SQ, UK

Editorial offices:
9600 Garsington Road, Oxford, OX4 2DQ, UK
The Atrium, Southern Gate, Chichester, West Sussex, PO19 8SQ, UK
111 River Street, Hoboken, NJ 07030-5774, USA

For details of our global editorial offices, for customer services and for information about how to apply for permission to reuse the copyright material in this book please see our website at www.wiley.com/wiley-blackwell

Library of Congress Cataloging-in-Publication Data
Gymnastics / edited by Dennis J. Caine, PhD, Keith Russell, PhD, Liesbeth Lim, MD.
     pages cm — (Handbook of sports medicine and science)
  Includes bibliographical references and index.
  ISBN 978-1-118-35758-3 (softback : alk. paper)—ISBN 978-1-118-35753-8—
ISBN 978-1-118-35754-5 (mobi)—ISBN 978-1-118-35756-9 (pdf)—
ISBN 978-1-118-35757-6 (pub) 1. Gymnastics. 2. Gymnastics injuries. 3. Gymnasts—Health and hygiene.
4. Sports medicine. I. Caine, Dennis John, 1949- II. Russell, Keith, 1944- III. Lim, Liesbeth.
  RC1220.G95G96 2013
  617.1'027644—dc23

                                                      2013007055

A catalogue record for this book is available from the British Library.

Wiley also publishes its books in a variety of electronic formats. Some content that appears in print may not be available in electronic books.

Cover image: Main image: © 2012 / Comité International Olympique (CIO) / HUET, John.
              Background image: © 2012 / Comité International Olympique (CIO) / HUET, John.

Cover design by OptaDesign.co.uk

Set in ITC Stone Serif Std 8.75/12pt by Aptara Inc., New Delhi, India
Printed and bound in Malaysia by Vivar Printing Sdn Bhd

1 2013

Contents

List of Contributors

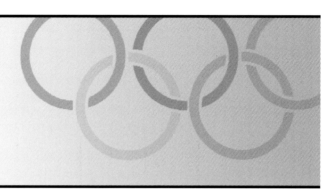

Stephen Aldridge, MA, MD
Consultant Orthopaedic Surgeon, Royal Victoria
Infirmary; Associate Clinical Lecturer, Newcastle
University, Newcastle upon Tyne, UK *and* Doctor,
British Gymnastics, Newport, UK

Neil Armstrong, PhD, DSc, DHC
Senior Deputy Vice-Chancellor, Professor of Paediatric
Physiology, Children's Health and Exercise Research
Centre, University of Exeter, Exeter, UK

Adam D.G. Baxter-Jones, PhD
Member Scientific Commission, Federation
Internationale de Gymnastique (FIG), Lausanne,
Switzerland *and* Acting Dean College of Graduate
Studies and Research and Professor of Kinesiology,
University of Saskatchewan, Saskatoon, SK, Canada

Elizabeth J. Bradshaw, PhD
Senior Lecturer, Centre for Physical Activity Across
the Lifespan, School of Exercise Science, Australian
Catholic University, Melbourne, VIC, Australia

Gert-Peter Brueggemann, PhD
Professor of Biomechanics and Head of Department,
Institute of Biomechanics and Orthopaedics, German
Sport University Cologne, Cologne, Germany

Dennis J. Caine, PhD
Professor and Interim Dean, College of Education and
Human Development, University of North Dakota,
Grand Forks, ND, USA

Daniel Courteix, PhD
Professor, Laboratory AME2P, Metabolic Adaptations to
Exercise in Physiological and Pathological Conditions,
Aubière Cedex, France *and* School of Exercise Science,
Australian Catholic University, Fitzroy, VIC, Australia

John S. Fuqua, MD
Professor of Clinical Pediatrics, Section of Pediatric
Endocrinology, Indiana University School of Medicine,
Indianapolis, IN, USA

Ina Garthe, PhD
Sports Nutrition Department, The Norwegian Olympic
and Paralympic Committee and Confederation of
Sport, Oslo, Norway

David Greene, PhD (ACU),
Deputy Head of School (NSW) and Senior Lecturer,
School of Exercise Science, Australian Catholic
University, Strathfield, NSW, Australia

Marita L. Harringe, PhD, PT
Lecturer, Department of Molecular Medicine and
Surgery, Stockholm Sports Trauma Research Center,
and Department of Neurobiology, Care Sciences
and Society, Division of Physiotherapy, Karolinska
Institutet, Stockholm, Sweden

Thomas Heinen, PhD
Visiting Professor, Institute of Sport Science, University
of Hildesheim, Hildesheim, Germany *and* Member of the
Scientific Commission of the Federation Internationale
de Gymnastique (FIG), Lausanne, Switzerland

Patria A. Hume, PhD
Professor Human Performance, Sport Performance Research Institute and Faculty of Health and Environmental Sciences, Auckland University of Technology, Auckland, New Zealand

Liesbeth Lim, MD
Former National Sports Physician of the Royal Dutch Gymnastics Federation, 1997–2012; Sports Physician, Sports Medical Advice Center Aalsmeer, Aalsmeer and Sports Medical Advice Center Annatommie (Centers for Orthopedics and Movement), Amsterdam, The Netherlands

Nanna Meyer, PhD, RD, CD
Assistant Professor, Beth-El College of Nursing and Health Sciences, University of Colorado and Senior Sport Dietitian, United States Olympic Committee, Colorado Springs, CO, USA

Larry Nassar, DO
USA Gymnastics National Medical Coordinator and Associate Professor and Team Physician, Department of Radiology, College of Osteopathic Medicine, Michigan State University, East Lansing, MI, USA

Geraldine Naughton, PhD
Professor of Paediatric Exercise Science, Director, Centre of Physical Activity Across the Lifespan, School of Exercise Science, Australian Catholic University, Fitzroy, VIC, Australia

Alan D. Rogol, MD, PhD
Professor of Clinical Pediatrics, Department of Pediatrics, Riley Hospital for Children, Indiana University School of Medicine, Indianapolis, IN,

and Professor Emeritus, University of Virginia, Charlottesville, VA, USA

Keith Russell, PhD
President, Scientific Commission, Federation Internationale de Gymnastique (FIG), Lausanne, Switzerland and Professor, College of Kinesiology, University of Saskatchewan, Saskatoon, SK, Canada

N.C. Craig Sharp, BVMS, PhD, DSc
Emeritus Professor of Sports Science, Centre for Sports Medicine and Human Performance, Brunel University, Uxbridge, UK

Jorunn Sundgot-Borgen, PhD
Professor, Department of Sports Medicine, The Norwegian School of Sports Science, Oslo, Norway

Konstantinos Velentzas, PhD
Lecturer, Department of Sport Science, Bielefeld University, Bielefield, Germany

Pia M. Vinken, Dipl Sport Sci, Expert Degree in Sportpsychology and Sportphysiotherapy
Lecturer, Institute for Sport Teaching Skills, German Sport University Cologne, Cologne and Lecturer, Institute of Sport Science, Leibniz University, Hanover, Germany

W. Jaap Willems, MD, PhD
Consultant Orthopaedic Surgeon, Shoulder/Elbow Unit Onze Lieve Vrouwe Gasthuis/de Lairesse Kliniek, Amsterdam, The Netherlands

Foreword by Dr Jacques Rogge

The various events of gymnastics have been important features of the Olympic Summer Games ever since the birth of the modern Olympic Movement at the 1896 Summer Games in Athens. The *Fédération Internationale de Gymnastique* (FIG) has been the governing body of competitive gymnastics since its foundation in 1881 and it is universally recognized as the oldest international sports organisation. Therefore, it is entirely appropriate that gymnastics is being added to the "Handbooks of Sports Medicine and Science" series published by the IOC Medical Commission.

The co-editors, Prof. Dennis Caine (USA), Prof. Keith Russell (Canada), and Dr Liesbeth Lim (The Netherlands), have developed a comprehensive outline and assembled a group of contributing authors who possess impressive credentials as regards experience, expertise, and authority, while working with athletes competing in gymnastics.

A wealth of information is presented by international authorities on the biological considerations of growth and maturation of the athletes. Extensive consideration is given to the issues of endocrinology, skeletal health, body mass management, and nutritional and energy needs. The biomechanical factors involved in injury and their roles as risk factors are emphasized. The final section includes the epidemiology of gymnastic injury, injury prevention, and the treatment and rehabilitation of injuries for the extremities, spine, trunk, and head. The comprehensive coverage is highly commendable.

We welcome this splendid addition to the Handbooks of Sports Medicine and Science series.

Jacques Rogge
IOC President

Foreword by Professor Bruno Grandi

Since the day I first stepped through the door of a gymnastics hall, I have intimately followed the evolution of the discipline from an educational and athletic standpoint. Some 60 years have afforded me an opportunity to familiarize myself with every area of the discipline—as a gymnast, coach, and judge—before ultimately occupying its highest administrative and political positions.

Well do I understand the emotion and sense of awe that permeate competitions, and I continue to be so inspired today. But that is just a small part of my interest in gymnastics. My loyalties have long been with the educational side of the discipline, and it is a joy for me to see this book published.

Today, more than ever before, people suffer from a lack of well-being that is noticeable at every level of society, particularly in the most developed countries. May this publication pave the way to finding solutions that our specialists can then pass on to the population. Growth, development, training, nutrition, and prevention: all issues are dealt with in this book, which at the same time reports on a certain state of affairs and brings field-specific knowledge to the cutting edge.

On behalf of the entire international gymnastics community, the FIG authorities, and our many gymnasts, I would like to extend my gratitude and compliments to the authors. Their contribution to the study and research of sustainable solutions is inestimable, for the greatest aspiration of any individual is his psychological and physical well-being.

With my compliments,

Prof. Bruno Grandi, President
Fédération Internationale de Gymnastique

Preface

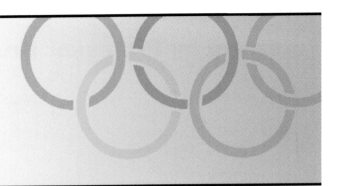

The Olympic sports of Artistic Gymnastics, Rhythmic Gymnastics, and Trampoline Gymnastics are very popular worldwide as evidenced by the extensive media attention surrounding the Olympics every 4 years. Gymnastics is a sport that is well known for its intense training regimen and, particularly among female gymnasts, the relatively young age of its participants. Extraordinary levels of athleticism and biomechanical loading during training and competition are characteristic of these sports. Participation in gymnastics is encouraging because physical activity clearly provides many health-related benefits to those who participate. However, increased involvement and difficulty of skills practiced at an early age, with the intense training required, exposes gymnasts to high performance demands and risk of injury. Our hope is to provide the reader with useful information to assist in the management and minimization of the risks associated with participation in gymnastics, and information that also optimizes the health and competitive performance of gymnasts.

The Handbook of Sports Medicine is an ongoing series of specialist reference volumes sponsored by the International Olympic Committee (IOC) and designed specifically for the use of professionals working directly with competitive athletes. The target groups for whom this handbook is written includes (1) interested medical doctors who have little or no training in sports medicine, as well as sports medicine professionals; (2) physiotherapists and other health-related professionals; (3) team coaches who have academic preparation in the basic sciences; and (4) knowledgeable gymnasts. The purpose of this volume is to present a comprehensive, state-of-the-art description of the medical and scientific aspects of Olympic gymnastics sports.

Part 1 of the book provides an introduction and information related to the evolution of gymnastics. Part 2 focuses on the growth and development aspects of gymnasts and includes chapters on growth and development, endocrinology, skeletal health of gymnasts, and energy needs and body weight management for gymnasts. Part 3 includes several chapters dealing with the training and performance aspects of gymnasts including gymnastics-specific biomechanics, physiology, and psychology. Finally, Part 4 deals with the sports medicine aspects of gymnastics. Chapters in this section include injury epidemiology, treatment and rehabilitation of common upper extremity injuries, treatment and rehabilitation of common lower extremity injuries, treatment and rehabilitation of common spine/trunk/head injuries, and a chapter on injury prevention.

From the outset, the editors worked to develop a plan for the book and uniformity across chapters. In November 2011, the co-editors met in Boston with Dr Howard Knuttgen, Harvard Medical School and Coordinator for Scientific Publications for the IOC, to develop an outline for the book and an approach that was consistent with other volumes in the IOC Handbook series. Each chapter in the book follows the same major sections:

- Introduction
- Review of the literature (using topic headings specific to the chapter subject)
- Further research
- Summary
- References
- Recommended reading

The number of references in each chapter is purposely limited given that the intent of each chapter, as far as possible, is to focus on generally accepted principles and more recent publications, yet including highly regarded older publications.

In closing, we wish to thank the authors for working diligently to provide up-to-date chapters, and to develop text consistent in format across the various chapters. We would also like to thank Dr Howard Knuttgen for his enthusiastic support and guidance throughout this project, as well as the Medical and Scientific Department of the IOC and the International Gymnastics Federation (FIG) for their enthusiastic support. Finally, we wish to thank the production and editorial team at Wiley-Blackwell for their helpful assistance and collaboration throughout this project.

Dennis J. Caine, PhD
Keith Russell, PhD
Liesbeth Lim, MD
2013

PART 1
INTRODUCTION

Chapter 1
The evolution of gymnastics

Keith Russell

Federation Internationale de Gymnastique (FIG), Lausanne, Switzerland *and*
College of Kinesiology, University of Saskatchewan, Saskatoon, SK, Canada

For most readers, the name "gymnastics" brings to mind those Olympic sports that gain wide media attention every 4 years. These include Men's Artistic Gymnastics (with its six apparatuses: floor exercise, pommel horse, rings, vault, parallel bars, and horizontal bar); Women's Artistic Gymnastics (with its four apparatuses: asymmetric bars, balance beam, vault, and floor exercise); Rhythmic Gymnastics with its lithe, flexible female gymnasts doing incredible manipulative skills with hand apparatus; and, of course, the acrobatically spectacular sport of Trampoline Gymnastics (TG). Collectively, these sports represent a very small percentage of the total gymnastics community. There are, in addition, several non-Olympic sports including Aerobic Gymnastics and Acrobatic Gymnastics plus a large family of recreational, educational, and exhibition forms of gymnastics that are grouped under the moniker Gymnastics for All. The word "gymnastics" comes to us from the ancient Greek verb "gymnazo" meaning to train naked, which is how young men in the 7th to 3rd centuries BC practiced the physical health and fitness part of their education in the outdoor "gymnasion," supervised by the trainers or "gymnastēs." The aristocratic young men devoted considerable time to practicing various athletic endeavors to be contested at religious festivals. They also received education in music, letters, and philosophy.

The word "gymnastics" is today an umbrella term, much the same as "aquatics," in that it encompasses not only a group of competitive sports but also many less formalized gymnastics activities in the fields of education, recreation, and fitness (Figure 1.1). These noncompetitive forms of gymnastics are showcased every year in gym festivals in many countries, some with over 100,000 participants. There is also the World Gymnaestrada held every fourth year with 20,000 participants. The Fédération Internationale de Gymnastique (FIG) is the world's oldest international sport governing body (incorporated in 1881 as the Fédération Européenne de Gymnastique) and has a contemporary stable of sports that includes the four Olympic sports plus two non-Olympic multicategory sports of Acrobatic Gymnastics and Aerobic Gymnastics. In addition, there are three competitive subdisciplines of TG that are not contested in the Olympic Games but are included in all other TG competitions: Tumbling, Double Mini-Trampoline, and Synchronized Trampoline.

Gymnastics-type movement was performed in the ancient Chinese, Mesopotamian, Indian, and Mediterranean cultures, which all left ample records of the importance they placed on this type of physical exercise and body movement. It was the Greeks of the Homeric and Classical eras, however, who had the most lasting influence on subsequent educational and medical gymnastics practice. Their emphasis on mind/body integration in the education of their youth would greatly influence educators 18 centuries later. Plato, whose original name

Gymnastics, First Edition. Edited by Dennis J. Caine, Keith Russell and Liesbeth Lim. © 2013 International Olympic Committee. Published 2013 by John Wiley & Sons, Ltd.

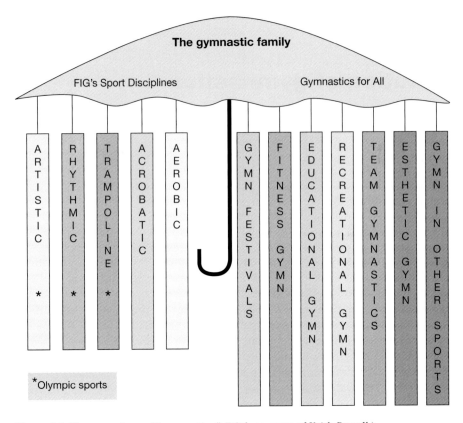

Figure 1.1 The many faces of "gymnastics." (With courtesy of Keith Russell.)

was believed to be Aristocles, was given the name Plato by his "gymnastai" Ariston of Argos because he had a broad (platon) and athletic chest (Yiannakis and Yiannakis, 1998).

The Romans followed the Greeks and continued many of their practices, but with more military emphasis. After the classical Greek era, the ensuing 10 centuries (the Middle Ages) had very little emphasis on sport, games, or the practice of integrating the mind and the body in education as extolled by the Greeks. It was not until the 1400s that we see a shift in thinking and a rebirth of the educational concepts introduced many centuries before by the Greeks. Let us trace how the contemporary sports and activities of gymnastics have coalesced via a fascinating and long journey through four primary ancestries: (1) the performing arts, (2) military training, (3) the medical professions, and (4) the education professions.

Gymnastics evolution from the performing arts

The earliest pictorial references to gymnastics activities come from paintings and engravings at several Egyptian sites. Most of them depict female performers tumbling and balancing and are dated from 2300 to 1000 BC (Touney, 1984). The tombs at Beni-Hassen show tumbling and ball passing and juggling skills that are surprisingly comparable to the contemporary sports of Tumbling and Rhythmic Gymnastics (Figure 1.2).

Around the same time, the Minoans, another great Mediterranean society centered on Crete, left many pictorial examples of performers vaulting and performing acrobatics on large adult bulls. Both male and female acrobats are illustrated and they appear to be paid professional performers (Gardiner, 1930). It would appear that subsequent

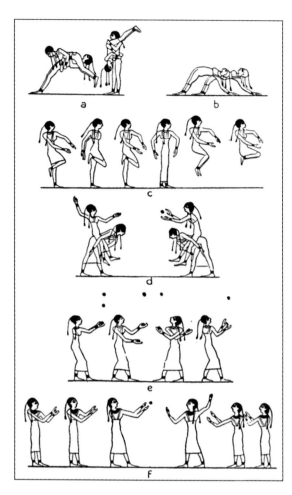

Figure 1.2 Ancient Egyptian gymnasts from tombs at Beni-Hassen (Source: Gardiner, E., Athletics in the Ancient World (1990) with permission from Oxford University Press.)

societies on mainland Greece took much of their reverence of athleticism and physical fitness from the Minoans and it became an integral part of Greek education. The Homeric poems describe Corfu artists combining acrobatics and dance with ball and musical accompaniment (Frantzopoulou *et al.*, 2011).

When we follow acrobatic performances through history, there is a clear thread of continuity running through them. The performances were often combined with dance and musical accompaniment, and are depicted in illustrations and text in both Western and Eastern civilizations. Chinese stone carvings from 1000 BC as well as 3rd century BC writing described acrobatic performances. By the

1st century BC, a combination of dance, acrobatics, and music called Juedixi was very popular in China. The circuses, traveling minstrel shows, and court performers throughout the world contained acrobatic performers and they often used a variety of devices to extend the acrobats' time in the air. The ancient Minoans used the momentum from grasping a bull's horns while being tossed in the air, while the Inuit of northern Canada used skins stretched between several throwers to toss one member high in the air to better see distant animals and also to entertain during celebratory events. The tossing of one acrobat by one or more others has a long tradition that continues in today's Acrobatic Gymnastics. Many aerial enhancement devices like teeterboards, Russian swings, trapezes, and contemporary devices like Double Mini-Trampoline and Trampoline have a clear genesis in the performing arts, and circuses had such devices that allowed performers to be propelled into the air. American inventor and performer George Nissen used his springing invention in a three-person traveling "rebound tumbling" act called the Three Leonardos soon after designing and building it in 1934. It was while traveling in Mexico that he learned that the Spanish word for diving board was trampolin. It is obvious that the sports of Trampoline, Tumbling, Acrobatic Gymnastics, and Rhythmic Gymnastics can trace part of their lineage directly to the various performing arts that have evolved over the millennia.

Gymnastics evolution from military training

There was an obvious appreciation for physical prowess in most ancient societies as a requisite for survival. The ancient Greek city-states developed a strong competition ethos that resulted in intercity competitions in many endeavors including physical activities like running, throwing, wrestling, and calisthenics. Many of these activities were associated with military prowess and are wonderfully described in Homer's epic poems the *Iliad* and the *Odyssey*. The Greek city-state competitions and regional athletic competitions evolved into large gatherings that culminated in four major games, one of which was the games at Olympia first documented in 776 BC. There was great debate in Greek literature about the value of so much time being devoted to training for these festivals, especially when the athletes became increasingly more professional and the rewards for winning multiplied (Manning, 1917).

The subsequent Roman Empire took these fitness arts to even greater sophistication but directed the training to military applications instead of purely athletic contests at religious festivals. One of the most influential medical writers in history was Claudius Galenus (Galen of Pergamon, 129–200 AD) who studied in the best medical schools in the Mediterranean region. He began his medical career treating the gladiators in his home city and was responsible for greatly reducing fatalities. Through this military medical exposure he learned much about training, rehabilitation, and the knowledge that physical fitness (gymnastics) was a natural and necessary part of life. Through his large body of publications he educated the entire world thereafter on Hippocratic theory and the practice of medicine (Machline, 2004).

It was not long after, that we see the first documentation on the use of wooden horses for military training. The first written description was a 375 AD description by Vegetius of a Roman legion training on them (Kaimakamis *et al.*, 2007). In the 6th and 7th century Europe, military skills on the wooden horse were considered one of the seven knightly virtues, and there are many references to such military training. Soldiers practiced mounting, dismounting, vaulting over, and weapon use while mounted on wooden practice horses. The practice moved from military venues to fencing academies to universities, and we see it today in the sport of Equestrian Vaulting as well as pommel horse, and vaulting in both Men's and Women's Artistic Gymnastics.

A similar military influence is apparent with "Indian" clubs. There are ancient Persian and Indian depictions of stone and wooden clubs being swung as part of physical training. The British soldiers in colonial India were very impressed with the physical robustness of practitioners of "Indian" club (jori) swinging. The British army incorporated this exercise into their training, combining it with Swedish gymnastics. The first book to appear in Europe describing Indian club exercises was Donald Walker's 1834 *British Manly Exercises*. This was followed a year later by another book *Exercises for Ladies Calculated to Preserve and Improve Beauty* in which Walker described the use of smaller, two pound Indian clubs he called "sceptres," which are the precursors of contemporary clubs in Rhythmic Gymnastics (Todd, 2010). Indian club swinging subsequently became an important part of physical education training in many countries.

Other examples of military antecedents to contemporary gymnastics sports are the obstacle courses on which soldiers trained. The balancing and locomotory activities on horizontal logs and beams, the strength demands of rope climbing, the trapeze swinging, and the pole vaulting across ditches all led to future sport events. These types of activities, together with massed group calisthenics, were regular parts of military training, and they evolved, via inter-academy competitions, into several of today's gymnastics apparatuses and competitive disciplines.

The 10 centuries following the Roman era (5th to 15th centuries) saw a decrease in intellectual and athletic pursuits that had been so prevalent during the Greek and Roman eras. There was, however, continual development of the military arts in which physical fitness and prowess were highly valued. During this time, the training of soldiers continued to employ and develop gymnastics-type skills and many military physical training instructors subsequently became the physical education teachers and sport masters in the public and private schools of Europe, thus establishing a prominent place for gymnastics in school physical education.

Gymnastics evolution from the medical professions

It is from the medical professions that we see the earliest writings on gymnastics. The word "gymnastics" was synonymous with purposeful exercise and could refer to running, physical preparation in general, or for wrestling and boxing. There were increasing references to "medical gymnastics" such as by Herodikos of Selymbria in the 5th century BC, and Galen's *De Sanitate Tuenda* in 1st century AD. Galen advocated the importance of exercise in the cultivation of both the mind and the body (Bakewell, 1997). As previously mentioned, Galen's writing on the virtues of exercise were little known during the Middle Ages in Europe, but were widely translated in Arabic and they strongly influenced Islamic medicine. It was physician Girolamo Mercuriale (or Hieronymus Mercurialis in Latin), who reintroduced Europeans to the teachings of the ancient Greeks. His book *De Arte Gymnastica* was the most influential book regarding this shift in medical thinking. Written in 1569 and reissued with elaborate illustrations of heavily muscled boxers, wrestlers, and gladiators in 1573, this book educated and influenced physicians and educators about the value of exercise, as taught by the Greeks (Figure 1.3). An earlier book, *Libro del Exercicio* by Spanish author Cristobal Méndez, was published in

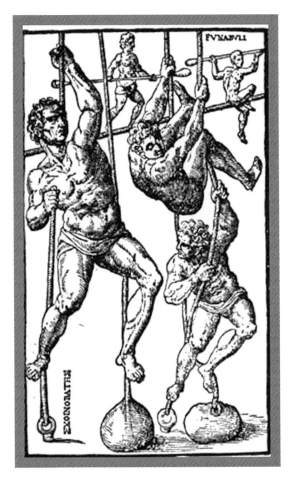

Figure 1.3 Gymnasts from Mercurialis's 1573 book. (Source: De Arte Gymnastica, Girolamo Mercuriale (1573).)

1553 and advocated exercise for health, but it was mainly for Spanish speaking general readers and was not widely known to the Latin reading intellectual classes of Europe (Machline, 2004).

About 100 years after Mercurialis, the Italian physiologist Giovanni Borelli (1608–1679) disputed Galen's principles of movement and linked movement to mechanical laws and to contracting muscles and, as such, is regarded as the father of biomechanics. His two books *De Motu Animalium I* (1680) and *II* (1685) changed forever the way physicians and educators viewed movement and exercise. The human body was now considered a series of mechanical levers moved by muscles, which were elastic, dynamic, and needed to be maintained to function effectively. Gymnastics practice was about to change.

These and similar publications fueled an intense interest in ancient Greek ideals and many publications appeared during the British Enlightenment period extolling the health benefits of regular exercise (medical gymnastics). The British medical writer Francis Fuller (the Younger) published *Medicina Gymnastica: A Treatise Concerning the Power of Exercise* in 1705 and the essayist and magazine founder Joseph Addison wrote in the magazine *Spectator* in 1711 that he exercised 1 hour every day with a dumbbell (cast iron bell silenced by removing the clapper). Fellow countryman and physician George Cheyne published the very popular book *Essay on Health and Long Life* (1724) in which he advocated a wide array of daily exercises (Batchelor, 2012). Medical gymnastics now had a more scientific footing and was gaining acceptance in the medical professions. This was bolstered by the 1741 Paris publication of *L'Orthopédia* by Nicolas Andry in which he highlights bone plasticity and rehabilitative properties in children. Thus, we see the births of biomechanics, physical therapy, physical education, and orthopedics all occurring at the same time, and central to all was "gymnastics." It is also a time of renewed emphasis on exercise and sport in public education. This was in part due to the revival of Greek educational philosophy, and in part to the medical professions' imprimatur. There was also the role public education was playing in bolstering a population of healthy military-ready youth in the climate of growing nationalism.

Gymnastics evolution from the education professions

The Renaissance period (1400–1600) also saw many educators such as the Italian Vitorrino da Feltre and the Swiss Johann Pestalozzi reintroducing the Greek model of education. These educators and philosophers, who are often grouped under the banner of "humanists," in turn influenced the Swiss Jean-Jacques Rousseau (1712–1778), and the German Johann Basdow (1724–1790) who both wrote extensively about "natural" education and strongly influenced our next group of four educators: GutsMuths, Vieth, Jahn, and Ling. It was this latter group who combined the scientific, medical, and educational changes into teaching systems, taxonomies of movement, and inventions of fitness apparatus that evolved into comprehensive systems of physical education (Figure 1.4). Now we can fill in the remaining parts of the history of present day gymnastics.

The very influential German teacher Johann GutsMuths (1759–1839) published *Gymnastik Fur Die Jugend* in 1793, which inspired many subsequent educators. GutsMuths outdoor gymnasium had many devices for physically developing his students including wooden vaulting horses, climbing ropes, trapezes, rope ladders, seesaws for hanging from, and balance beams. Another German teacher Gerhard Vieth (1763–1836) published an encyclopedia of physical education in 1794 that included passive activities and active activities such as climbing, mounting, and vaulting over wooden horses (Kaimakamis *et al.*, 2007).

A third German teacher and soldier, Freidrich Jahn (1778–1852), using similar apparatus and methods, had the greatest influence of all by organizing turnvereins, or gymnastics clubs, which spread all over Europe and the world. Jahn visited GutsMuths in 1807 and later opened an open-air gymnasium (a turnplatz) in Berlin's Hasenheide from 1811 to 1819. He expanded GutsMuths' systematic approach and developed exercises and skills to be performed on the various apparatuses. He is credited with widely popularizing the apparatus that would subsequently define Artistic Gymnastics.

Another very influential educator who studied GutsMuths and visited the German schools was Pehr Henrik Ling (1776–1839) from Sweden. Ling, who was a fencing master in his home country, developed a very different style of gymnastics that incorporated some apparatus, but mostly consisted of rhythmical and free-flowing calisthenics (Figure 1.5). He designed

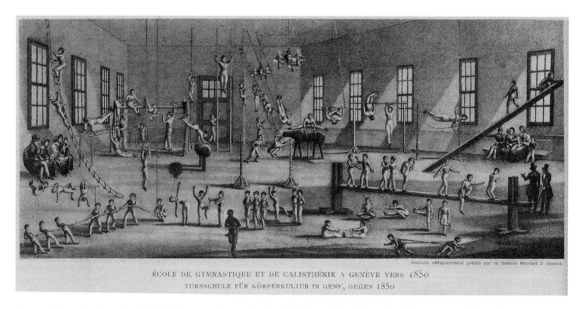

ÉCOLE DE GYMNASTIQUE ET DE CALISTHÉNIE À GENÈVE VERS 1850
TURNSCHULE FÜR KÖRPERKULTUR IN GENF, GEGEN 1850

Figure 1.4 Swiss turnschule 1850. (Source: Huguenin A., *100 Years of the International Gymnastics Federation 1881–1981*, FIG, Moutier, Switzerland 1981 with permission from Fédération Internationale de Gymnastique.)

exercises and routines to systematically develop all anatomical movements. His system was used around the world in both educational and military training and from his influence we can trace floor exercise and the balance beam style of early Women's Artistic Gymnastics. Likewise, the practice of Swedish (Ling)-style gymnastics in female physical education colleges and institutions, especially when combined with music and dance, can be seen as the antecedent of the sports of Rhythmic Gymnastics and Aerobic Gymnastics. This marriage of dance, music, and gymnastics thus has deep roots in educational practices, as well as the performing arts. When combined with the military and medical influences we now have a full picture of the genesis and evolution of the contemporary sports and activities of gymnastics.

Gymnastics in the Olympic Games

The concept of athletic festivals, in the tradition of the ancient games in Greece, has had many modern rebirths. Rühl (1997) identified 13 different "Olympic Games" prior to the IOC Olympics of 1896. A few were one-off events such as the 1844 Montreal Olympic Games and the 1853 New York Olympic Games, but the rest were repeating events in Drehberg Germany, Rondeau France, Ramlösa Sweden, Lake Palić Serbia plus five different "Olympic" festivals in England including a local festival started in 1850 in the small Shropshire town of Much Wenlock under the leadership of Dr William Penny Brookes. In 1859, just 2 months after the newly named Wenlock Olympian Games took place (and still runs annually), the first of the so-called Zappas Olympic Games was launched in Athens Greece. These "Zappas Games," funded by Greek business magnate Evangelis Zappas, were modern versions of the ancient games. The first two games in 1859 and 1870 (20,000 spectators) included, amongst other apparatuses, the ancient gymnastics competitions in pole climbing and balancing. In the 1875 Zappas Games, the German gymnastics apparatuses of parallel bars and horizontal bar were added, but since not all the program could be completed, no awards were given. The next, and the last, of these games in 1889 was quite small with only

30 pretrained athletes, and included competition in mast and rope climbing as well as pole long leap (pole vault) and there was also an exhibition of mass gymnastics by 100 school children (Rühl, 2004).

During this same time period in England, Dr Penny Brookes organized a national version of his Wenlock Olympian Games—the National Olympian Games—which were held in London in 1866 and three successive years in different cities in England. These Olympian Games included an extensive gymnastics component, which is not surprising given the other two major organizers. One was John Hulley the gymnasiarch of the Liverpool Gymnasium and promoter of another Olympic Festival that ran for 6 years in and around Liverpool commencing in 1862. The other was Ernst Ravenstein the president of the German Gymnastics Society of London. These same three men were amongst the small group of founders of the National Olympian Association in 1865, and which was a forerunner of the British Olympic Association. Ravenstein and Hulley were also co-authors of two gymnastics books.

In 1890, the young French academic Pierre Frédy, Baron de Coubertin paid a visit to Much Wenlock to witness the Olympian Games. This was one of Coubertin's many trips to the United Kingdom to study how British schools encouraged sports and games in physical education. In Dr Penny Brookes, Coubertin found an advocate for reestablishing the Olympic Games as an international event incorporating modern sports. Four years later Coubertin organized an international conference in Paris that formed the International Committee of the Olympics, which, in turn, spearheaded the first Olympic Games under the auspices of the IOC in Athens in 1896.

It should not be forgotten that in addition to these "Olympic" events there were also many large gymnastics festivals (turnfests) in German speaking Europe. GutsMuths reflects in his book that they were like "...revived Olympic Games" (Borgers, 2003). The first Deutsches Turnfest was held in Coburg Germany in 1860 with 970 gymnasts and grew so rapidly that the 1863 Turnfest in Leipzig had 20,000. The year 1860 was also when Miroslav Tyrš founded the first Sokol club in Prague. The Czech Sokol movement was similar to the German Turnverein movement and it quickly spread throughout the Slavic world and beyond Europe. They too initiated a large gymnastics festival, called a Slet, in 1882 and by the end of the century they were hosting 10,000–12,000 gymnasts. There were also similar large gymnastics festivals occurring in Scandinavia as well as multisport, multinational athletic exhibitions and competitions occurring in conjunction with the growing number of national and international trade and commerce fairs that eventually evolved into the world fairs. Not surprisingly, the first three IOC Olympic Games were integrated and organized under the programs of world fairs.

In the evolution of contemporary gymnastics, there was considerable debate regarding the virtues of the German versus the Swedish styles of gymnastics, and both of them versus the English sports approach in education. Coubertin was a strong believer in the English approach to physical education but he believed the German style of gymnastics was superior to the more medically oriented Swedish system "... German gymnastics ... is energetic in its movement, based on strict discipline and, in a word, military in its essence" (Coubertin, 1892). Thus, we see in the first IOC Olympic Games in Athens in 1896 the inclusion of the German gymnastics apparatus of horizontal bar, parallel bars, pommelled horse, rings, horse vault, and rope climb, but there was also group synchronized competitions on horizontal bar and parallel bars. In the Paris Olympics of 1900, the gymnastics competition consisted of 16 different types of apparatus including compulsory and voluntary routines on the same apparatus used in the 1896 Olympics. In addition, there were freestanding exercise, pole climb, combined jumps (high jump, long jump, pole vault), and a weight lifting competition. The battle between the Swedish and German styles played out in the next several Olympics with some interesting twists and turns. In the 1904 St. Louis Olympics, there were actually two separate gymnastics competitions held several months apart. The Turnverein (German) competition was held first and then 4 months later the Swedish gymnastics competition. The events listed in the official results include horizontal bar, parallel bars, pommelled horse, rings, vault, 100-yard run, long jump, and shot put. The latter three were called the triathlon and these scores were added

to the other scores to determine the combined all around champions. Also listed were the specialty apparatuses of rope climb and club swinging.

In the 1908 London Olympics, there were no individual apparatus medals, so athletes had to compete on all seven (heptathlon): (1) horizontal bar, swinging; (2) horizontal bar, slow movements; (3) parallel bars; (4) rings, stationary; (5) rings, swinging; (6) pommelled horse; and (7) rope climb. There was also, however, a Swedish-style team mass exercise competition of 16–40 competitors doing free exercise or exercises with hand apparatus with a maximum time limit of 30 minutes.

In 1912 in Copenhagen and again in 1920 in Antwerp, there were only the four German gymnastics apparatuses of horizontal bar, parallel bars, still rings, and pommelled horse that were summed to determine the individual all around medal, but there were also three separate team competitions. One was the apparatus team competition, another was the Swedish gymnastics team competition, and the third was a free team competition.

The 1924 games in Paris saw compulsory and voluntary routines being performed on the same four apparatuses used in the previous two Olympics plus voluntary skills on rope climb, side horse vault (no pommels), and long horse vault (interestingly by vaulting over a high jump bar before contacting the horse). From this date on, there have been individual apparatus awards given in each Olympic competition. There was also a group "drill" routine that was added into the team total. Five countries performed demonstrations of their particular styles of group gymnastics (men's groups and women's groups) and they included the Danish men's group formed 4 years earlier by Neils Bukh. This group introduced a fresh and artistically influential approach to the Scandinavian style of gymnastics (Figure 1.5). They subsequently traveled extensively internationally and strongly influenced the male aesthetic in subsequent gymnastics generations and had a particularly strong influence in Japan where universities still compete in this style of men's team "rhythmic" gymnastics. Danish demonstration teams still tour extensively.

In Amsterdam in 1928, rope climb was deleted and compulsory and voluntary routines were performed on the same four apparatuses as in the previous years

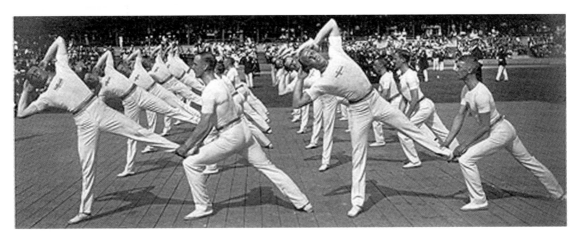

Figure 1.5 Scandinavian-style group gymnastics. (Reprinted with permission from Olympic Museum Collections.)

plus a compulsory vault over side horse with pommels and a voluntary vault over long horse. This was the first Olympics in which women officially competed in gymnastics even though there had been women's gymnastics group exhibitions in most of the former Olympics. For the women, there was only a team award that was decided by adding the cumulative scores from voluntary team routines on vault (jumps), drill with or without hand apparatus, and exercises on the apparatus. It is not clear what apparatuses were competed since "Each country is entirely free in its choice of exercices (sic), apparatus and jumps" (Official Report, 1928 Olympic Games). It is possible, from viewing the pictures in the official report, that one team chose group rope climbing. This could, however, also have been an exhibition group.

Women did not compete in gymnastics in the 1932 Olympics in Los Angeles, where the men had an unusually large selection of apparatus. Still rings were replaced with flying rings, and the all around and team competitions used scores from the usual four apparatuses (flying rings instead of still rings) plus long horse vault. All apparatuses were awarded medals including the Indian clubs, rope climb, tumbling, and individual freehanded exercise. This latter was Swedish-style calisthenics without hand apparatus, thus "freehanded," and was to become one of the six permanent apparatuses in subsequent Olympic competitions. It has also been variously called free exercises, freestanding exercise, and floor exercise.

The Berlin 1936 Olympics saw the standardization of the men's apparatus to the current six: (1) floor exercise, (2) pommel horse, (3) still rings, (4) vault, (5) parallel bars, and (6) horizontal bar. The women competed on individual apparatus for the first time, even though only a team score was awarded medals. They also competed in two group routines, one with and one without "portable" (hand) apparatus. Interestingly, the official Olympic report shows the Polish team using long bows as their "portable" apparatus. Again it is not clear if this is a competitive or a display group. They competed compulsory and voluntary routines on three apparatuses: (1) balancing beam, (2) vault, and (3) parallel bars (on which the compulsory routine was done on uneven bars but it appears that, at least, some of the voluntary routines were done on the even parallel bars, as per the men's apparatus).

In the 1948 London Olympics, the men's apparatuses were the same as in Berlin 1936 Olympics, and the women again had only team awards, but interestingly the women competed on swinging rings (compulsory routines only). The other women's apparatus included compulsory and optional routines on balance beam and pommelled side horse vault plus two group routines, one with and one without hand apparatus.

The 1952 Helsinki Olympics program included the six contemporary apparatuses for men and the four contemporary apparatuses for women (except vault was listed as long horse, not side horse) in both compulsory and optional routines. The women also competed on an optional routine in the Swedish-style gymnastics group competition with hand apparatus. Medals were given for individual apparatus, individual all around, and team.

The exact same apparatuses were contested in the 1956 Melbourne Olympics, and subsequent Olympics, but Melbourne would be the last time, under the banner of Artistic Gymnastics, that the women would compete in a Swedish-style group competition with hand apparatus.

Contemporary Olympic gymnastics

The Swedish-influenced group gymnastics and gymnastics with hand apparatus continued to evolve and develop and was strongly influenced by modern dance personalities like Emile Jaques-Dalcroze of Switzerland and American dancer Isadora Duncan as well as by the Rhythmic Gymnastics styles evolving in the Soviet Union, Finland, and Estonia. The sport of modern gymnastics came under FIG's umbrella in 1961 and changed its name to Rhythmic Sportive Gymnastics and had its first world championship in 1963 (Figure 1.6). It was then "reintroduced" into Olympic competition in the 1984 Olympics as the sport of Rhythmic Gymnastics.

A similar evolutionary process was happening with another group of sports that joined the FIG in 1999 as TG. These include Trampoline (individual and synchronized pairs), Tumbling, and Double Mini-Trampoline. Trampoline (individual male and female) was added to the Olympic program in 2000.

Summary

In summary, whether it is the competitive sports of gymnastics or the large massed group displays seen at the quadrennial World Gymnaestrada, or the recreational gymnastics class in the local municipal hall, all can trace their existence back to the performing arts, military training, medical professions, or educational professions. It has been a fascinating journey that continues to evolve at a rapid pace.

In the past 20 years, when compared to changes in other sports over the same time, change in gymnastics has been extraordinary. The apparatuses have undergone, and are still undergoing, extensive modifications that have changed gymnastics sports as radically as fiberglass poles have changed pole vaulting. Consider the recent adaptations only in the single sport of Artistic Gymnastics, where increasing elasticity has occurred in all apparatus—springy floor exercise area; padded and slightly sprung balance beams; sprung-top and much wider vaulting tables

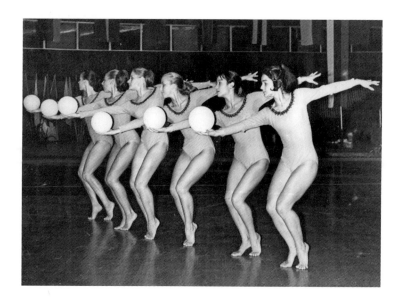

Figure 1.6 1969 Bulgarian Rhythmic World Championship team. (With courtesy of Vera Marinova-Atkinson.)

instead of narrow vaulting horses; spring-loaded ring suspension on frames designed to bow and recoil; thicker landing mats; much thinner, hollow fiberglass rails on parallel bars and asymmetric bars; higher and much wider separation of asymmetric bars; and adjustable springs on vaulting boards. These modifications have produced radically different gymnastics skills. Now, prepubertal gymnasts around the world commonly perform skills that Olympic champions were incapable of performing only a few years ago!

Trampoline has added the brand new evaluation component of measuring bounce height (air time) that has an immediate influence on performance. In addition, the non-Olympic disciplines of Acrobatic and Aerobic Gymnastics are also evolving rapidly. Aerobic Gymnastics recently added two new competitive categories aerobic dance and aerobic step to its competitive roster. The other discipline under the FIG's direction is Gymnastics for All, and it too has recently made a major change in its program by adding the new international Gym For Life Challenge competition, which pits individual clubs against one another in a world championship of exhibition gymnastics.

This rapid evolution has, however, also brought changes that are more difficult to evaluate as being favorable or unfavorable. Younger than normal gymnasts began to appear at the Dortmund World Championships in 1966, and by 1975 Nadia Comaneci won every gold medal except one at the European Championships. She was 13 years old. At the Montreal Olympics in 1976 we had the two 14 year olds Nadia Comaneci and Nellie Kim take the spotlight with their incredible level of performance. This trend has been recently reversed by the imposition of a minimum age of 16 for Olympic competition. This increase in age, while positive, has opened the possibility that the most successful female Artistic Gymnastics competitors may be those who are actually much later maturers than was previously the case, as evidenced by the fact that the average height and weight of the female Olympic gymnasts has not changed, even though the age has increased. Perhaps changes in the judging rules will be needed to decrease the advantage of small prepubertal female Artistic gymnasts.

In Rhythmic Gymnastics, there has been a trend for increased flexibility that now crosses over into contortion and this has generated great discussion within the ranks of FIG officials. This trend has partially been ameliorated by recent rule changes giving less reward for it, but the debate continues.

The following trends are realities of contemporary gymnastics, and all need continual monitoring and debate:
• The ages of gymnasts training at high levels has progressively decreased.
• The training hours, notably for young children, have increased dramatically.
• The skill difficulty levels have increased exponentially, which results in greater forces being sustained by the body, for longer periods of time, at younger ages.
• Injury rates, especially growth plate injuries, seem higher than previously reported (Kolt and Kirkby, 1999, Kolt and Caine, 2010).
• Subjective evaluation of athletes contains the inherent pitfalls of nationalistic bias.
• The importance of, and meaningful use of, music has diminished.
• Rule makers are predominantly from the ranks of judges with little input from the coaching community.
• Skill convergence in Women's Artistic and Rhythmic Gymnastics has led to overuse injuries.

Yes, there are challenges in the world of gymnastics, but the 5000-year-old adventure continues with no signs of stagnation. The many forms of gymnastics are wonderful foundations to other physical pursuits, and are amongst the most exciting sports to perform and to watch. The marriage of artistry and sport is not an easy union. However, the outcomes are well worth the struggle and the many forms of gymnastics deliver innumerable positive outcomes.

Acknowledgment

The author would like to thank John Atkinson and Hardy Fink for making helpful suggestions.

References

Bakewell, S. (1997) Medical gymnastics and the cyriax collection. *Medical History*, **41** (4), 487–495.

Batchelor, R. (2012) Thinking about the gym: Greek ideals, Newtonian bodies and exercise in early eighteenth century Britain. *Journal of Eighteenth-Century Studies*, **35** (2), 185–197.

Borgers, W. (2003) From the temple of industry to Olympic arena: the exhibition tradition of the Olympic Games. *Journal of Olympic History*, **11** (1), 7–21.

Coubertin, P. (1892) Quoted on p. 436, Weiler, I. (2004) The predecessors of the Olympic movement, and Pierre de Coubertin. *European Review*, **12**, 427–443.

Frantzopoulou, A., Douka, S., Kaimakamis, V., Matsaridis, A., and Terzoglou, M. (2011) Acrobatic gymnastics in Greece from ancient times to the present day. *Studies in Physical Culture and Tourism*, **18** (4), 337–342.

Gardiner, E. (1930) *Athletics in the Ancient World*. Oxford University Press.

Kaimakamis, V., Anastasiou, A., and Duka, S. (2007) An outline of the development of the gymnastic horse from the roman times to the age of humanists. *Studies in Physical Culture and Tourism*, **14** (1), 47–51.

Kolt G. and Caine, D. (2010) Gymnastics, Chapter 12. In: *Epidemiology of Injury in Olympic Sports*, pp. 144–160. Blackwell Publishing.

Kolt, G. and Kirkby, R. (1999) Epidemiology of injury in elite and sub-elite female gymnasts: a comparison of retrospective and prospective findings. *British Journal of Sports Medicine*, **33**, 312–318.

Machline, V. (2004) Cristobal méndez medical ideas about the influence of joy and pleasure (rather than humor) upon health. *Revisita de Humanidades. Tecnologico de Monterrey*, **17**, 115–128.

Manning, C. (1917) Professionalism in Greek athletics. *The Classical Weekly*, **11** (10), 74–78.

Olympic Games (1928) General Regulations – Gymnastics. IOC website. URL http://doc.rero.ch/record/28731 [accessed on February 11, 2013].

Rühl J. (1997) The Olympian Games at Athens in the year 1877. *Journal of Olympic History*, Fall, 26–34.

Rühl J. (2004) Olympic Games before Courbertin. In: John E. Findling and Kimberly D. Pelle (eds), *Encyclopedia of the Modern Olympic Movement*, p. 3. Greenwood Publishing Group.

Todd, J. (2010) The strength builders: a history of barbells, dumbbells and Indian clubs. *The International Journal of the History of Sport*, **20** (1), 65–90.

Touney, A. (1984) History of sport in ancient Egypt. In: Proceedings of the International Olympic Academy, pp. 85–90.

Yiannakis, T. and Yiannakis, S. (1998) The meaning of names in Greek antiquity, with special reference to Olympic athletes. *The International Journal of the History of Sport*, **15** (3), 103–114.

PART 2
GROWTH AND DEVELOPMENT ASPECTS

Chapter 2
Growth, maturation, and training

Adam D.G. Baxter-Jones

Federation Internationale de Gymnastique (FIG), Lausanne, Switzerland *and*
College of Graduate Studies and Research and Professor of Kinesiology, University of Saskatchewan, Saskatoon, SK, Canada

Introduction

Concern over possible growth inhibition effects of competitive sports has been and continues to be a source of much debate. In recent years, parents, coaches, sport administrators, sports medicine practitioners, and the broader public has been alarmed by reports of potentially harmful effects of intensive physical training beginning at a young age in the growing athlete. Most of the attention has been centered on the observed short stature and later maturation of female Artistic Gymnastics. Although, short stature has also been reported in female Rhythmic gymnastics, the evidence is less equivocal. Very little has been written about the female trampoline athlete. The size and maturation of male gymnasts have not been placed under similar scrutiny, although studies have suggested that their growth deterioration may be more marked compared to females. The major concerns are that training may reduce growth potential and possibly delay pubertal maturation. On the other hand, claims have also been expressed for the positive influences of intensive training for sport on the growing and maturing individual, such as improved bone health.

Interest in the effects that physical activity and/or exercise have on a child's growth and maturation has a long history. At the beginning of the 20th century, D'Arcy Thompson (1917) wrote his classic treatise *On Growth and Form* suggesting that exercise was a direct stimulus to growth (Thompson, 1942). In 1964, James Tanner published *The Physique of the Olympic Athlete* in which he concluded that "the basic body structure must be present for the possibility of being an athlete to arise." Other authors who have subsequently measured the growth and development of young athletes have agreed with this statement and concluded that body size is likely genotypic (nature) and probably reflects selection at a relatively young age for the size demands of the sport (Malina, 1994). This suggests that nature rather than nurture is the driving force behind the observed size differences in sports. However, a number of studies, especially with aesthetic sports such as gymnastics, have suggested that when heavy training regimens are started at a young age, the growth (Theintz et al., 1993) and maturation (Daly et al., 2000) of the child may be adversely affected (nurture).

In female gymnastics, particular attention has to be paid to the fact that the age, and thus size, of artistic women gymnastic champions, such as Larisa Latynina (who won Olympic gold at 22 years of age in 1956) and Věra Čáslavská (who won Olympic medals at 22 years in 1964), has declined over the decades. At the 1972 Olympics Olga Korbut won Olympic gold at 17 years of age and in 1976 Nadia Comaneci won at the age of 14 years. In 1987 the mean age at the world championships was 13 years and height and weights reflected the prepubertal body type. In 1997 the minimum competition age

Gymnastics, First Edition. Edited by Dennis J. Caine, Keith Russell and Liesbeth Lim. © 2013 International Olympic Committee. Published 2013 by John Wiley & Sons, Ltd.

was raised to 16 years and the average age at the 2008 world championships was 18.8 years. However the height and weights in 2008 were similar to those observed in 1987. Thus, the nature versus nurture debate continues. However, before discussing the evidence for and against this argument, it should be pointed out that one common element often overlooked is the natural variations in the timing and tempo of growth and maturation observed within a normal healthy population.

Growth, maturation, and development

All children experience three interacting processes: (1) growth, (2) maturation, and (3) development. Often these terms are treated as the same; yet, these terms refer to three distinctive processes that occur in the daily lives of children and youth for approximately the first two decades of life.

Growth specifically refers to the increase in the size of the body as a whole and of its parts. Thus, as young children grow, they become taller and heavier, they increase in lean and fat tissues, their organs increase in size, and so on. Different parts of the body grow at different rates and different times. For example, in normal healthy children heart volume and mass follow a growth pattern similar to body weight, while lung size and bone mass grow in proportion to height. The different rates and timing of growth in the body and its parts result in changes in body proportions, that is, the relationship of one part of the body to another. The legs, for example, grow faster than the trunk during childhood; hence, the child becomes relatively longer legged.

Maturation refers to progress towards the biologically mature state. It is an operational concept because the mature state varies with body systems. Maturation differs from growth in that although various biological systems mature at different rates, all individuals reach the same endpoint and become fully mature. In contrast, there are wide variations in endpoints of growth, that is, adult stature, physique, and so on. Maturation, that is, the process of maturing, has two components, timing and tempo. The former refers to when specific

maturational events occur, for example, age when menarche is attained, age at the beginning of breast development, age at the appearance of pubic hair, or age at maximum growth during the adolescent growth spurt. Tempo refers to the rate at which maturation progresses, for example, how quickly or slowly an individual passes from initial stages of sexual maturation to the mature state. Timing and tempo vary considerably among individuals. Studies of growing children commonly focus on sexual and skeletal maturation.

Development refers to the acquisition of behavioral competence, that is, the learning of appropriate behaviors expected by society. It is culture specific. As children experience life at home, school, church, sports, recreation, and other community activities, they develop cognitively, socially, emotionally, morally, and so on. Children and adolescents learn to behave in culturally appropriate manners.

It is important to recognize that the three processes, growth, maturation, and development, occur simultaneously and interact. Growth and maturation are characterized by individual variation and, although under genetic and neuroendocrine control, environmental factors may also have an influence. Physical activity, especially intensive training for sport, is often indicated as one such environmental factor. The demands of specific sports are superimposed upon those associated with normal growth, maturation, and development. Although widely discussed and to a lesser extent systematically investigated, the exact role of regular training is yet to be determined. Nevertheless, concern is periodically expressed about potentially negative influences of intensive training on the growth and maturation of elite young female athletes in some sports. To understand fully the effects of training on a gymnast's growth and maturation one has to first have a clear understanding of the growth process itself.

The curve of growth

One of the most famous records of human growth is that of a boy known simply as de Montbeillard's son. Between 1759 and 1770 the Count Philibert Gueneau de Montbeillard successively measured his son at approximately 6-month intervals. Although tabulated in 1778, that data was not plotted in the form of a chart until 1927, by R.E. Scammon (Figure 2.1). This is known as a height distance or height for age curve.

Growth can be thought of in terms of a journey, the curve in Figure 2.1 describes the distance traveled from birth to 18 years of age; from the figure you can see that a child's height at any particular age is a reflection of how far that child has progressed towards the mature adult state. With data collected approximately every 6 months this clearly illustrates that growth is not a linear process. That is to say we do not gain the same amount of height during each calendar year. Figure 2.1 also illustrates the fact that between birth and 18 years of age the distance curve is made up of a number of different shaped curves with different slopes. Relatively rapid growth is observed in infancy, which gradually declines by 5 years of age, that is, the slope of

the line decreases. This is followed by steady growth in childhood (between 5 and 10 years of age) and then rapid growth during adolescence (between 10 and 16 years of age). Finally, very slow growth is observed as the individual approaches an asymptote at 19 years of age. Although this distance curve shows the continuous rate of magnitude of change with age, in terms of our journey it only tells us where we are at any particular point in time. No information is provided as to how we reached this point; thus the distance point is largely dependent on how much the child has grown in all proceeding years.

What is more useful is a measure of growth that describes the speed of our journey at any one point in time. To get an idea of speed, the data has to be expressed in terms of a rate of growth (centimeter per year) (Figure 2.2). Velocity of growth is a better reflection of the child's state at any particular time than the distance achieved.

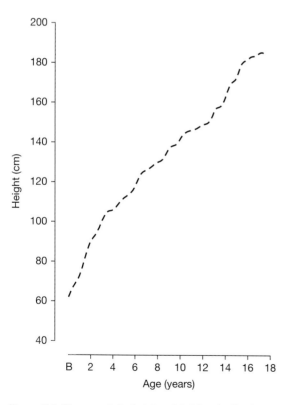

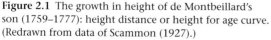

Figure 2.1 The growth in height of de Montbeillard's son (1759–1777): height distance or height for age curve. (Redrawn from data of Scammon (1927).)

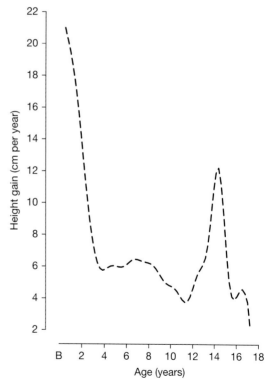

Figure 2.2 The growth in height of de Montbeillard's son (1759–1777): velocity curve (Redrawn from data of Scammon (1927).)

From the curve you can see that following birth two distinct increases in growth rates occur. The first of these is the juvenile or mid-growth spurt occurring between 6 and 8 years of age. The second, more dramatic, increase occurs between 11 and 18 years and is called the adolescent growth spurt. Whilst the juvenile growth spurt varies in magnitude between individuals, it occurs at roughly the same age both within and between sexes. The adolescent growth spurt, however, varies in both magnitude and timing within and between the sexes. Males enter their adolescent growth spurt, on average, almost 2 years later than females and have a slightly greater magnitude of height gain (Figure 2.3). This extra 2 years of growth prior to adolescence, in combination with a greater magnitude of growth during adolescence explains in part the increased final adult height and relatively longer legs observed in males. At the same time, other skeletal changes occur that result in gender difference in adulthood, such as wider shoulders in males and wider hips in females. Males also demonstrate rapid increases in muscle mass whilst females accumulate greater amounts of fat, thus as a result of natural biological development by the end of adolescence males are stronger.

Growth in stature

Stature is made up of sitting height (distance from the sitting surface to the top of the head) and leg length, or subischial length (distance between the hip joint to the floor). The exact landmark of the hip joint is sometimes hard to locate so leg length is most often calculated by subtracting sitting height from standing height. Stature varies during the course of the day, with greater readings in the morning that decrease throughout the day. Shrinkage during the day occurs because the intervertebral discs become compressed as a result of weight bearing, thus the diurnal variation may be as much as 1 cm or more.

During the first year of life, infants grow at a fast rate, approximately 25 cm per year, in fact during the first 6 months of life the velocity may be even faster, around 30 cm per year (Figure 2.3). During the second year of life there is growth of another 12–13 cm in stature. This accelerated growth means that by 2 years of age boys have attained approximately 50% of their adult stature. Girls are always closer to their mature status, even at birth, than boys and reach 50% of their final adult stature by 18 months of age. From then on there is a steady deceleration in growth, dropping to a rate of about 5–6 cm per year before the initiation of the adolescent growth spurt. Between 6.5 and 8.5 years, there is a small but distinct increase in growth rate, known as the juvenile or mid-growth spurt. During adolescence the maximum velocity of growth is known as peak height velocity (PHV). Girls, on average, attain PHV approximately 2 years earlier than boys with their onset of PHV occurring between 8.2 and 10.3 years (Figure 2.4). On average PHV is reached between 11.3 and 12.2 years. Corresponding ages for boys are 10.0–12.1 years and 13.3–14.4 years. By PHV individuals have attained 92% of their adult height.

Upon reaching final adult height males are on average 13 cm taller than females, however up until the initiation of PHV the sex differences in height are small (Figure 2.4). Therefore, boys achieve their

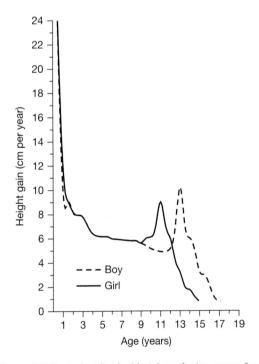

Figure 2.3 Typical-individual height–velocity curves for boys and girls, representing the velocity of the typical boy and girls at any given instance. (Redrawn from data of Malina *et al.* (2004).)

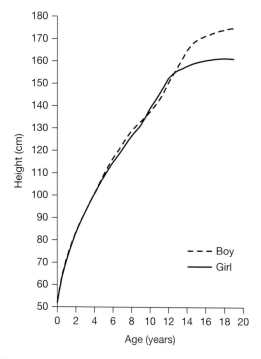

Figure 2.4 Typical-individual distance curves for boys and girls (Redrawn from data of Malina *et al.* (2004).)

height advantage during the adolescent period. Specifically, boys on average experience about 2 years more preadolescent growth, approximately 5 cm per year, than girls. This is roughly 10 cm of growth that girls do not experience. Boys also achieve a slightly greater (on average 2 cm) magnitude of height at PHV. Both of these growth differences cause males, on average, to have a greater adult stature. Girls stop growing in stature by about 16 years of age and boys by about 18 or 19 years of age. However, these ages may be spuriously young as many growth studies stop measuring youth at 17 or 18 years of age, and it is known that many youth, especially males, continue to grow into their early to mid 20s.

These curves of growth in height reflect the growth patterns found in all healthy children who live in a normal environment. As mentioned, individuals will differ in absolute height of growth velocity (i.e., adult heights) and in the timing of the adolescent growth spurt; however, to reach their destined final height each individual will go through a similar pattern of human growth.

Patterns of growth

Statural growth, as demonstrated in Figure 2.4, shows only one of several patterns of growth found within the human body. Different parts of the body grow at different rates and different times. It has been proposed that all tissues and systems follow four patterns of growth: (i) neurological (e.g., brain and head), (ii) reproductive (e.g., reproductive organs), (iii) lymphoid (e.g., lymph glands, tonsils, and appendix) and (iv) general (e.g., stature and heart size). Brain and head growth (neural tissue) exhibits the most rapid early growth. At birth a child's head is roughly half its adult size. From birth there is steady growth up until 7 years of age; by 8 years of age neural tissue growth is almost complete. In contrast, reproductive tissue does not really start to increase in size until 12 to 14 years of age. The reproductive curve includes primary sex characteristics (e.g., uterus, vagina and fallopian tubes in females; prostate and seminal vesicles in males) and secondary sex characteristics (e.g., breasts in females, facial hair in males, and axillary and pubic hair in both sexes). The reproductive curve shows some growth during infancy followed by reduced growth during childhood; by 10 to 12 years of age reproductive organs are only 10% of their adult size. During adolescence (puberty) there is a rapid growth in genital tissues. The general curve of growth includes many tissues and systems in the body, such as skeletal tissue, the respiratory system, and the digestive system. As illustrated by the shape of stature shown in Figure 2.4, the general curve follows a sigmoid curve of growth and reflects a rapid growth during infancy and early childhood, steady growth during mid-childhood, and rapid growth during early adolescence.

Development of shape

In contrast to changes in size, which just show a child's progression in terms of a percentage of adult status, the concept of change in shape reflects the changes in proportionality of body segments from infancy to adulthood. As already indicated, there is a twofold increase in head size from birth to maturity; however, other segments show different patterns. The trunk increases threefold, the arms fourfold and the legs at maturity are five times their length at birth. These changes illustrate that there is a head–trunk–legs gradient. In early fetal growth the head is fastest growing, in infancy trunk growth accelerates, and in childhood leg growth accelerates. Other gradients of growth are also observed; within the limbs, during childhood and adolescence, growth occurs distal to proximal. For example, the hand and feet experience accelerated growth first, followed by the calf and the forearm, the hips and the chest, and lastly the shoulders. Thus, during childhood there may be a period where children appear to have large hands and feet in relation to the rest of their body. However, once the adolescent growth spurt has ended, hands and feet are a little smaller in proportion to arms, legs, and stature. Most body dimensions, with the exception of subcutaneous adipose tissue and the dimensions of the head and face, follow a growth pattern similar to that of stature; however, there are wide variations in the timing of growth spurts. From childhood to adolescence, the lower extremities (legs) grow faster than the upper body (trunk). This results in sitting height contributing less to stature as age progresses. During the adolescent growth spurt the legs experience a growth spurt earlier than the trunk. Thus, for a period during early adolescence a youth will have relatively long legs, but the appearance of long-leggedness disappears with the later increase in trunk length. Sex differences in leg length and sitting height are small during childhood. For a short time during the early part of adolescence, girls, on average, have a slightly longer leg length than boys, due to girls experiencing adolescence on average 2 years earlier. By about 12 years of age boys' leg length exceeds girls, but boys do not catch up in sitting height until about 14 years of age. The longer period of preadolescent growth in boys is largely responsible for the fact that men's legs are longer than women's in relation to trunk length.

Biological maturity

As indicated previously, there is wide variation amongst children both within and between genders as to the exact timing and tempo of maturation. Therefore, to adequately distinguish the effects of physical activity or exercise on a group of children,

biological maturity needs to be controlled. When considering how to assess biological maturation it is first important to understand that 1 year of chronological time does not equal 1 year of maturational time. Whilst every individual passes through the same stages of maturity they do so at differing rates, resulting in children of the same chronological age differing in their degree of maturity; this is reflected in Figure 2.5. The graphs illustrate the growth of two girls (A and B), both 11 years of age; however, what is not apparent is the fact that they differ considerably in their degree of maturity. At 11 years of age they are similar in height (girl A is 156 cm; girl B 158 cm); however, the second bars reflect the same individuals at 35 years of age and indicate that adult heights are significantly different (girl A is 181 cm; girl B is 165 cm). It is therefore apparent that at 11 years of age girl B is very close to her final adult height, 7 cm of growth remaining, and thus close to full maturity. In contrast, at 11 years of age girl A still had 25 cm of growth to go and thus was less mature at 11 years of age. This illustrates the point that the size of an individual is not an accurate indicator of maturity. Certainly, in very general terms, size is associated with maturity, in that a bigger individual is likely to be chronologically older and thus be more mature than a smaller individual. However, it is well recognized that size does not play a part in the assessment of maturity.

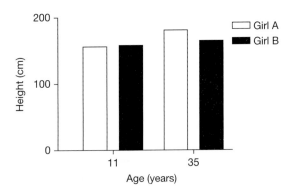

Figure 2.5 Two girls measured at the same chronological ages (11 and 35 years). At 11 years of age, girl A has 25.2 cm of growth in stature remaining and girl B 6.5 cm of statural growth remaining. (Data taken from two individuals who participated in the Saskatchewan Growth and Development Study (1964–1998).)

To adequately control for maturity an indicator of maturity needs to be identified. The maturity indicator chosen should be any definable and sequential change in any part of the body that is characteristic of the progression of the body from immaturity to maturity. The most commonly used methods to assess maturity are: skeletal maturity, sexual maturity, biochemical and hormonal maturity, somatic or morphological maturity, and dental maturity.

The interrelationships among the various indicators of biological maturation are complex, because only skeletal maturity and percentage of adult stature span the entire maturation period from birth to adulthood. During puberty a number of other indicators become apparent, such as somatic and sexual maturity, both of which are related to skeletal maturity. In girls, the first event to be noticed is the start of breast development: the time when prepubertal girls in breast stage 1 enter breast stage 2, the advent of the breast bud. This occurs on average around 11.0 years of age (range 9.0 to 13.0 years). The onset of pubic hair development is a little later, although in about one-third of girls pubic hair appears before the breast bud. Menarche, the first menstrual period, occurs relatively late in puberty, between 12.8 and 13.2 years, typically just past PHV. When menarche occurs most girls are in breast stage 4 and pubic hair stages 3 or 4; however, some girls can be in pubic hair stage 1 and others in pubic hair stage 5. The relationship between menarche and PHV is much stronger, occurring at the time of maximum deceleration of height velocity.

Beginning testicular enlargement is usually the first sign of puberty in boys; accompanied by changes in the texture and color of the skin of the scrotum, this occurs on average around 11.5 years of age. A little later the penis starts to enlarge and pubic hair starts to appear. Acceleration of penis growth begins on average at about 12.5 years (range 10.5–14.5 years) with completion of growth by 14.4 years (range 12.5–16.5 years). It is therefore possible for a late-maturing boy to start penis growth after the earliest maturer has completed it. On average, pubic hair development starts around 12 years of age (stage 2) and is completed by 15 years of age (stage 5). The adolescent growth spurt starts on average at around 12.5 years, a year after the first signs of testicular enlargement, and reaches its peak (PHV) at around 14 years of age, when genitalia development is between stages 4 and 5, and pubic hair between stages 3 or 4. Facial hair appears somewhat later, as does the breaking of the voice, a relatively late pubertal event (Tanner, 1989).

Training and growth and maturation

Training refers to the systematic, specialized practice for a specific sport or sport discipline for most of the year or to specific short-term experimental programs. Training programs are ordinarily specific (e.g., endurance running, strength training, sport skill training, etc.), and vary in intensity and duration. Although early studies suggested that training increased the rate of growth, particularly in the height of males, the results were limited. The apparent acceleration in height observed in some studies was likely related to the earlier biological maturation of the young male athletes studied and sampling variation rather than the intensity of the training program. More recently, the literature examining the potential effects of training for sport on maturation has concentrated on female athletes, particularly the age at which menarche is attained.

Sport participation and training for sport have no apparent effect on growth in height or the rate of growth in height in healthy, adequately nourished children and adolescents. With few exceptions, athletes of both sexes in a variety of sports have, on average, heights that equal or exceed data for nonathletes. Exceptions among athletes are gymnasts, participants in a sport in which successful participants present shorter heights than average. This trend probably reflects the selection criteria of the sport. The smaller size of elite gymnasts is evident long before any systematic training starts, and is in part familial, that is, gymnasts have parents who are shorter than average. When parental stature was used to predict adult target height in a group of male gymnasts, swimmers, and soccer and tennis players, it was found that gymnasts had significantly lower target heights than the other sports (Baxter-Jones et al., 1995). There is also a size difference between those who persist in the sport and those who drop out, with those who drop out attaining greater height. Some studies have attributed low body weight and later sexual maturation of female artistic gymnasts to excessive energy expenditure and/or insufficient energy intake (Georgopolous *et al.*, 2004). These observations speak to concerns related to dietary monitoring and manipulation, and increased risk of disordered and pathologic eating behaviors among some elite adolescent female gymnasts. However, it is important to take into account that although female gymnasts have lower weights than reference data, in general their weights are appropriate for their shorter heights.

Short-term longitudinal studies of athletes in several sports in which the same youngsters are followed on a regular basis over time (volleyball, diving, distance running, basketball) indicate rates of growth in height that, on average, closely approximate rates observed in nonathletic children and adolescents. The growth rates observed were within the range of normally expected variation among youth. Studies investigating the interactions between club-level sports training for gymnasts, figure skaters, and runners, compared to controls, found that club-level sports training did not affect growth or maturation during puberty. However, others suggest an opposite view, with some studies suggesting that gymnasts were failing to obtain full familial height. However, decreasing predicted adult height during puberty is a characteristic of slow or late maturation, confirmed by the late onset of menarche in such subjects. Other studies of gymnasts, over longer time periods, have also observed lags in adolescent growth, but then report subsequent catch-up growth and thus no differences in attained adult heights (Erlandson *et al.*, 2008). In contrast to height, body mass can be influenced by regular training for sport, resulting in changes in body composition. Training is associated with a decrease in fatness in both sexes and occasionally with an increase in fat-free mass, especially in boys. Maintenance of reduced levels of fatness depends on continued, regular activity or training (or caloric restriction, which often occurs in sports like gymnastics, ballet, figure skating, and diving in girls and wrestling in boys).

When training is significantly reduced, fat tends to accumulate.

Biological maturation and regular training

Does regular training for and participation in sport influence the timing and tempo of biological maturation? As noted earlier, there is a wide range of normal variation among youth in the timing and tempo of biological maturation. It is a highly individual characteristic that often shows a tendency to run in families; that is, mothers and their daughters may both be early or late maturing. Short-term longitudinal studies of girls in several sports have indicated similar gains in skeletal maturation in both athletes and nonathletes. On average, skeletal age proceeds in concert with a child's chronological age. It should be noted that in later adolescence, differences in maturity status among participants at younger ages are reduced and eventually eliminated as skeletal maturity is attained by all individuals.

Available data indicated no effect of training for sport on the age at PHV and growth rate of height during the adolescent spurt in boys and girls. It has been suggested that intensive training may delay the timing of the growth spurt and stunt the growth spurt in female gymnasts. Unfortunately, the data are insufficient to warrant such a conclusion. Many confounding factors are not considered, especially the rigorous selection criteria for gymnastics, marginal diets, short parents, and so on. Female gymnasts, as a group, show the growth and maturation characteristics of short, normal, slow-maturing children with short parents. Interestingly, male gymnasts also present consistently short statures and late maturation, but these trends are not attributed to intensive training.

Longitudinal data on the sexual maturation of girls who are regularly active or training for sport are not extensive. The available data are largely cross-sectional so that it is difficult to make clear statements on potential effects of training for sport. The limited longitudinal data for girls active in sport compared to nonathletic girls indicated no effect of training on the timing and progress of breast and pubic hair development. Mean intervals for progression from one stage to the next or across two stages of secondary sex characteristics are similar for active and nonactive youth, and are well within the range of normal variation in longitudinal studies of nonathletes. The interval between ages at PHV and menarche for girls active in sport and nonactive girls also does not differ. This interval (1.2–1.5 years) is similar to those for several samples of nonathletic girls.

Most discussions of the potential influence of training on sexual maturation focus on the later mean age at menarche, which was often observed in female athletes (Malina, 1994). Typically, training for sport was indicated as the factor responsible for the later mean age at menarche, with the inference that training "delayed" menarcheal onset. Unfortunately, most studies of athletes do not consider other confounding factors known to influence menarche. For example, there is a familial tendency for later maturation in athletes. Mothers of athletes in several other sports attained menarche later than mothers of nonathletes, and sisters of elite swimmers and university athletes attained menarche later than average. In addition, age at menarche in athletes varies with the number of children in the family. Athletes from larger families attain menarche later than those from smaller families. Thus, allowing for the many factors known to influence menarche, it is exceedingly difficult to implicate sport training per se as the causative factor for later menarche in female athletes.

Sport selection

As continually emphasized in this chapter, sport is extremely selective and exclusive at elite levels. Most community-based programs emphasize mass participation. Other programs have as their objective the identification and subsequent training of young athletes with potential for success in regional, national, and/or international competition. In these programs, the selection/exclusion process begins early and appears to be a closed one, excluding many children from entering sport at a later age.

Much time and effort has been spent trying to identify the particular physical and psychological characteristics that contribute to the selection and development of athletic talent. The debate often focused on the relative contributions of genetic, environmental, and social factors. From the research available it would appear that training does not affect growth and maturation. It is more likely that young athletes select themselves, or are selected by coaches and sport systems, into their specific sports. This finding implies that, in general, sporting success in the young athlete has a large genetic component and that the differences observed in growth and maturation between athletes and nonathletes are mainly the result of nature rather than nurture. Genetic considerations in growth, maturation, and performance are discussed in more depth elsewhere.

The young, potentially talented athlete has to be introduced to her sport. A major limiting factor to organized sport participation is the availability of local resources, in particular human resources in the form of adults to coach, supervise, and administer programs. Parental support, both in terms of time and finance, is very important. In a study of young British athletes, parents played the main role in introducing children into sport. Furthermore, most of these parents participated in sport themselves when they were younger. Similarly, among university athletes in the United States, parents were most often indicated as the primary persons responsible for getting them involved in sport, and the majority of these athletes had one or both parents involved in sport at the high school level or above.

Economic considerations are an additional factor. Young athletes often travel considerable distances to get to a training facility and are dependent on their parent(s) for transport. Further, the cost of intensive training can be considerable and in the most part is met almost exclusively by parents. Systematic training in sports such as gymnastics, swimming, diving, tennis, and figure skating are often limited to private clubs and require a substantial economic investment by parents and possibly sponsors. Economic considerations are, therefore, likely to limit access to sports for children and adolescents in many countries.

Further research

Because children of the same age do not all follow the same tempo and timing of biological maturity (i.e., there are early, average, and late maturers) it is essential to consider growth and maturity confounders when studying training adaptations in gymnastic populations. The research available is currently limited to research in artistic gymnasts, especially female populations. What is lacking is research on male gymnasts, trampoline gymnasts, as well as rhythmic gymnasts. Future studies should consider working with these populations to investigate whether they show patterns of growth and maturation observed in female artistic gymnasts. Whatever population is chosen, it is important to remember that interpretation of training effects on young gymnasts is hampered by study designs. The majority of studies are cross-sectional in nature, are small in sample size, start at too late an age, use athletes with low levels of training, and do not measures all the variables known to influence growth and maturation. To address questions related to training effects on gymnasts growth and development, studies have to be longitudinal in nature; this is because the effects of normal growth and development may mask or be greater than the training effects. Studies have to start prior to commencement of gymnastics training (i.e., 4–6 years of age) and have comparison groups of similar aged children who are not training. Since gymnasts tend to demonstrate patterns of growth that represent slow-developing late maturers with familial short stature it is important that comparison groups of nongymnasts also demonstrate these growth characteristics. A measure of maturity is essential for all studies, preferably one that incorporates measures of the endocrine system. Finally, studies also have to measure other variables known to affect growth such as dietary intake, family size, training hours, training intensity, and the training environment.

Summary

Much of the existing literature related to the effects of training on the growth and maturation in gymnastics deals with artistic female gymnasts, with only a few studies addressing male gymnasts, rhythmic gymnasts, and trampoline gymnasts. Since research related to gymnasts in general is dealing with a biased sample of self-selected individuals it is important to first consider the normal variations in growth and maturation observed in the general population. Before considering the effect of training, the following generalizations related to normal growth and development should be considered:

- Although all young people follow the same pattern of growth from infancy to full maturity there is considerable variation both between and within sexes, in the timing and magnitude of these changes.
- Within an age group, early maturers are on average taller and heavier and have a larger fat-free mass (especially boys) and fat mass (especially girls) than late maturers.
- Indicators of skeletal, sexual, and somatic maturation are moderately to highly correlated during adolescence; however, no one indictor gives a complete description of the tempo of growth and maturation.
- From available data, it would appear that adult height of male and female artistic gymnasts are not compromised by training at a young age and more likely reflect selection and retention factors into the sport.
- Gymnastics training does not appear to attenuate segmental growth or pubertal maturation. However, some gymnasts do report height increments below normal ranges for age and maturation but when followed serially appear to reach predicted targets.

References

Baxter-Jones, A.D.G., Helms, P., Maffulli, N., and Preece, M. (1995) Growth and development of male gymnasts, swimmers, soccer and tennis players: a longitudinal study. *Annals of Human Biology*, **22**, 381–394.

Daly, R.M., Rich, P.A., Klein, R., and Bass, S.L. (2000) Short stature in competitive prepubertal and early pubertal male gymnasts: the result of selection bias or intense training? *Journal of Pediatrics*, **137**, 510–516.

Erlandson, M.C., Sherar, L.B., Mirwald, R.L., Maffulli, N., and Baxter-Jones, A.D.G. (2008) Growth and maturation of adolescent female gymnasts, swimmers, and tennis players. *Medicine and Science in Sports and Exercise*, **40**, 34–42.

Georgopolous, N.A., Theodoropoulou, A., Leglise, M., Vagenakis, A.G., and Markou, K.B. (2004) Growth and skeletal maturation in male and female artistic gymnasts. *Journal of Clinical Endocrinology and Metabolism*, **89**, 4377–4382.

Malina, R.M. (1994) Physical growth and biological maturation of young athletes. *Exercise and Sport Science Reviews*, **22**, 389–433.

Scammon, R.E. (1927) The first seriatim study of human growth. *American Journal of Physical Anthropology*, **10**, 329–336.

Tanner, J.M. (1964) *The Physique of the Olympic athlete*. George Allen and Unwin Ltd, London.

Tanner J.M. (1989) *Foetus into Man*. Castlemead Publications, London.

Theintz, G.E., Howald, H., Weiss, U., and Sizonenko, P.C. (1993) Evidence for a reduction of growth potential in adolescent female gymnasts. *Journal of Pediatrics*, **122**, 306–313.

Thompson, D.A.W. (1942) *On Growth and Form*. University Press, Cambridge.

Recommended reading

Baxter-Jones, A.D.G., Maffulli, N., and Mirwald, R.L. (2003) Does elite gymnastics competition inhibit growth and maturation? Probably not! *Pediatric Exercise Science*, **15**, 373–382.

Boas, F. (1930) Observations on the growth of children. *Science*, **72**, 44–48.

Caine, D., Bass, S.L., and Daly, R. (2003) Does elite competition inhibit growth and delay maturation in some gymnasts? Quite possibly. *Pediatric Exercise Science*, **15**, 360–372.

Cameron, N. (2002) *Human Growth and Development*. Academic Press, Elsevier Science, San Diego, CA.

Hall, S.S. (2006) *Size Matters*. Houghton Mifflin Company, Boston, MA.

Malina, R.M., Baxter-Jones, A.D.G., Armstrong, N., Beunen, G.P., Caine D, Daly, R.M., Lewis, R.D., Rogol, A.D., Russell, K. (2013). Role of intensive training on growth and maturation in artistic gymnasts. Sports Medicine, in press.

Malina, R.M., Bouchard, C., and Bar-Or, O. (2004) *Growth, Maturation, and Physical Activity*, 2nd edn. Human Kinetics Books, Champaign, IL.

Malina, R.M. (1998) *Sports and Children*, pp. 133–138. Williams and Wilkins Asia-Pacific, Hong Kong.

Tanner, J.M. (1962) *Growth at Adolescence*. Blackwell Scientific Publications, Oxford.

Ulijaszek, S.J., Johnston, F.E., and Preece, M.A. (1998) *The Cambridge Encyclopedia of Human Growth and Development*. Cambridge University Press, Cambridge.

Chapter 3
Endocrinology

John S. Fuqua[1], Alan D. Rogol[2,3]

[1]Section of Pediatric Endocrinology, Indiana University School of Medicine, Indianapolis, IN, USA
[2]Riley Hospital for Children, Indiana University School of Medicine, Indianapolis, IN, USA
[3]University of Virginia, Charlottesville, VA, USA

Introduction

The endocrine system consists of numerous complex axes, each of which interacts with the others, and through which the organism maintains homeostasis. These axes include the growth hormone (GH)/insulin-like growth factor-1 (IGF-1) axis, the hypothalamic-pituitary-gonadal (HPG) axis, the hypothalamic-pituitary-thyroid (HPT) axis, and the hypothalamic-pituitary-adrenal (HPA) axis (Figure 3.1). Each is self-regulating through a negative feedback response of its end product hormones on the regulating trophic hormones. Thus, in the normal state, increasing serum levels of cortisol, the end product of the HPA axis, suppress the production of corticotropin releasing hormone (CRH) in the hypothalamus and maintain relatively stable circulating concentrations of cortisol. Although each axis has its own regulatory mechanism(s), perturbation of one axis typically produces changes in the others. Alterations in the organism's steady state may be the result of injury, infection, stress, or exercise. Thus, athletes in training represent a dynamic of changing and interacting hormones that may have major effects on training outcomes. Female gymnasts in particular may reach high levels of training and competition during adolescence. Additionally, with age and maturation the endocrine axes change both qualitatively and quantitatively, leading to significant challenges to our understanding of the age-related physiology.

In this chapter, we shall review the GH/IGF-1, HPG, and HPA axes, initially focusing on developmental changes that occur as a child ages and matures and then moving to a discussion of the effects of exercise on these systems. We shall then review our current understanding of factors influencing energy balance in the individual, particularly the factors controlling food intake, hunger, and satiety in the exercising adolescent. Finally, we shall discuss the interplay between neuroendocrine mechanisms regulating energy balance and maturation of the HPG axis.

Although there is a large amount of data on these systems in normal individuals and a significant amount in athletes, there are not many data specific to gymnasts. We shall cover these where available.

Hypothalamic-pituitary axes

GH/IGF-1 axis

GH is produced in the somatotropes of the anterior pituitary gland under the control of two hypothalamic regulatory hormones, GH releasing hormone (GHRH) and somatostatin, with GHRH stimulating production and somatostatin inhibiting it (Figure 3.2). Once released, circulating GH interacts with its receptors on the cell membranes of

Gymnastics, First Edition. Edited by Dennis J. Caine, Keith Russell and Liesbeth Lim. © 2013 International Olympic Committee. Published 2013 by John Wiley & Sons, Ltd.

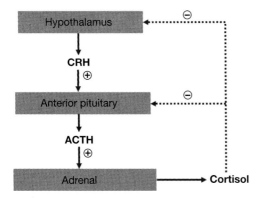

Figure 3.1 Hypothalamic-pituitary-adrenal (HPA) axis. Corticotropin releasing hormone (CRH) secreted by the hypothalamus stimulates pituitary release of adrenocorticotropic hormone (ACTH). This in turn stimulates secretion of cortisol by the adrenal gland. Cortisol has negative feedback effects on the pituitary and hypothalamus to regulate its secretion. There are numerous inputs to the hypothalamus that influence circulating cortisol levels (not shown).

GH-responsive tissues. In the liver, GH stimulates secretion of IGF-1 from hepatocytes, resulting in the majority of circulating IGF-1. Additional IGF-1 is produced locally within many tissues. Both circulating and locally produced IGF-1 are anabolic, acting through the IGF-1 receptor on many different tissues to increase cell growth, inhibit cell death, and promote cellular differentiation. GH

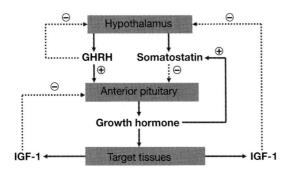

Figure 3.2 Regulation of growth hormone (GH) secretion occurs via the positive effects of GH releasing hormone (GHRH) and the negative effects of somatostatin. GH leads to target tissue release of insulin-like growth factor-1 (IGF-1), which provides regulatory control via its effects on GHRH and somatostatin release.

also stimulates secretion of IGF-2, which is thought to be mainly related to fetal growth and perhaps tissue repair. GH also has direct effects independent of IGF-1 and IGF-2. Acting through the GH receptor, GH stimulates cartilage growth and differentiation and promotes bone growth, increases lipolysis in adipose tissue, and stimulates amino acid uptake in muscle. IGF-1 acts in a negative feedback fashion to decrease pituitary GH release. Additionally, many neurotransmitters and neuropeptides also play roles in GH production, many of which are also active in regulating other endocrine axes, the hypothalamic stress response, and energy intake. An example of this is ghrelin, a peptide produced in the stomach that has potent orexigenic (appetite stimulating) properties. Although the physiologic relevance of this is unclear, ghrelin also acts to increase GH secretion (see Section "Neuroendocrine regulation of appetite/satiety"). In boys, GH secretion increases during mid-puberty, and the mean daily GH concentration correlates with growth rate (Figure 3.3). Exercise also influences the GH/IGF-1 axis. In gymnastics, initiation of intense exercise may reduce circulating IGF-1, possibly through the effect of higher levels of inflammatory cytokines. Prolongation of the exercise results in recovery of IGF-1 levels, possibly related to a decline in inflammation. These levels potentially reach concentrations above baseline.

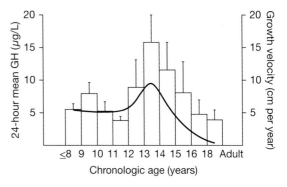

Figure 3.3 Results from Martha *et al.* (1989) of a cross-sectional study of growth hormone (GH) secretion in healthy males of normal stature. The mean 24-hour GH concentration increased in late puberty and then declines into adulthood. Superimposed is the standard height velocity curve for this age range, showing the relationship of GH secretion to linear growth rate. (Copyright 1989, The Endocrine Society.)

Hypothalamic-pituitary-gonadal axis

Perhaps more than any other endocrine axis, the HPG axis changes dramatically over the lifespan. In a reproductively mature individual, gonadotropin releasing hormone (GnRH) is produced in the hypothalamus and secreted into the hypothalamic-pituitary portal system in a pulsatile fashion. Control of GnRH secretion is poorly understood, but involves numerous inputs communicating nutritional status, physical and emotional stress, and other factors (see Section "HPG axis in adolescence"). In the pituitary gland, the pulsatile effect of GnRH promotes synthesis and secretion of the gonadotropins, luteinizing hormone (LH), and follicle stimulating hormone (FSH). In the male, LH promotes testosterone production from testicular Leydig cells, and FSH increases Sertoli cell and seminiferous tubule growth and leads to increased testicular volume. In the female, estrogens,

primarily estradiol, promote breast development, changes in distribution of adipose tissue, and cause proliferation of the endometrium. The physical changes of puberty are assessed using the Tanner stages of pubertal maturation (Table 3.1). Testosterone causes the well-known increases in muscle mass and strength in addition to normal male pubertal development. In the mature female, LH and FSH have complex and variable effects that lead to estrogen secretion and ovulation. In general, the sex steroids (estrogens and testosterone) act via negative feedback effects to suppress gonadotropins, particularly LH. The exception to this is the transient positive feedback effect of estradiol that causes a surge in LH production and triggers ovulation in the mid-portion of the menstrual cycle. Testicular Sertoli cells and ovarian granulocytes secrete inhibins, a class of hormones that act centrally to suppress FSH secretion (Figure 3.4).

Table 3.1 Tanner stages of pubertal maturation.

Breast development in females	
Stage	Physical characteristics
1	Prepubertal
2	Breast budding, elevation of both breast and nipple as a small mound
3	Continued enlargement of both breast and areola without separation of their contours
4	The areola and nipple form a secondary mound projecting above the contour of the breast
5	Adult shape, areola and nipple recessed to the contour of the breast

Pubic hair development in males and females	
Stage	Physical characteristics
1	Prepubertal
2	Sparse growth of long, lightly pigmented hairs at the base of the penis in males or the mons veneris/labia majora in females
3	Additional darkening and coarsening of hair, spreading over the pubic symphysis
4	Adult in character but has not spread to the lower abdomen in males or to the medial surface of the thighs in males and females
5	Adult in distribution, extension to the lower abdomen in males and/or the medial surface of the thighs in males and females

Genital development in males	
Stage	Physical characteristics
1	Prepubertal
2	Enlargement of the testes and scrotum, thinning and reddening of the scrotal skin, penis remains prepubertal
3	Further growth of testes and scrotum, enlargement of the penis in length and width
4	Further growth of testes and scrotum with pigmentation of the scrotal skin, further enlargement of the penis with maturation of the glans
5	Testes, scrotum, and penis are adult in size and shape

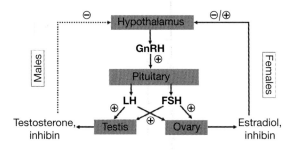

Figure 3.4 Hypothalamic-pituitary-gonadal (HPG) axis in males (left) and females (right). Gonadotropin releasing hormone (GnRH) stimulates pituitary release of the gonadotropins [luteinizing hormone (LH) and follicle stimulating hormone (FSH)]. LH is the primary stimulus for testicular testosterone secretion, while both FSH and LH are required for normal ovarian estradiol production. In males, testosterone provides negative feedback for LH secretion, while inhibin suppresses FSH release. The situation in females is more complicated, as estradiol can inhibit GnRH release, but can also provide positive feedback during the mid-point of the menstrual cycle.

Hypothalamic-pituitary-adrenal axis

Cortisol is a naturally occurring corticosteroid (glucocorticoid) that has wide-reaching and complex actions that influence nutrition and energy distribution, immune function, and growth. It is the product of the adrenal cortex and is produced under the trophic influence of pituitary-derived adrenocorticotropic hormone (ACTH). ACTH production is stimulated by hypothalamic CRH and vasopressin. As is the case for the GH/IGF-1 and HPG axes, the HPA axis also receives many other inputs, including the light/dark cycle, feeding schedules, immune regulation, and many neurotransmitters that mediate the effects of exercise and physical and psychic stress.

Hypothalamic-pituitary function in childhood

As discussed in the preceding section, hypothalamic-pituitary function varies over the lifespan. In utero, GH is relatively unimportant, as evidenced by individuals with Laron dwarfism caused by loss of the GH receptor. Such infants are within 10% of normal size at birth and only begin to demonstrate growth

failure in the first few months after birth. However, IGF-1 and IGF-2 are critical for fetal growth, as is insulin. During infancy and childhood, IGF-2 seems to be less important, although IGF-1, insulin, and thyroid hormone become critical for growth. In the male fetus, testosterone plays a critical role in the development of normal male internal and external genitalia and likely has effects to "masculinize" the brain and lead to male-typical behavior patterns. Sex steroids in the female fetus do not appear to be involved in physical development, although in both males and females, the transient surge of sex steroids in the first 6 months after birth ("minipuberty of infancy") may play roles in later gonadal function. Neither estradiol nor testosterone is produced in large amounts during later infancy or childhood.

Between the age of about 3 years and the onset of puberty, linear growth continues at a relatively constant velocity (see Chapter 2) under the continuing influence of the GH/IGF and thyroid axes. The HPG axis, which had been active at a low level for approximately 6 months in boys and as long as 2 years in girls, remains quite suppressed until the onset of puberty (see Section "HPG axis in adolescence"). However, the HPA axis changes its activity usually between the ages of 6 and 8 years. There are no differences in the secretion of ACTH or cortisol or the salt-retaining hormone, aldosterone; however, the inner zone of the adrenal cortex (zona reticularis) begins to increase in size in both sexes and to secrete the adrenal androgen precursors, dehydroepiandrosterone (DHEA) and its sulfate (DHEA-S), and androstenedione. This zone continues to proliferate, and the levels of these androgen precursors increase until late adolescence/young adulthood, likely under the influence of a pituitary factor distinct from ACTH. These morphological and biochemical changes are translated into a low magnitude and quite variable mid-childhood (~8 years old) growth spurt and the outward signs of adrenarche: pubic and axillary hair and axillary sweating ("pubarche").

The GH/IGF-1 system remains pulsatile throughout this period of growth and likely reflects the level and distribution of body fat and lean body mass, only to show a remarkable augmentation as very early pubertal maturation ensues (see Section "GH/IGF-1 axis in adolescence").

During this time between the "minipuberty" of infancy and the onset of puberty, the HPG axis is active at very low circulating concentrations of gonadotropins and sex steroid hormones. This state is likely due to the exquisite sensitivity of the GnRH-secreting neurons to feedback from the minute (compared to pubertal) levels of the sex steroid hormones. As puberty unfolds, this sensitivity to negative feedback lessens and the hypothalamus and pituitary begin to secrete GnRH and gonadotropins, respectively—at first at night and then during the day as well (see Section "HPG axis in adolescence"). This altered HPG activity underlies the physical changes of pubertal maturation.

Effects of physical activity on the endocrine system in prepubertal children

Physical activity (PA) refers to any body movement produced by the skeletal muscle that results in a substantial increase over resting energy expenditure. It has historically been viewed as important for healthy growth, but the type, frequency, intensity and duration required to support growth are not known with certainty. Nutrition (and energy balance) is presumably the non-pituitary, non-sex-steroid-mediated mechanism that surveys the "size" of the child and signals that an adequate supply of energy is available to promote and sustain the processes of growth and maturation.

Three maturity indicators have been used in studies of young athletes—(1) skeletal age (SA), (2) secondary sexual characteristics, and (3) the adolescent growth spurt in height. Among these, the SA is the only one appropriate for the prepubertal child or for longitudinal studies beginning prepubertally and finishing during or after pubertal maturation.

Few data are available in athletes less than 10 years of age. Most data from boys note a spectrum including some with advanced or delayed SA compared to age-matched controls. After the age of 10–11 years and until mid- to late puberty, the male athletes who continued to participate were more likely to be skeletally advanced (Figure 3.5). Adolescent gymnasts were the single exception among male athletes, for they were likely to present with delayed SA.

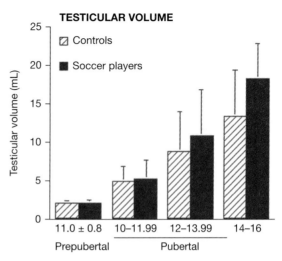

Figure 3.5 Male competitive soccer players were more advanced in puberty and were taller than age-matched controls. In this cross-sectional study (Cacciari *et al.*, 1990), 175 boys, aged 10–16 years, were compared to 224 boys who had never participated regularly in sports. The athletes were more advanced in all measures of pubertal maturation, including testicular volume. Testicular volume did not differ in prepubertal athletes and controls, but in pubertal subjects, mean testicular volume was 3 mL greater in athletes than controls, suggesting more rapid maturation in athletes. Bone age was more advanced, and the differences in height between athletes and controls did not persist when corrected for bone age. (With kind permission from Springer Science and Business Media.)

For the females, most athletes were noted to have an average SA for chronological age and to grow and mature (SA) at a physiologic pace. Once again, the exception was peripubertal artistic gymnasts; for, as noted in boys, there was a spectrum from early to late SA during childhood, but from the peripubertal ages onward, competitive athletes were more likely to have modest delays in SA. In the main, these data are based on cross-sectional studies. In the few longitudinal studies, gains in skeletal and chronological ages were similar in both boys and girls. Given the available data, one may conclude that training for sport does not influence skeletal maturation as noted at the hand and wrist. Selection for specific sport is apparently the most important factor influencing delayed or advanced SA.

Hypothalamic-pituitary function in adolescence

The onset of adolescence is marked by dramatic changes in endocrine systems, particularly in the HPG and GH/IGF-1 axes. These changes do not occur in isolation, but the two systems are intimately connected, with increased secretion of sex steroids and increased action of GH together having synergistic effects on physical maturation.

HPG axis in adolescence

The mechanism that signals the onset of pubertal maturation remains unknown but involves a decrease in negative feedback inhibition of gonadotropin secretion. The earliest neuroendocrine manifestation of puberty is the production of kisspeptin from hypothalamic neurons. Kisspeptin alters release of GnRH from the hypothalamus, stimulating the amplitude and pulse frequency of secretion. In the prepubertal child, GnRH is released in low amplitude pulses at a relatively low frequency. In the early stages of puberty, pulse amplitude increases and frequency increases to every 1–2 hours, primarily at night. As maturation progresses, these changes extend into the daytime hours. Along with GnRH secretion, LH and FSH production also increase, initially during the night. Early in puberty, serum levels of FSH are typically higher than those of LH, but this reverses as puberty ensues.

In the female, FSH promotes early follicular development in the ovary, and in conjunction with LH leads to gradually increasing secretion of the major circulating estrogen, estradiol. Estradiol concentrations in early puberty are quite low and vary with time of day, peak levels occurring in the morning hours. Estradiol is maintained at higher levels throughout the day as puberty progresses, and begins to show monthly cyclicity well before the onset of menstrual periods. With increasing gonadotropin stimulation, ovarian follicle development progresses and estradiol-induced proliferation of the uterine lining (endometrium) occurs. Near the end of puberty, typically at breast Tanner stage 4, part or all of the endometrium is sloughed, leading to menarche. Often, episodic endometrial loss occurs before ovulation begins and this non-ovulatory bleeding may be irregular and unpredictable. Additional gonadotropin exposure leads to establishment of dominant follicles and large increases in estradiol secretion. As the hypothalamus matures, the classic negative feedback effect on LH by estradiol is reversed at high levels, leading to a spike in LH secretion that stimulates ovulation and progesterone secretion. The ruptured follicle becomes the corpus luteum and continues progesterone and estradiol secretion for several days. As progesterone and estradiol levels subsequently fall, FSH increases and promotes follicle development for the next cycle. Eventually, progesterone and estradiol concentrations are insufficient to maintain the endometrium, and a normal menstrual period ensues.

In the male, increasing LH production in the nighttime hours results in testicular Leydig cell secretion of testosterone. In the early stages of puberty, this is primarily a nightly and early morning phenomenon. However, although daytime testosterone concentrations increase with progression of puberty, there continues to be a diurnal variation in testosterone levels into young adulthood. Serum concentrations of testosterone increase from <10 ng/dL before puberty to 300–900 ng/dL in adulthood, with the most rapid rise occurring between Tanner stages 2 and 3. FSH promotes development of the Sertoli cells and seminiferous tubules, which comprise the majority of the testicular volume. Testicular volume increases from 1–3 mL before puberty up to 15–25 mL in adulthood. Spermatogenesis begins early in pubertal development, between Tanner stages 2 and 3, although normal sperm concentration, morphology, and motility are often not established until the end of puberty. Throughout puberty in males, a portion of testosterone and androstenedione is converted to estradiol, which plays a major role in the promotion of body growth (see next section).

GH/IGF-1 axis in adolescence

The hallmark of adolescent growth is the pubertal growth spurt. The timing and magnitude of the growth spurt varies between boys and girls, and both are extremely variable between individuals. In the average girl, the growth spurt begins around age 9, reaches its maximum velocity of 8.3 cm per year between breast Tanner stages 2 and 3, and accounts for a total growth of 28 cm. Boys have later and larger growth spurts, with the take-off beginning at an average age of 11 years, peaking at a height velocity of 9.5 cm per year, and accounting for 30–31 cm of total growth. In both boys and girls, the pubertal growth spurt accounts for 17% of adult height. Prepubertal growth involves relatively greater growth of the extremities. Thus, a teen with delayed puberty has longer legs in proportion to total height.

During the pubertal growth spurt, large increases are noted in the serum concentrations of both GH and IGF-1, mediated largely by the higher levels of sex hormones as reviewed above. Thus, patients lacking gonads, but with intact pituitary glands, do not experience growth spurts. Interestingly, studies of males with a defective estrogen receptor or the inability to synthesize estradiol have demonstrated that, even in males, estrogens are specifically required for the increased GH/IGF-1 axis activity and increased height velocity during puberty. Additionally, these individuals also illuminate the requirement of estrogens for growth plate maturation, cessation of growth, and accrual of normal bone mass in males as well as females.

Ovarian-derived estrogens in females and estrogens produced from conversion of testosterone to estradiol in males act to increase GH secretion from the pituitary gland (Figure 3.6). In the liver, the higher GH activity stimulates secretion of IGF-1

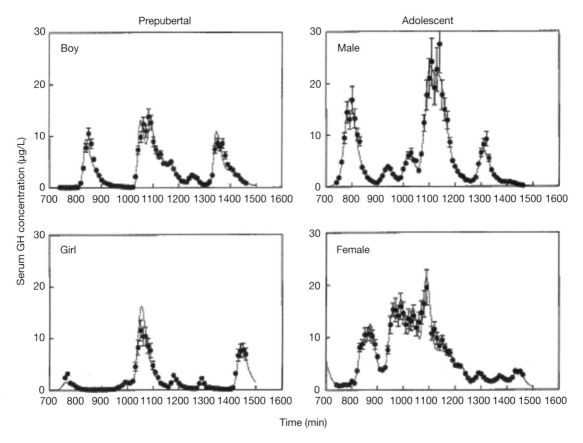

Figure 3.6 Growth hormone (GH) is secreted from the anterior pituitary in an irregular pulsatile pattern, with the first pulse usually corresponding to stage III/IV sleep. The panels on the left show typical secretory patterns from a prepubertal boy and girl. The panels on the right are from a boy and girl in later puberty and demonstrate larger pulses, but not necessarily greater pulse frequency. (Source: Veldhuis, *et al.* (2000). Copyright 2000, The Endocrine Society.)

into the circulation, where it is delivered to target tissues. Additionally, estrogens increase local (autocrine and paracrine) production of IGF-1 in peripheral tissues, including the growth plates of long bones. This higher circulating and locally derived IGF-1 leads to chondrocyte proliferation and hypertrophy, thus increasing the rate of long bone growth. Increasing estrogen concentrations in later puberty lead to ossification of the cartilage, termed growth plate senescence, and linear growth ceases.

Testosterone has limited, GH-independent effects on bone development. Acting via the androgen receptor on osteoblasts, testosterone increases cortical bone thickness and strength, protecting against osteoporosis. The androgen receptor is also present in the growth plates, and testosterone may have a modest direct contribution to linear growth independent of the GH/IGF-1 axis and without conversion to estradiol.

Stress response

The HPA axis is activated by stress, whether physical or psychological. The increased cortisol production acts in concert with the sympathetic nervous system. The teleological objective is to meet the increased demand for energy in somatic tissues and to dampen the threat or perceived threat to homeostasis.

If the challenge (stress) of total energy imbalance (deficit) is significant enough, the HPG axis is down-regulated. This is more noticeable in girls to keep the HPG axis in the prepubertal state, with the clinical condition of delayed pubertal maturation, or if menarche has occurred, with the clinical condition of secondary amenorrhea. The latter is marked by diminished pulsatile GnRH (and LH) release along with a relative nighttime predominance of LH pulses, as in early to mid-pubertal maturation. Less well described are the additional effects of energy deficit to dampen the HPT axis, which may also contribute to the disruption of the HPG axis.

As the energy deficit becomes chronic, IGF-1 levels decrease with a concomitant rise in GH levels as the feedback loop is opened, resulting in a state of partial GH insensitivity. This has also been noted in some male athletes in sports that maintain weight classes (weight-restricted), such as wrestling.

Many previous reports of "stress" endocrinology have employed multiple samples of blood or urine. These may be quite invasive for athletes who are training or especially competing. There are now some early reports analyzing levels of stress hormones in saliva, particularly cortisol and some androgen precursors. Because it is uncommon for the steroid binding (carrier) proteins to be found in saliva, the assays require additional sensitivity given that it is the free fraction of the circulating hormone that is measured. The collection procedure is relatively straightforward and stress-free, an important point for those who attempt to measure psychological stress, not only of physical training but also of the anticipation of competition. An example of this is Georgopoulos et al. (2011), who demonstrated loss of diurnal variation of salivary cortisol excretion in male and female elite artistic gymnasts.

Neuroendocrine regulation of appetite/satiety

Energy balance

The neuroendocrine regulation of appetite/satiety is just part of the overall balance in total energy. Athletes in the aesthetic sports attempt to limit caloric intake at a time when energy expenditure is high. Nutrition studies of female gymnasts report mean energy intakes that are 275–1200 kcal lower than recommended. Even after accounting for the differences in precision of the various self-reported food intakes, it is evident that many female gymnasts eat too little (Caine et al., 2001). Experimentally, this has been studied by Loucks and Thuma (2003), who noted decreasing LH pulsatility in runners as their energy balance turned negative by decreasing intake from 45 kcal/kg lean body mass to 10 kcal/kg lean body mass (Figure 3.7). This is similar to the cross-sectional study of Ackerman and colleagues (2012) noted below. Others have noted increasing cortisol secretion as well as an additional factor that diminishes GnRH release in those who exercise at an energy deficit. These perturbations are likely integrated at the anterior hypothalamus through neurons that respond to leptin,

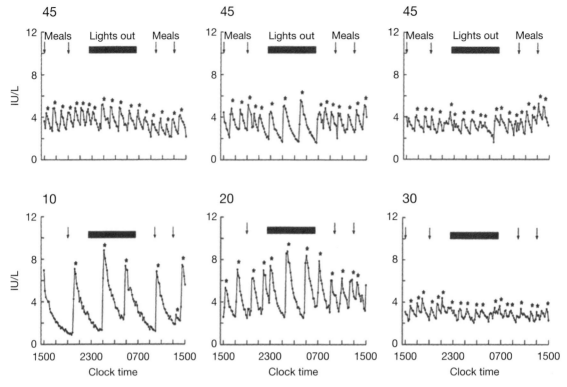

Figure 3.7 Effects of energy availability on luteinizing hormone (LH) pulsatility. Results of a study of 29 healthy sedentary young women who underwent supervised exercise and a controlled diet yielding energy availability of 45 kcal/kg lean body mass per day (Loucks & Thuma, 2003). Energy intake was then restricted to provide availabilities of 30, 20, or 15 kcal/kg per day. The top frames show serum concentrations of LH measured every 10 minutes for 24 hours at baseline for three representative subjects, with normal pulsatility. The bottom frames show the same measurements following restriction of energy availability. Below a threshold of 30 kcal/kg per day, LH pulsatility was disrupted, with decreased pulse frequency and increased amplitude. (Copyright 2003, The Endocrine Society.)

ghrelin, and peptide tyrosine tyrosine (peptide YY, PYY). The mechanism that diminishes gonadotropin release as a consequence of the energy deficit involves kisspeptin and proopiomelanocortin (POMC) neurons.

The neuroendocrine regulation of appetite and satiety is incompletely understood, but many publications over the last 10 years have expanded our knowledge. Current concepts involve a balance of inputs from two key hormones, leptin and ghrelin (see Sections "Leptin" and "Ghrelin"), that provide competing feedback to the CNS regarding peripheral fat stores. Intriguingly, both leptin and ghrelin also are intimately involved in the HPG axes and are thought to integrate energy balance with reproductive function.

Leptin

Leptin was discovered in 1994. It is a product of adipose tissue, and serum leptin concentrations are directly proportional to body fat stores. Leptin acts in the hypothalamus to suppress appetite via its actions on neurotransmitters including melanocyte stimulating hormone, neuropeptide Y, and agouti-related peptide. That leptin is active in long-term body weight regulation was demonstrated by animal models of leptin deficiency as well as a few children with mutations in the genes for leptin or its receptor. Such individuals have early onset severe obesity (within the first year of life), and administration of exogenous leptin results in suppression of appetite and weight loss. The vast majority of obese individuals, however, have elevated leptin concentrations, reflecting a resistance to its action that is not well understood.

Leptin also influences other neuroendocrine processes, including the HPA and HPG axes. Leptin is required for normal reproductive function, and both leptin-deficient animals and humans lack normal GnRH and gonadotropin secretion, and they do not enter puberty normally. Replacement of leptin in leptin-deficient humans also leads to the initiation of pubertal maturation, accelerates GnRH pulsatility, and stimulates pituitary gonadotropin secretion. Thus, leptin appears to be one of the links between adiposity and the triggers of puberty. Strenuously exercising young women often have secondary amenorrhea due to decreased energy availability related to increased energy expenditure and decreased energy intake. Serum leptin concentrations may be one of the mediators of this phenomenon. Administration of leptin for 36 weeks to 10 female athletes with hypothalamic amenorrhea led to resumption of menses in 70%, compared to 22% of women receiving placebo (Chou *et al.*, 2011). Those subjects receiving leptin also demonstrated increases in serum markers of bone formation and with longer term treatment increased their bone mineral density. In elite gymnasts, serum leptin concentrations are lower than those of the general population and are directly correlated with BMI and percent body fat. Leptin concentrations in this group are comparable to those seen in females with anorexia nervosa (Matejek *et al.*, 1999).

Ghrelin

Ghrelin was discovered in 1999 as a small molecule promoter of GH secretion. Although it does act via its receptor on GH-secreting cells of the pituitary gland, it arguably has more important actions in body weight regulation. Ghrelin is produced in the gastric mucosa, and its release is stimulated by gastric emptying and inhibited by food intake. It has potent orexigenic actions, acting in the hypothalamus via the neurotransmitters neuropeptide Y and agouti-related peptide. Levels of ghrelin increase during fasting and decrease during feeding, but ghrelin also appears to function in the long-term regulation of body weight as well. Serum

concentrations of ghrelin are inversely proportional to body mass index and increase with weight loss. Ghrelin appears to functionally antagonize leptin's actions in the hypothalamus, with each providing checks and balances against the other.

Like leptin, ghrelin is also involved in regulation of the reproductive system. There are relatively few human data, so our picture of how this works in humans is incomplete. In animals, ghrelin leads to decreases in GnRH secretion and gonadotropin production, thus acting inversely to leptin. Limited human data support this action. Elevation in circulating ghrelin delays puberty in rats and appears to have a sexually dimorphic effect, with males being affected more than females. Whether this is true in humans is unknown. Ghrelin also acts locally in the gonads. Again, human data are limited, but in the rat testis, ghrelin decreases testosterone production within the Leydig cell. In the ovary, ghrelin is produced by multiple cell types but seems to be most abundant in the corpus luteum. It may act in the ovary to decrease estradiol and progesterone production. What is not clear at present is whether these effects of ghrelin are mediated by circulating hormone or by locally produced (paracrine) hormone. Studies of gymnasts have revealed higher plasma concentrations of ghrelin compared to age-, sex-, and BMI-matched controls (Parm *et al.*, 2011). Although it is teleologically appealing to think that high-circulating ghrelin resulting from energy deprivation acts to inhibit gonadal function, thus limiting reproductive function in times of starvation, evidence for this is lacking at present.

Interaction of appetite regulatory systems and control of pubertal maturation

Thus, leptin and ghrelin seem to have opposing effects on both appetite/satiety and reproductive function. While leptin acts as a satiety signal and inhibits food intake, ghrelin acts to signal hunger and increases food intake. Furthermore, leptin has a stimulatory role in HPG axis activity and promotes pubertal maturation and reproductive function, while ghrelin appears to decrease both hypothalamic and gonadal activity and has negative effects on reproduction. Both leptin and ghrelin act via the arcuate and paraventricular nuclei in the hypothalamus and may deliver opposing effects on mediators such as neuropeptide Y, galanin-like peptide, and kisspeptin to influence GnRH, gonadotropin, and sex steroid production in addition to their more established effects on appetite and feeding.

There are some data to show that the human chronic stress response in athletes involves interplay among all of the hormones noted above and likely many more in other areas of the hypothalamus. Work by Kluge *et al.* (2007) demonstrated that higher ghrelin levels and lower leptin secretion are associated with diminished LH pulsatile release in amenorrheic adolescent athletes compared to either a control group or a group of eumenorrheic athletes. Ackerman and colleagues (2012) noted that ghrelin infusion suppresses the secretion of LH in healthy adults, and leptin has been noted to partially restore menstrual cycles in women (including athletes) with hypothalamic amenorrhea. In addition, leptin administration permits pubertal maturation in children with congenital leptin deficiency. Synthesizing all of these data into a central *hypothesis*, one may note that the diminished pulsatile release of LH has, as a proximate cause, an increased stress response that not only modifies the HPA axis (up-regulation) but also intersects with the energy homeostasis system, at least through the increase in ghrelin and the decrease in leptin. There are few data for the very delayed-maturing gymnasts who are the subject of this review. The extant data for other athletes by no means prove this mechanism but lay the groundwork for focused clinical trials.

Future research

Descriptive data for anthropometry, pubertal development, and basal hormone levels (with reference to the HPG and GH/IGF-1 axes) have been published and reviewed above. Future research should focus on the dynamic aspects of the regulation and interconnectivity of these axes. There are many connections to the hormones of appetite and energy regulation that will produce another level of complexity among these axes and energy homeostasis. It is becoming clearer that bone is no longer a passive bystander awaiting gravitational or muscle-activated loading. A new whole animal physiology, including metabolic actions within the bony compartment, will inform the homeostatic functions with the classical feedback loops to define both the "basal" state and the "biologically selected" gymnasts along with the responses to their training and competition. A more complete understanding of the effects of the forces on the structural compartments of bone will follow from the more recent use of new imaging techniques, particularly peripheral quantitative computed tomography (pQCT).

Summary

The endocrine system consists of numerous complex axes, including the GH/IGF-1, HPA, and reproductive systems. Each is self-regulating through a negative feedback response of its end product hormones on the regulating trophic hormones, resulting in maintenance of homeostasis. Alterations in this steady state may be the result of injury, infection, stress, or exercise. Thus, athletes in training represent a dynamic of changing and interacting hormones that may have major effects on training outcomes. Female gymnasts in particular may reach high levels of training and competition during adolescence and may be particularly susceptible to adverse endocrine effects. Gymnasts experience a reduction in IGF-1 concentrations with acute exercise that subsequently return to baseline, and long-term body growth does not appear to be impaired. The HPA axis is activated by physical or psychological stress. The GH/IGF-1, HPA, and the reproductive axes appear to exert many of their effects through energy balance, acting via the neuroendocrine regulation of appetite and satiety. Some athletes in aesthetic sports attempt to limit caloric intake at a time when energy expenditure is high, thus leading to a state of negative energy balance. Two key hormones, leptin and ghrelin, appear to provide competing feedback to the CNS regarding peripheral fat stores, reflecting energy balance. Both leptin and ghrelin also are intimately involved in the HPG axis and are thought to integrate energy balance with reproductive function.

In elite gymnasts, serum leptin concentrations are lower than those of the general population, which may lead to the secondary amenorrhea seen in strenuously exercising young women as a reflection of decreased energy availability related to increased energy expenditure and decreased energy intake. Studies of gymnasts have also revealed higher concentrations of ghrelin resulting from energy deprivation, and high-circulating ghrelin appears to inhibit gonadal function, although studies in humans are limited. The higher ghrelin levels and lower leptin secretion are associated with diminished LH pulsatile release in amenorrheic adolescent athletes. Additional research should focus on the interrelationship of these systems.

References

Ackerman, K.E., Slusarz, K., Guereca, G., Pierce, L., Slattery, M., Mendes, N., Herzog, D.B., and Misra, M. (2012) Higher ghrelin and lower leptin secretion are associated with lower LH secretion in young amenorrheic athletes compared with eumenorrheic athletes and controls. *American Journal of Physiology, Endocrinology, and Metabolism*, **302**, E800–E806.

Cacciari, E., Mazzanti, L., Tassinari, D., Bergamaschi, R., Magnani, C., Zappulla, F., Nanni, G., Cobianchi, C., Ghini, T., Pini, R., and Tani, G. (1990) Effects of sport (football) on growth: auxological, anthropometric and hormonal aspects. *European Journal of Applied Physiology and Occupational Physiology*, **61**, 149–158.

Caine, D., Lewis, R., O'connor, P., Howe, W., and Bass, S. (2001) Does gymnastics training inhibit growth of females? *Clinical Journal of Sports Medicine*, **11**, 260–270.

Chou, S.H., Chamberland, J.P., Liu, X., Matarese, G., Gao, C., Stefanakis, R., Brinkoetter, M.T., Gong, H., Arampatzi, K., and Mantzoros, C.S. (2011) Leptin is an effective treatment for hypothalamic amenorrhea. *Proceedings of the National Academy of Science of the United States of America*, **108**, 6585–6590.

Georgopoulos, N.A., Rottstein, L., Tsekouras, A., Theodoropoulou, A., Koukkou, E., Mylonas, P., Polykarpou, G., Lampropoulou, E., Iconomou, G., Leglise, M., Vagenakis, A.G., and Markou, K.B. (2011) Abolished circadian rhythm of salivary cortisol in elite artistic gymnasts. *Steroids*, **76**, 353–357.

Kluge, M., Schussler, P., Uhr, M., Yassouridis, A., and Steiger, A. (2007) Ghrelin suppresses secretion of luteinizing hormone in humans. *Journal of Clinical Endocrinology and Metabolism*, **92**, 3202–3205.

Loucks, A.B. and Thuma, J.R. (2003) Luteinizing hormone pulsatility is disrupted at a threshold of energy availability in regularly menstruating women. *Journal of Clinical Endocrinology and Metabolism*, **88**, 297–311.

Martha, P.M., Jr., Rogol, A.D., Veldhuis, J.D., Kerrigan, J.R., Goodman, D.W., and Blizzard, R.M. (1989) Alterations in the pulsatile properties of circulating growth hormone concentrations during puberty in boys. *Journal of Clinical Endocrinology and Metabolism*, **69**, 563–570.

Matejek, N., Weimann, E., Witzel, C., Molenkamp, G., Schwidergall, S., and Bohles, H. (1999) Hypoleptinaemia in patients with anorexia nervosa and in elite gymnasts with anorexia athletica. *International Journal of Sports Medicine*, **20**, 451–456.

Parm, A.L., Jurimae, J., Saar, M., Parna, K., Tillmann, V., Maasalu, K., Neissaar, I., and Jurimae, T. (2011) Plasma adipocytokine and ghrelin levels in relation to bone mineral density in prepubertal rhythmic gymnasts. *Journal of Bone and Mineral Metabolism*, **29**, 717–724.

Veldhuis, J.D., Roemmich, J.N., and Rogol, A.D. (2000) Gender and sexual maturation-dependent contrasts in the neuroregulation of growth hormone secretion in prepubertal and late adolescent males and females–a general clinical research center-based study. *Journal of Clinical Endocrinology and Metabolism*, **85**, 2385–2394.

Recommended reading

Caspersen, C.J., Powell, K.E., and Christenson, G.M. (1985) Physical activity, exercise, and physical fitness: definitions and distinctions for health-related research. *Public Health Reports*, **100**, 126–131.

Chrousos, G.P. (2009) Stress and disorders of the stress system. *Nature Reviews Endocrinology*, **5**, 374–381.

Dungan, H.M., Clifton, D.K., and Steiner, R.A. (2006) Minireview: kisspeptin neurons as central processors in the regulation of gonadotropin-releasing hormone secretion. *Endocrinology*, **147**, 1154–1158.

Eliakim, A. and Nemet, D. (2010) Exercise training, physical fitness and the growth hormone-insulin-like growth factor-1 axis and cytokine balance. *Medicine Sports and Science*, **55**, 128–140.

Malina, R. and Rogol, A. (2011) Sport training and the growth and pubertal maturation of young athletes. *Pediatric Endocrinology Reviews*, **9**, 440–454.

Pauli, S.A. and Berga, S.L. (2010) Athletic amenorrhea: energy deficit or psychogenic challenge? *Annals of the New York Academy of Sciences*, **1205**, 33–38.

Strobel, A., Issad, T., Camoin, L., Ozata, M., and Strosberg, A.D. (1998) A leptin missense mutation associated with hypogonadism and morbid obesity. *Nature Genetics*, **18**, 213–215.

Chapter 4
Skeletal health of gymnasts

Daniel Courteix[1,2], David Greene[3], Geraldine Naughton[2]

[1]Laboratory AME2P, Metabolic Adaptations to Exercise in Physiological and Pathological Conditions, Aubière Cedex, France
[2]School of Exercise Science, Australian Catholic University, Fitzroy, VIC, Australia
[3]School of Exercise Science, Australian Catholic University, Strathfield, NSW, Australia

Introduction

Gymnastics is a sport characterized by early intensive practice. It can represent the most demanding sport in which excellence in performance is reached during childhood and early adolescence. Childhood and adolescence are periods of enormous skeletal growth (at the end of adolescence, the major part of adult bone mass is acquired). Continuous processes of bone resorption and formation are characteristic features of the bone tissue in the entire human body and produce a constant turnover during the life span.

The balance between bone resorption and formation involves changes in the size, shape, and material properties of bone that determine skeletal strength. Moreover, skeletal changes (tempo of growth in bone size, mass, and density) evolve differently within different regions of the skeleton and within the trabecular and cortical compartments. Although genetic factors determine the major part of the variability in skeletal development, modifiable factors related to lifestyle and disease can influence bone health.

Gymnastics, First Edition. Edited by Dennis J. Caine, Keith Russell and Liesbeth Lim. © 2013 International Olympic Committee. Published 2013 by John Wiley & Sons, Ltd.

Factors involved in skeletal growth: sensitive period from childhood to adulthood

During skeletal growth, the balance of cellular activity occurs in favor of net bone formation. At the time of peak bone mass, the osteoclastic bone resorption is exactly matched by the osteoblastic bone formation. Peak bone mass is the amount of bone tissue accrued during childhood and adolescence and present at the end of the skeletal maturation. Beyond sex and racial differences in skeletal development, large variability exists among individuals in bone size, geometry, and mass. After the heritable factors that account for an estimated 60–80% of the variability, growth and sex hormones play an essential role during adolescence.

A number of hormones affect bone modeling and remodeling. Endogenous circulating estrogens and androgens independently exert positive effects on bone growth, development, and mineral acquisition in both male and female adolescents. Hormonal deficiencies or receptor abnormalities are associated with lower than expected bone mass. The growth hormone (GH) regulates directly the bone size and mass. Endogenous GH and insulin-like growth factor-1 (IGF-1) increase dramatically during puberty, augmented by the increasing concentrations of sex steroids. The action of GH on bone is mainly mediated through IGF-1, which positively affects bone turnover by stimulating osteoblast proliferation and differentiation. The bone remodeling cycle is directly influenced by endocrinopathies (e.g., thyroid or parathyroid hormone and cortisol) or indirectly via their effects on the sex steroids.

The peripubertal period is characterized by major hormonal changes. This stage of development seems particularly sensitive to the factors involved in building the skeleton. It has been shown that, in females, incremental gains in bone mass are particularly pronounced over a 3-year period, generally from 11 to 14 years of age. The rate of gain dramatically slows after 16 years of age and/or 2 years after menarche. In males, the gain in bone mass is particularly high over a 4-year period, generally from 13 to17 years; after which time, the rate of gain markedly attenuates. However, in males, bone growth remains significant between 17 and 20 years for lumbar spine and mid-femoral shaft regions.

Genetic potential for bone health can be reached only when diet, physical activity, and hormone production are adequate. Specifically, this includes an environment with sufficient intake of protein, efficiency of calcium and vitamin D absorption, an "above threshold" response to biomechanical stimuli, and other mechanisms that influence the skeletal development. The skeletal effect of calcium and vitamin D in children and adolescents is an issue that has been extensively researched. However, skeletal loading during physical practice, with respect to exercise modalities, is the most effective stimulus for improving the bone mineral accrual. Activities characterized by weight bearing or impact loading are known to have an osteogenic action on the skeleton. There is evidence to suggest that the capacity of bone to adapt its mass to such activity is greatest during puberty. Artistic Gymnastics is a dynamic sport, habitually exposing young gymnasts to training programs higher in volume and intensity than other sports for children of a similar age. Artistic Gymnastics from an early age is associated with a similar peak in bone mineral accrual in prepubertal female participants. It represents one form of physical activity that is particularly effective for the acquisition of bone mass in children.

Most physical activity interventions in children occur in the school setting. The interventions involve adding weight-bearing physical activity to children's lifestyle. The greatest "window" for responsiveness appears to occur at and around the time of puberty. But habitual exposure to gymnastics is associated with pronounced advances in bone parameters even prior to puberty.

Mechanisms of adaptive responses of bone to exercise

Experimental studies report that movement (mechanical) opportunities could determine over 40% of post-natal bone strength. The skeleton responds to the mechanical stimuli by inducing or inhibiting bone modeling and remodeling, a process that keeps peak strains within a safe physiological range. Such a mechanism is associated with the mechanostat theory that proposes a negative feedback system to explain the adaptation of bone by homeostatic control of peak strains. This process depends on the characteristics of the loading. The modalities for rendering the stimuli "osteogenic" consist of high-magnitude, high-frequency, and unusually disseminated strains. The mechanical load needed to stimulate osteogenesis decreases as the strain magnitude and frequency increase. The mechanosensitivity of bone cells is saturated after a few cycles of loading but can recover after rest; thus, separating loading into short bouts with periods of rest optimizes the response to loading. As a result, many of the demands of gymnastics can be interpreted as highly likely to be adequately stimulating bone growth.

Exercise as a stimulus for bone site

The evidence base of research supporting the positive effects of physical activity on bone strength continues to increase. The nature and frequency of exposure determine the potential ability for a sport to be more or less osteogenic. For example, weight lifters display higher bone mineral content (BMC) and bone mineral density (BMD) than runners or swimmers, although factors relating to the bias of self-selection may in part explain these findings. Weight-bearing or impact-loading exercises are essential for stimulating bone accretion, but loading is site specific.

Among the best examples of exercise loading on specific sites are reports from young tennis players who displayed marked side-to-side differences in arm bone mass and density (favoring the dominant arm), in comparison with age-matched controls (Haapasalo *et al.*, 1998). A less documented mechanism to increase bone strength is the redistribution of the bone mass to the regions submitted to high mechanical strains. Further, in prepubertal children, the increased bone density induced by gymnastic training in the stressed sites of the body could be related to a decreased skull bone mass. Courteix *et al.* (1999) report that the contribution of the head BMC to the whole body was significantly lower in gymnasts (25%) than in swimmers (28%) and controls (29%). Similar observations were found in astronauts during weightlessness conditions. In the gymnastics population, the bone mass increased at the head (+4.2%) and decreased at the pelvis (–7.4%), and femoral neck (–5%). This gradient in bone mass changes may be related to fluid shifts occurring in microgravity.

Exercise during growth is important because of the associated changes in bone geometry that translate to greater increases in bone strength than an increase in bone mass alone (Ducher *et al.*, 2009a; Figure 4.1). A study performed in school children highlighted how the prepubertal skeleton develops in response to the repetitive training it experiences

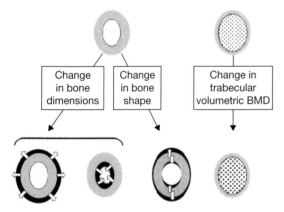

Figure 4.1 Potential changes in bone mass and shape that underpin the exercise-induced increase in bone strength in children and adolescents. The different mechanisms depicted are not mutually exclusive and in many instances, are combined. Changes in bone dimensions and bone shape are the preferential mechanisms in long bone shafts in response to exercise during growth. In long bone ends that are rich in trabecular bone, the increase in bone size is limited, and thus, exercise alternatively promotes an increase in trabecular volumetric density (trabecular vBMD). (Source: Ducher *et al.* (2009a).)

when participating in regular gymnastics (Ducher *et al.*, 2009). At diaphyseal sites these differences are predominantly in the bone and muscle geometry and not density. Conversely, at trabecular sites, the differences are increased density rather than geometry.

Comparisons of site-specific loading in young jockeys (mean age 19 years) with age-matched controls showed lower bone strength at the tibia. However, at other occupationally specific sites such as the radius, jockeys showed greater bone strength and trabecular density, independent of bone size (Wyner, 2010).

Specificity of gymnastics in upper and lower limbs

As a widely practiced activity by very young athletes, gymnastics has been studied extensively. Many gymnastics skills have been analyzed to determine the specific impact loading exerted on the skeleton. Ground reaction forces to both the upper and lower extremity have previously been recorded. Often, advanced level skills can generate forces of up to 13–14 times body weight on young highly trained gymnasts. Few intermediate skills have been assessed, with forces varying from 2 to 4 times body weight for the wrists and 10 times bodyweight for the ankles. Estimates of national and international gymnasts' upper and lower body ground reaction forces confirmed higher forces in the more experienced, skilled gymnasts.

Video analysis of the frequency of gymnastic-specific movements has been also used to estimate gymnastics loading. Gymnastic-specific movements including static, swing, and impact movements have been used to quantify the frequency of gymnastics loading during different phases of training, for male international level gymnasts. In this study (Burt *et al.*, 2010), gymnastics training was associated with, on average, 102 and 217 impacts per session on the upper and lower extremities, respectively with peak magnitudes of 4 and 10 times body weight.

One can point out that the wrist is subjected to forces in gymnastics that can exceed two to four times body weight. Therefore, the regular use of the upper extremities to support body weight subjects the wrist joint to recurrent impacts and loading. Wrist pain is common among artistic gymnasts of both sexes.

Estimates of wrist pain in these participants range from 46 to 79% (Mandelbaum *et al.*, 1989). In addition, more than 50% of young, beginning to mid-level, gymnasts also experience wrist pain. Cross-sectional surveys indicate that approximately 45% of gymnasts report pain of at least 6 months' duration.

There may be many possible causes of wrist pain in young gymnasts including dorsal wrist impingement, triangular fibrocartilage complex, and ulnar impaction syndrome (DiFiori *et al.*, 2006). However, because nearly all gymnasts enter the sport at a young age, the growth plates of the wrist are also potential sites for injury. Roy *et al.* (1985) described a stress reaction in a series of young gymnasts (Figure 4.2). Since then, there have been multiple case reports and case series describing stress injury to the distal radial physis. The cause of physeal injury in this setting may be a compromise of the metaphyseal and/or epiphyseal blood supply and may, infrequently, result in premature partial or complete closure of the epiphysis (DiFiori, 2006). The reports of distal radial physeal arrest are consistent with experimental studies in which prolonged intensive physical loading is associated with inhibition of linear bone growth. These findings suggest repetitive physical loading in excess of tolerance limits as a principle etiological factor in distal radius physeal injury and growth disruption. Unfortunately, other potential etiological factors such as nutrition, technique, and equipment have not been well studied.

In summary, repetitive loading of the wrist joint in young gymnasts is frequently associated with wrist pain, and injury to the distal radial physis occurs in some individuals. However, the relationship between these events and the development of positive ulnar variance is less clear.

Skeletal responses to mechanical loading at pre-, peri-, and post-pubertal stages

The osteogenic benefits obtained from exercise during growth are maturity- and sex-dependent. Exercise interventions seem to be most effective

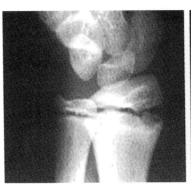 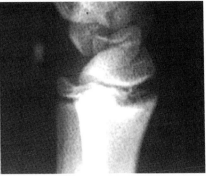

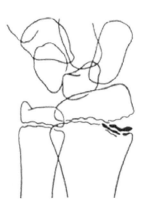 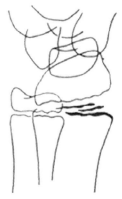

Figure 4.2 Radiographs and line drawings of the wrist of a symptomatic young gymnast. Changes of the distal radial epiphysis include widening of the radial margin, fragmentation, cystic changes and irregularity of the metaphyseal margin, and a beaked effect of the distal aspect of the epiphysis. (Source: Roy S, Caine D, Singer KM (1985) with permission from SAGE Publications.)

when initiated during pre- or early puberty. It is thought that exercise may preferentially affect the surface of bone that is undergoing apposition during growth. Before puberty, the skeleton reveals the capacity of responding to loading by adding more bone on the periosteal surface than would normally occur through growth-induced periosteal apposition.

Several studies have suggested that the skeletal response to activity varies by pubertal stage. A 6-year longitudinal study (Saskatchewan bone mineral accrual study; Bailey et al., 1999) showed that active children gained more bone during the 2 years surrounding peak bone velocity than inactive children (from 10 to 40% depending on the skeletal site). In this study the accrual rates for the different maturation stages were not assessed.

A cross-sectional Finnish study analyzed the relationship between maturity and BMD in child and adolescent female racquet sport players and maturity-matched controls (Haapasalo et al., 1998). In this study, the side-to-side BMD differences were measured at the proximal humerus, humeral shaft, and distal radius. The differences were significantly greater in players than controls at Tanner stages 3, 4, and 5. There were no differences between players and controls at Tanner stage 1, while the girls differed at the humeral shaft for Tanner stage 2. A potential correlation between training volume and intensity, and maturation stages could bias such observations, but it seems that after stage 3 the association of training and bone gain suggest a synergistic effect of pubertal hormone activity and mechanical loading in explaining the bone accretion.

Knowing the stage of development at which bone is most responsive to mechanical constraints offers an attractive possibility to enhance bone mass to benefit children by means of a physical activity program.

Ironically, as age increases in the majority of children, and girls in particular, physical activity decreases. Intuitively, establishing good physical activity patterns prior to puberty appears appropriate. Promoting sports such as gymnastics with great attraction for girls and well-established

musculoskeletal benefits would seem to be a developmentally appropriate strategy.

Differential effects of gymnastics on bone mass, density, geometry, architecture, and bone strength index

Gymnastics training is unique in generating high mechanical loading to the skeleton of very young children. Most of the studies have focused on competitive female participants. Recently, studies have extended to recreational gymnasts, using longitudinal follow-up designs. In these studies, a large range of participants has been analyzed, from 4 to 17 years old. Indeed, this age span includes peripuberty in which bone is highly responsive to loading stimulations. As such, gymnastics provides an excellent model for assessing the effects of weight-bearing physical activity on bone mineral development.

Bone mineral density

To date, there is evidence for an osteogenic effect of gymnastic training, specifically via bone mass and density.

From cross-sectional studies, girls training regularly in gymnastics for 2 or more years have displayed a higher BMD than their untrained counterparts at specific skeletal sites. Prepubertal girls who participated in elite level gymnastics had greater BMD at the mid-radius, distal radius, lumbar spine, femoral neck, and Ward's triangle than age-matched peers. In contrast, prepubertal female swimmers failed to show differences in BMD values when compared with age-matched nonswimmers (Courteix et al., 1998; Figure 4.3). These differences may be attributable to the intermittent high-impact ground reaction forces, such as jumping and tumbling that are involved in gymnastics, as opposed to the generation of muscular forces in a low-gravity environment such as swimming.

Some studies have assessed the link between the volume (duration and intensity) of training and the magnitude of improvement in bone mass gain.

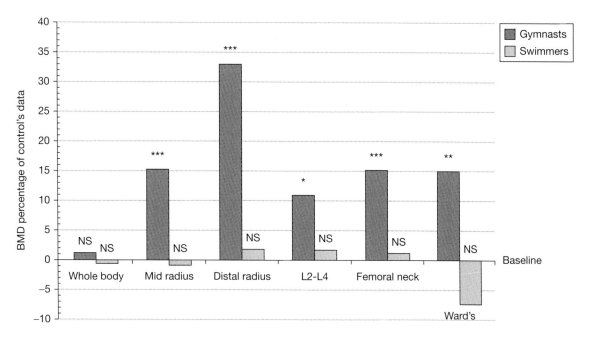

Figure 4.3 BMD values for gymnasts and swimmers, expressed as a percentage of control values. *$p < 0.05$; **$p < 0.01$; ***$p < 0.001$; NS, difference between groups is not statistically significant. (Source: Courteix *et al.* (1998) with permission from Springer Science + Business Media.)

Results indicate that the higher the volume of practice, the greater the enhancement of bone mass.

Longitudinal studies have reported that areal BMD increased 30–85% more rapidly in young female gymnasts than in sedentary children. One study compared the bone mineral accrual of high-level versus recreational participation in gymnastics by 4–10-year-old girls (Erlandson *et al.*, 2011b). The findings suggest that recreational and precompetitive gymnastics participation is associated with greater BMC. This study emphasizes the ability of low-level gymnastics participation to positively influence bone accretion. Therefore, participation in gymnastics even through school physical education programs should be promoted for all children.

The association of sports participation to longitudinal changes in BMD in collegiate female athletes aged 18–29 years was explored in gymnasts, runners, swimmers, and controls, in two cohorts followed-up for either an 8-month or a 12-month period (Taaffe *et al.*, 1997). These results pointed out the highest BMD values in gymnasts. During follow-up, the gymnasts were the only participants to exhibit positive gains at both the lumbar spine and femoral neck.

Beyond the use of dual energy X-ray absorptiometry (DXA) in investigating the bone density of skeleton, recent investigations have also used more precise methods to explore the changes of shape, size, and geometry within bone compartments.

Although BMD is one of the most important factors contributing to bone strength, it cannot explain alone how the bone tissue organization evolves under the constraints. Other factors including geometry and microarchitecture are involved in explaining bone strength.

Geometry

The mechanical behavior of bone not only depends on its material properties but also largely depends on the spatial distribution of bone material within the given structure. Geometric factors such as external diameter and cortical thickness can significantly influence bone strength. The outer diameter of long bone can, for example, predict up to 55% of the variation in bone strength.

Most bone geometric research in retired gymnasts have been performed at the forearm, with results often showing greater indices of total bone size and strength in gymnasts than controls.

In a recent cross-sectional study, the geometry of 173 gymnast and control participants, 8–17 years old, was analyzed using the hip structural analysis technique (Dowthwaite *et al.*, 2012). Maturity, assessed by the stages described by Tanner, was taken into account in this study. Maturity-specific comparisons suggested site-specific skeletal adaptation to loading during growth, with greater advantages at the radius than the proximal femur. At the radius, gymnasts' advantages included greater bone width, cortical cross-sectional area (CSA), and cortical thickness; in contrast, at the femoral neck, gymnasts' bone tissue CSA and cortical thickness were greater, but bone width was narrower than in nongymnasts.

Although hip structural analysis provides interesting additional data, it remains limited by its two-dimensional techniques. Peripheral quantitative computed tomography (pQCT) provides three-dimensional (3D) analyses in regions of interest to bone loading such as the tibia and radius. Devices such as pQCT are included among instruments capable of providing more informative 3D analyses of bone geometry at the "macroarchitectural" level.

Macroarchitecture: bone strength

Bone geometry can be an important component of the quantitative assessment of bone. Understanding bone strength at the macroarchitectural level involves the characteristics of shape and structural integrity, particularly from data acquired for cortical bone.

It is also possible to acquire microarchitectural characteristics to improve the understanding of bone geometry at a more precise level and include information about trabecular volume, trabecular spacing, and connectivity. Microarchitectural analyses will be discussed later in this chapter.

Devices such as the pQCT provide macrostructural characteristics such as cortical area, CSA, and density. However, one of the most interesting components of bone geometry is bone strength. Essentially, bone strength is the product of bone structure (size and shape) and material properties (density). Using estimates obtained from a pQCT device, bone strength at a specific site is calculated by first dividing the cross-sectional moment of inertia by 0.5 of the subperiosteal width and then multiplying the quotient by the cortical density.

In a comparison of well-trained adolescent female athletes, gymnasts showed 60% and 53% greater bone strength at the distal and proximal tibia, respectively, than their nonactive peers (Greene *et al.*, 2012). Independent of bone size, bone strength differences can be found. Weight-bearing bones in small people can continue to develop strength by laying down cortical bone on the inside surface and/or through improving cortical density.

For example, when tibial bone characteristics of young apprentice jockeys were compared with age-matched peers, the apprentice jockeys showed lower bone strength at the tibia than controls. However, greater bone strength was apparent at the radius of the jockeys than the controls. Site-specific loading adaptations are therefore well supported by macroarchitectural estimates of bone strength.

Longitudinal results from recreational and competitive gymnasts who were tracked for 6 months just prior to, or in the early stages of, puberty, showed the greatest bone strength gains in the radius of the gymnasts who were most exposed to gymnastics over this period of time. From the longitudinal results, we can also improve our understanding of how dose-responsive musculoskeletal adaptations can occur from participating in sports such as gymnastics.

Measures of bone strength have also been used in combination with body weight and forearm length to estimate fracture risk in the radius and ulna of gymnasts. Greater bone strength to weight ratios were found in 6–11-year-old gymnasts than non-gymnasts at the proximal ulna than radius (Burt *et al.*, 2011). This has also been shown in retired elite gymnasts. The traditional measurement site of the radius may therefore be underestimating the magnitude of exercise-induced skeletal adaptations that can be associated with participating in sports such as gymnastics.

Microarchitecture

Access to parameters of bone quality has improved in recent years with the refinement of bone imaging techniques. Using high-resolution pQCT (HR-pQCT) or magnetic resonance imaging, 3D images of the radius and tibia with a high resolution can be readily achieved. This provides in vivo access to parameters such as percentage of bone volume (BV/TV), cortical thickness (Ct.Th), trabecular number (Tb.N), trabecular thickness (Tb.Th), and trabecular separation (Tb.Sp).

Trabecular bone microarchitecture is an important skeletal feature that identifies individuals with fracture risk as well as, or better than, BMD. The unique study (Modlesky *et al.*, 2008) that investigated the trabecular bone microarchitecture, such as apparent trabecular bone volume to total volume (appBV/TV), trabecular number (appTb.N [mm^{-1}]), trabecular thickness (appTb.Th [mm]), and trabecular separation (appTb.Sp [mm]) using magnetic resonance imaging in young female artistic gymnasts exhibit higher appBV/TV (14%) and appTb.N and lower appTb.Sp (14%) than controls (Figure 4.4).

Skeletal health of gymnasts after training cessation

The exercise-induced skeletal benefits obtained during growth cannot be considered clinically important unless they are maintained into late adulthood, when fractures occur. Intuitively, this would seem unlikely because the mechanostat theory predicts a decrease in bone strength if exercise is reduced or ceased in adulthood.

A recent paper from the University of Saskatchewan's *Pediatric Bone Mineral Accrual Study* presents the results of a 14-year follow-up in gymnasts and nongymnasts in whom higher bone mass was previously reported (Erlandson *et al.*, 2011a). At the start of the study, the participants were premenarcheal. The last bone measurements were performed 10 years after the retirement or cessation of training, that is, 14 years after the first investigation. Ten years after retirement, gymnasts had maintained similar (and superior) size-adjusted total body, lumbar spine, and femoral neck BMC differences ($p < 0.05$) (13%, 19%, and 13%, respectively) when compared with nongymnasts. Therefore, bone mass benefits first observed in premenarcheal gymnasts were still apparent even after the long-term removal of the gymnastics loading stimulus.

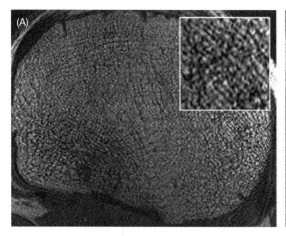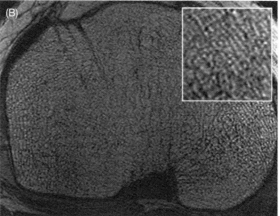

Figure 4.4 High-resolution magnetic resonance images of the proximal tibia of a female collegiate artistic gymnast **(A)** and a female control **(B)**. There is a greater amount of trabecular bone (black) and less marrow (white) in the gymnast's proximal tibia, which is highlighted by the magnified subregions presented at the top right of each image. (Source: Modlesky *et al.* (2008) with permission from Springer Science + Business Media.)

The literature brings evidence that past gymnastics training is associated with greater bone mass and bone size in women some years after retirement. Skeletal benefits are site specific, with greater geometric adaptations (greater bone size) in the upper compared with the lower limbs. Further investigations with pQCT revealed that the greater bone mass of the retired gymnasts was associated with greater bone size, cortical CSA, and trabecular volumetric density in the radius, and greater CSA and trabecular volumetric density at the tibia.

These results support the theory that structural adaptations obtained during growth may be maintained until senescence. This can be explained by the fact that the mature skeleton is thought to lose bone mass essentially through remodeling on the endosteal envelope, and to a much lower extent on the periosteal envelope, thereby preserving bone size and strength.

Further research (with questions still to be answered or to be investigated)

1 Gymnastics is usually considered one of the most osteogenic sports, its practice induces great magnitude and frequency of constraints on upper and lower limbs. Therefore, if naturally these impacts can induce a better bone strength, reducing the risk of fracture later in life, one can consider that the soft tissues and the joints could also be improved or altered by these high stresses.

   The question to be investigated is to determine the effects of intensive gymnastic training, on joints and conjunctive tissues, and whether the consequences on the joints and connective tissue could induce deleterious side effects on the children' health.

2 Female gymnasts frequently present with overt signs of hypoestrogenism, such as late menarche or menstrual dysfunction. Primary amenorrhea has been found in approximately 15–20% of elite female gymnasts, while episodes of secondary amenorrhea were reported in 40–60% of this population. There are discrepancies in the results concerning the effects of hormonal disorders on bone tissue. One recent study reported greater lumbar spine BMC and BMD as well as trabecular volumetric density and bone strength in the peripheral skeleton of former gymnasts without a history of menstrual dysfunction, but not in those who reported either primary or secondary amenorrhea (Ducher et al., 2009b). Another study reported that mechanical forces generated by high-impact loading and muscular contraction during gymnastics training had powerful osteogenic effects, which could counteract the increased bone resorption resulting from oligo-amenorrhea and amenorrhea observed in the gymnasts (Burt et al., 2010). Other researchers have attempted to determine whether hypoleptinemia occurring in rhythmic gymnasts, and probably resulting from the energy deficits observed in such population, may negatively impact on bone health; the authors concluded that high-impact training is able to counterbalance bone effects usually encountered in young females with abnormal hormonal responses.

The question would be: can we advance the understanding of the mechanisms of higher bone mass and properties observed in gymnasts despite the presence of amenorrhea, oligo-amenorrhea, and hypoleptinemia?

Summary

In summary, children participating in the sport of gymnastics have the potential to benefit from a very osteogenic environment created by habitual, intermittent, and relatively high-intensity loading of the musculoskeletal system. Although the understanding is incomplete, loading (impact forces) of up to 2–4 times body weight has been identified at the wrists and 10 times body weight loading has been estimated at the ankles during performances of fundamental gymnastics skills. Without the support of bone enhancing hormones that promote bone modeling and remodeling during puberty, significant advances in bone health parameters can be observed in prepubertal gymnasts. It is postulated that pubertal hormonal activity in combination with gymnastics training may be optimal for the musculoskeletal health of many, but not all, gymnasts. Although limited, there is also evidence that some of the benefits associated with gymnastics measured during the peripubertal stage of development, can be maintained into adulthood. The evidence of the effectiveness of gymnastic participation for the musculoskeletal health of children is strengthened by the availability of precise devices such as DXA and, more recently, pQCT. However, more randomized controlled trial and longitudinal studies are required. Research on dose responsiveness showing greater adaptations with more intense gymnastics participation remains imperfect due to the limited number of studies involving recreational participants and because of the confounding potential of musculoskeletal maladaptation (injuries) with increased exposure to gymnastics. Wrist injuries among gymnasts remain highly prevalent. Multiple and developmentally important factors such as associative changes to joints and connective tissue, and hormones associated with menstrual function (and dysfunction) require further investigation if we are to more completely understand the impact of gymnastics on the musculoskeletal health of young females.

References

Bailey, D.A., McKay, H.A., Mirwald, R.L., Crocker, P.R., and Faulkner, R.A. (1999) A six-year longitudinal study of the relationship of physical activity to bone mineral accrual in growing children: the university of Saskatchewan bone mineral accrual study. *Journal of Bone and Mineral Research*, **14**, 1672–1679.

Burt, L., Ducher, G., Naughton, G., and Greene, D.A. (2011) Skeletal differences at the ulna and radius between pre-pubertal non-elite female gymnasts and non-gymnasts. *Journal of Musculoskeletal and Neuronal Interactions*, **11**(3), 227–233.

Burt, L.A., Naughton, G.A., Higham, D.G., and Landeo, R. (2010) Quantifying training load in pre-pubertal artistic gymnastics. *Science of Gymnastics Journal*, **2** (3), 5–14.

Courteix, D., Lespessailles, E., Obert, P., and Benhamou, C.L. (1999) Skull bone mass deficit in prepubertal highly-trained gymnast girls. *International Journal of Sports Medicine*, **20**, 328–333.

Courteix, D., Lespessailles, E., Peres, S.L., Obert, P., Germain, P., and Benhamou, C.L. (1998) Effect of physical training on bone mineral density in prepubertal girls: a comparative study between impact-loading and non-impact-loading sports. *Osteoporosis International*, **8**, 152–158.

DiFiori, J.P. (2006) Overuse injury and the young athlete: the case of chronic wrist pain in gymnasts. *Current Sports Medicine Reports*, **5**, 165–167.

DiFiori, J.P., Caine, D.J., and Malina, R.M. (2006) Wrist pain, distal radial physeal injury, and ulnar variance in the young gymnast. *American Journal of Sports Medicine*, **34**, 840–849.

Dowthwaite, J.N., Rosenbaum, P.F., and Scerpella, T.A. (2012) Site-specific advantages in skeletal geometry and strength at the proximal femur and forearm in young female gymnasts. *Bone*, **50**, 1173–1183.

Ducher, G., Bass, S., and Karlsson, M.K. (2009a) Growing a healthy skeleton: the importance of mechanical loading. In: *Primer on the Metabolic Bone Diseases and Disorders of Mineral Metabolism*, pp. 86–90. John Wiley & Sons, Inc.

Ducher, G., Eser, P., Hill, B., and Bass, S. (2009b) History of amenorrhoea compromises some of the exercise-induced benefits in cortical and trabecular bone in the peripheral and axial skeleton: a study in retired elite gymnasts. *Bone*, **45**, 760–767.

Erlandson, M., Kontulainen, S., Chilibeck, P., Arnold, C., Faulkner, R., and Baxter-Jones, A. (2011a) Higher premenarcheal bone mass in elite gymnasts is maintained into young adulthood after long-term retirement from sport: a 14-year follow-up. *Journal of Bone and Mineral Research*, **27** (1), 104–110.

Erlandson, M.C., Kontulainen, S.A., Chilibeck, P.D., Arnold, C.M., and Baxter-Jones, A.D. (2011b) Bone mineral accrual in 4- to 10-year-old precompetitive, recreational gymnasts: a 4-year longitudinal study. *Journal of Bone and Mineral Research*, **26**, 1313–1320

Greene, D.A., Naughton, G.A., Bradshaw, E., Moresi, M., and Ducher, G. (2012) Mechanical loading with or without weight-bearing activity: influence on bone strength index in elite female adolescent athletes engaged in water polo, gymnastics, and track-and-field. *Journal of Bone and Mineral Metabolism*, **30** (5), 580–587.

Haapasalo, H., Kannus, P., Sievanen, H., Pasanen, M., Uusi-Rasi, K., Heinonen, A., Oja, P., and Vuori, I. (1998) Effect of long-term unilateral activity on bone mineral density of female junior tennis players. *Journal of Bone and Mineral Research*, **13**, 310–319.

Mandelbaum, B.R., Bartolozzi, A.R., Davis, C.A., Teurlings, L., and Bragonier, B. (1989) Wrist pain syndrome in the gymnast. Pathogenetic, diagnostic, and therapeutic considerations. *American Journal of Sports Medicine*, **17**, 305–317.

Modlesky, C.M., Majumdar, S., and Dudley, G.A. (2008) Trabecular bone microarchitecture in female collegiate gymnasts. *Osteoporosis International*, **19**, 1011–1018.

Roy, S., Caine, D., and Singer, K.M. (1985) Stress changes of the distal radial epiphysis in young gymnasts. A report of twenty-one cases and a review of the literature. *American Journal of Sports Medicine*, **13**, 301–308.

Taaffe, D.R., Robinson, T.L., Snow, C.M., and Marcus, R. (1997) High-impact exercise promotes bone gain in well-trained female athletes. *Journal of Bone and Mineral Research*, **12**, 255–260.

Wyner, P. (2010) Musculoskeletal health of male and female apprentice jockeys. *Journal of Science and Medicine in Sport*, **12**, e119.

Recommended reading

Bachrach, L.K. and Asbmr (2009) Skeletal development in childhood and adolescence, Chapter 14. In: *Primer on the Metabolic Bone Diseases and Disorders of Mineral Metabolism*, pp. 74–79. John Wiley & Sons, Inc.

Greer, F.R., Krebs, N.F., Committee on Nutrition, and American Academy of Pediatrics (2006) Optimizing bone health and calcium intakes of infants, children, and adolescents. *Pediatrics*, **117**, 578–585.

Kohrt, W.M., Bloomfield, S.A., Little, K.D., Nelson, M.E., and Yingling, V.R. (2004) American College of Sports Medicine Position Stand: physical activity and bone health. *Medicine and Science in Sports and Exercise*, **36**, 1985–1996.

Keller, M.S. (2009) Gymnastics injuries and imaging in children. *Pediatric Radiology*, **39** (12), 1299–1306.

Chapter 5
Energy needs and weight management for gymnasts

Jorunn Sundgot-Borgen[1], Ina Garthe[2], Nanna Meyer[3]

[1]Department of Sports Medicine, The Norwegian School of Sport Science, Oslo, Norway
[2]Sports Nutrition Department, The Norwegian Olympic and Paralympic Committee and Confederation of Sport, Oslo, Norway
[3]Beth-El College of Nursing and Health Sciences, University of Colorado *and* United States Olympic Committee, Colorado Springs, CO, USA

Introduction

Gymnastics requires gracefulness, speed, power, and coordination. Gymnastics is supposed to be aesthetically appealing. A finite balance between strength and body composition is required so that routine movements can be performed gracefully. Thus, it is important for gymnasts at the elite level, representing all the four disciplines of Olympic gymnastics (e.g., Rhythmic, Men's and Women's Artistic, and Trampoline), to maintain a lean physique and strength for both performance and aesthetic reasons. Optimal nutritional practices are critically important for training and top performance during competition. It is particularly important that young gymnasts consume sufficient energy and nutrients to meet the demands of growth, training, and tissue maintenance. Dietary assessments of high level gymnasts at different age groups indicate that many of these athletes consume less than the recommended amount of energy and some nutrients for their age and training load (Jonnalagadda *et al.*, 1998; Michopoulou *et al.*, 2011).

Studies indicate that delayed menarche, menstrual dysfunction, and eating disorders are common among female gymnasts, which may impact growth, development, and athletic performance. It is clear that all of these factors are influenced by the gymnasts' nutritional status. Therefore, in this chapter, the nutritional demands of male and female gymnasts are explored, including the potential risks and consequences of restrictive eating. In addition, recommendations related to optimal energy and nutrient intake and healthy weight control are included.

Energy requirements for gymnasts

Energy intake

Energy intake (EI) should support the variability of the gymnast's annual training and competition plan to bring dedicated months and years of training to fruition with expected performance outcomes. How much the athlete needs to eat is not easily estimated, especially considering the four different disciplines of Olympic gymnastics. Examining the literature on doubly labeled water (DLW) studies, conducted in athletes participating in various sports in free-living conditions, shows that energy expenditure can be quite high but variable among sports.

What these studies also show is that there is a mismatch between total daily energy expenditure (TDEE) and EI in the absence of weight loss, indicating the inherent bias of dietary assessment methods to underreporting (Hill and Davies, 2001). Underreporting is especially of concern in populations focused on body mass and weight loss and should also be expected in gymnasts (Hill and Davies, 2001).

Gymnastics, First Edition. Edited by Dennis J. Caine, Keith Russell and Liesbeth Lim. © 2013 International Olympic Committee. Published 2013 by John Wiley & Sons, Ltd.

For the practitioner working with gymnasts, assessing TDEE in athletes also comes with a variety of complications. At the least complex level, the sport dietitian can select physical activity levels (PALs) or physical activity coefficients (PA) in calculations deriving energy expenditure requirement (EER) and/or multiples of resting metabolic rate (RMR). RMR can be measured or assessed. Practitioners are advised to use lean body mass if possible when estimating RMR in athletes. Other quick approaches include reference tables summarizing energy cost for a given person relative to weight and sport. More time-consuming, burdensome, and complex approaches are assessment techniques that involve PA records using metabolic equivalents for 24 hours or less (e.g., detailing exercise energy expenditure, EEE).

Energy requirements to support daily training for female and male athletes exercising approximately 90 minutes per day or less may need to be around 45 kcal kg^{-1} per day and 50 kcal kg^{-1} per day, respectively. This may be a helpful target for those working with athletes and is similar to what is suggested by Manore *et al.* (2007).

Using EI data from dietary records in combination with stable body weight has also been recommended as a tool for determining energy needs of athletes.

That these data can accurately reflect energy requirement of athletes should not be assumed and several factors should be considered when using dietary intake data to estimate TDEE in gymnasts. As mentioned above, underreporting of dietary intake occurs in individuals and groups. Especially in sports such as the gymnastic disciplines that emphasize leanness and thinness, it should be expected that EI is underreported. Other issues of using EI to gauge energy needs in athletes relate to energy efficiency. For example, reported EI of gymnasts do not seem to be very high (Jonnalagadda *et al.*, 1998; Michopoulou *et al.*, 2011). Does this mean that gymnasts have grown accustomed to long-term underfeeding? If true, reported EI is expected to meet the newly established, however, suppressed TDEE.

There are a few other approaches to evaluate whether a gymnasts eats enough, without having to assess two highly biased variables, EI and TDEE. First, evaluating changes in body weight and composition for the purpose of nutritional, and especially caloric,

adequacy can be an effective approach, especially if used over time. However, in athletes with disordered and/or restrictive eating, energy efficiency may again complicate the professional's ability to evaluate the athlete using body weight and composition. While no follow-up studies have confirmed this, Duetz *et al.* (2000) showed a significant association between the energy deficits incurred throughout the day and percent body fat. This study compared gymnasts to runners and showed that runners who appeared to graze throughout the day had less body fat than gymnasts who seem more prone to energy restriction throughout the day. Interestingly, both groups experienced a similar energy deficit at the end of the day, but grazing versus dieting for prolonged periods of time was associated with lower body fat levels in runners versus gymnasts (Duetz *et al.*, 2000). Thus, it is possible that gymnasts who chronically diet are at greater risk for low RMR and increased fat storage to preserve energy. These athletes are also expected to be more resistant to a weight loss program, and thus, may struggle more to attain and maintain a lean physique.

Another valuable tool to evaluate adequacy of EI is menstrual regularity, as menstrual dysfunction may indicate a low EI, high EEE, or a combination of the two. A diet reduced in calories may simply be too low to meet all physiologic functions beyond what is necessary for exercise. This concept is referred to as energy availability (EA) and is derived by EEE subtracted from EI. For female athletes in particular, reducing EI, while continuing with hard training poses a risk due to the link between low EA and menstrual dysfunction. Thus, an irregular or absent menstrual cycle may well indicate that the athlete is not consuming enough calories to meet the demands of the sport and daily energy needs for growth and repair. Menstrual dysfunction is one of the components of the female athlete triad (Nattiv *et al.*, 2007). While an athlete not eating enough may jeopardize endocrine function, she/he is also at risk for acute effects that may interfere with performance, including glycogen depletion, micronutrient deficiencies, and fatigue. Manore *et al.* (2007) proposed the following guidelines for maintaining EA in exercising women during various phases of weight loss, maintenance, growth, and recovery (Table 5.1). These values can be used

Table 5.1 Recommended levels of energy availability for female athletes during various phases of training, competition, growth and weight maintenance.

	Weight loss (kcal kgFFM^{-1} d^{-1})	Maintenance (kcal kgFFM^{-1} d^{-1})	Growth/intense training or racing (kcal kgFFM^{-1} d^{-1})
Energy availability	30–45	45	>45

Source: Manore et al., 2007.
FFM: fat-free mass

to evaluate at least a female athlete's EI relative to various phases of training, competition, and/or growth. To date, there are no recommendations for male athletes, although it may be that similar targets apply due to the relative expression (i.e., body weight) of these values.

Taking into consideration the methodological challenges and the limitations related to EI data, Table 5.1 shows that EI in gymnasts varies and EI reported is well below expected requirement, although this is dependent on gender, age, performance level, and gymnastic discipline. Some studies report that the adolescent gymnast has adequate intake, however, the majority of the studies report insufficient EI and daily energy deficits in both adolescent and older female gymnasts (Jonnalagadda et al., 1998; Michopoulou et al., 2011). There are very few data on male gymnasts. However, from the studies reviewed it seems that male gymnasts report a more adequate EI. While the low reported EI in female gymnasts may reflect underreporting or energy efficiency issues, it may also be due to their attitudes about diet and body image. There are several concerns regarding a low EI, especially in athletes with heavy training loads. Low EI will, in most cases, lead to insufficient macro- and micronutrient intakes. When low EI is reported, it also commonly shows a lower than optimal carbohydrate and protein intake.

Carbohydrates

Carbohydrates provide energy for performance and recovery and exhibit a protein sparing effect. Gymnasts undergoing moderate, repetitive, skill-based training require a carbohydrate intake of at least 3 g kg^{-1} per day (Burke et al., 2011) and up to 5–6 g kg^{-1} per day if subjected to higher training loads (Burke et al., 2011). Most gymnasts, training

5–6 hours per day, need a carbohydrate intake of between 5 and 6 g kg^{-1} per day, which in absolute terms ranges from 250 to 300 g of carbohydrate per day for a female athlete weighing 50 kg. For carbohydrate, reduced intakes (~3 g kg^{-1} per day) in gymnasts are not problematic, as long as the athlete understands the importance of increasing carbohydrate with greater training intensity or volume. Carbohydrate adequacy is essential for the maintenance of glycogen stores and the ability to recover from training on a daily basis. Depleting glycogen stores during heavy training may pose both performance and health risks to the athlete. Obviously, when needed, weight loss and body composition manipulations should be attempted during off-season and low-intensity training phases. However, this is not always possible nor is it practical. Therefore, utmost attention should be paid to carbohydrate adequacy and a minimum level of 3 g kg^{-1} per day (Burke et al., 2011) should be met by both artistic and rhythmic gymnasts. While dietary assessment methods can help evaluate carbohydrate intake, performance indices along with subjective ratings of fatigue, mood state, hours of sleep, in combination with interdisciplinary approaches to monitor performance and health in the athlete can help evaluate overall stress and risk for underrecovery and overtraining related to carbohydrate inadequacy.

Protein

When it comes to protein intakes in gymnasts there are no specific recommendations. The recommended daily allowance (RDA) of protein for the general population is set at 0.8 g kg^{-1} per day and the adequate macronutrient distribution range (AMDR) suggests 10–35% of EI coming from protein. Athletes and active individuals have greater protein needs due to the importance of muscle growth and repair (Phillips and Van Loon, 2011) and this includes gymnasts. Protein recommendations have recently focused on optimizing post-exercise muscle protein synthesis (Phillips and Van Loon, 2011). Optimal protein intake may now be expressed relative to a meal based on recent research by Moore *et al.* (2009) who studied protein intake post-resistance exercise in a dose-response protocol. The optimal intake to maximize muscle fractional synthetic rate after exercise appears to fall within a range of 20–25 g. However, further analyses show that a relative protein intake of 0.25 g kg^{-1} per meal may be a more practical approach and would also prevent an excess intake in lighter athletes. Using these dynamic recommendations throughout the day, total daily protein intake still ranges from 1.2 to 1.6 g kg^{-1} per day, which is in line with current recommendations (Phillips and Van Loon, 2011). Thus, for a gymnast weighing 50 kg, a protein intake of 12–15 g spread over two post-exercise snacks and 15–20 g over three meals will equate to ~80 g (1.6 g kg^{-1}) per day. To be specific, a gymnast of that body mass could target 12–15 g of protein post-exercise to support recovery processes before eating lunch or dinner 1–2 hours later. It is likely that nutrient intakes will vary and protein ingestion may exceed 15–20 g for a dinner, especially if a piece of fish, meat, or poultry (25–30 g per 100 g) is combined with carbohydrate-rich sources such as pasta. This should not be of concern, however, and is usually compensated for by breakfast and lunch that are somewhat lower in protein.

The physiological demand of gymnastics is met by both aerobic and anaerobic means. In addition, gymnasts are generally strong as they need to generate a high level of power. Rhythmic gymnasts' physique, however, tends to be less muscular, as this discipline requires less strength and power compared to artistic gymnasts. Many daily training hours dictate a protein intake similar to strength and power athletes and on the order of 1.6 g kg^{-1} per day. In addition, dieting athletes or athletes with low EI may minimize loss of lean body mass if there is a relatively high protein intake. Further, adequate protein intake is considered important in low-energy diets due to the thermogenic and satiety-inducing effects.

Protein intake post-exercise has the ability to enhance recovery and repair of muscle tissue. Timing of intake, type of protein, and the addition of other macronutrients such as carbohydrate have all been investigated (Phillips *et al.*, 2011). Using the strategy discussed above (0.25 g kg^{-1} per meal) should also be beneficial for gymnasts, especially after hard training sessions as protein intake post-exercise enhances the ability to repair and rebuild muscle tissue. A thorough dietary assessment should provide the basis for recommendations given to athletes regarding daily protein requirements.

Fat

There are currently neither specific fat recommendations nor an RDA set for the general public or the active individual. The AMDR for fat is 20–35% of EI. Athletes should aim to distribute their fat calories among saturated and unsaturated fat and consume essential fatty acids as recommended by the dietary reference intakes (DRIs). Thus, nutrition education for gymnasts should include the discussion of the type of fats known to provide health and performance benefits. For gymnasts, carbohydrate and protein should be a priority due to the type of activity and appearance; however, fat intake should not be lower than 15–20% of total EI.

Vitamins and minerals

Although vitamins and minerals are not a source of energy, they play a vital role in energy metabolism and overall health. RDAs for vitamins and minerals are defined to prevent nutrient deficiencies and are not determined based on PALs (see "Recommended reading"). In general, athletes have adequate intakes of vitamins and minerals as long as EI is appropriate. However, B vitamins, calcium, vitamin D, iron, some antioxidants (e.g., vitamin C and E, beta carotene, and selenium), zinc, and magnesium can be of concern, especially in gymnasts. Athletes who may present with compromised micronutrient status are those who restrict energy for weight control and/or performance, eliminate one or more food groups due to dietary regimens, restrictions, or fear of calories, or who consume unbalanced diets characterized by low micronutrient density.

Studies including gymnasts show that intake of iron, copper, potassium, calcium, magnesium, zinc, vitamin A, several B vitamins, and vitamin D and E are compromised in these low-energy diets. Actually, some studies report inadequate micronutrient intakes in adolescent gymnasts, despite a relatively high EI. This shows that a well-planned eating (i.e., meals) and fueling (before, during, and after exercise) strategy should be followed when restricting EI to ensure adequate intakes. A gymnasts' food intake should be rich in nutrients, while low in energy (calories). This requires careful attention when selecting foods and snacks. Finally, most micronutrients are available through dietary sources with the exception of vitamin D, which is best obtained from the sun. Due to the indoor nature of gymnastics, these athletes are at risk for vitamin D deficiency and thus, should be screened for low vitamin D status and adequately treated if deficiency exists.

In summary, nutritional habits of gymnasts are often suboptimal considering their daily training regimen. Sport nutrition professionals should ensure that athletes meet energy requirements. Low EI leads to both acute and chronic adaptations, some of which affect performance, while others may compromise the health and growth of the athlete. Gymnasts should ingest sufficient carbohydrate and protein to ensure daily performance in the gym and rapid recovery post-exercise. Gymnasts should eat a diet rich in nutrients but low in energy density to meet all micronutrient requirements. Finally, gymnastics occurs indoors with little sunlight. All indoor athletes are at greater risk for vitamin D deficiency and should be screened. The next section will focus on the prevalence and risks of disordered eating and eating disorders in the sport of gymnastics.

Dieting and disordered eating in gymnasts

The prepubertal physique confers a performance advantage for gymnasts. Given the biological changes in both male and female athletes during adolescence, it is important to remember that the body in young growing female athletes develops in a direction against the ideal body in gymnastics—being as lean as possible. This may intensify perceptions of self-appearance and performance. Gymnasts start practicing sports by the age of 3 or 4 years of age, and already at age of 5–7 years, girls competing in gymnastics, report greater weight concerns than girls in nonaesthetic sports and nonathletic girls (Davison et al., 2002). As a result, a number of elite female Artistic and Rhythmic Gymnastics teams report the use of self-prescribed diets and pathogenic weight control methods. While more reported in female athletes, inadequate nutritional intake and the use of pathogenic weight control methods are also experienced in some male gymnasts. Female elite gymnasts often display low estradiol levels, hypoleptinemia, reduced body fat mass, insufficient caloric intake, and retarded menarche, while the pubertal development of male gymnasts remains almost unaltered. Long-term inadequate energy and nutrient intakes during the growth period could result in delayed pubertal development and retarded growth. However, there is presently only limited epidemiological evidence of reduced growth or delayed pubertal development in gymnasts. It is difficult to prove that gymnasts experience inadequate growth because of the selection for late-maturing females into the sport. Therefore, the study has yet to be conducted that would provide an estimate of the incidence rate of inadequate growth among female gymnasts.

The consequences of long-term low energy availability (LEA), such as amenorrhea and the imbalance in bone remodeling, are more severe for the adolescent athlete since the lag time of adequate bone formation interferes with reaching a high peak bone mass, adequate stature, and the normal development of the reproductive system. While a long-term process, studies demonstrate a catch-up effect for bone growth and body mass when caloric intake is normalized in young athletes suffering from LEA (Caine et al., 2001).

Although dieting is considered an important risk factor for the development of eating disorders, it is not necessarily dieting per se that triggers disordered eating or eating disorders. Controlled weight loss interventions in elite athletes seem not to increase the risk for disordered eating or eating disorders when guided by a professional sports dietician (Garthe *et al.*, 2011). However, athletes who are still growing should not diet, but be guided how to optimize EI and nutrient intake. Risk factors for eating disorders can be divided into two categories: (1) The pathogenesis of eating disorders is multifactorial with cultural, individual, family, and genetic/biochemical factors all playing a role. (2) There are sports-related factors such as personality factors, experienced pressure to lose weight leading to restricted eating, body dissatisfaction, early start of sport-specific training, injuries, the impact of coaching behavior, and sports regulations (Nattiv *et al.*, 2007). The reason why some athletes, including gymnasts, cross the line from dieting to serious clinical eating disorders is currently unknown. However, it has been reported that dieting and the desire to be leaner to improve performance is associated with the development of eating disorders in adolescent athletes and that regulations, such as in gymnastics, might indirectly increase the risk for eating disorders (Sundgot-Borgen and Garthe, 2011). Prospective controlled studies, examining risk and trigger factors for eating disorders in athletes, do not exist, and thus, the true risk factors for clinical eating disorders in aesthetic sports are not yet known.

Optimizing energy intake and body composition

In order for coaches to adequately perform a supportive function, many need factual information on nutrition and optimal body composition, risks and causes of disordered eating, menstrual (dys)function for females and hormonal changes in males, and psychological factors that both negatively and positively affect health and athletic performance. The authors suggest that all gymnastic disciplines should have position statements with guidelines related to optimizing nutrition and body composition and how to recognize symptoms associated with disordered eating and components of the triad. Dieting and weight issues should never be initiated from the coach, but be presented according to the athletes wish. Coaches should avoid putting pressure and/or telling an athlete to lose weight. Most gymnasts are fit and lean, but

often want to reduce weight. In such a case the coach and health care team should motivate the athlete to improve strength and power rather than encouraging weight loss. The focus should be on optimal nutrition and performance enhancement via nondieting strategies including better eating strategies, maintenance of optimal health, as well as improved mental and psychological approaches to training and competition. Health care providers should educate gymnasts and coaches that weight loss does not necessarily lead to improved athletic performance. Furthermore, since athletes are eager to perform, it is important to inform them about the side effects of undereating and inconsistent eating behavior. If the coach is concerned about an athlete's eating behavior, body image, and/or weight or body fat level, he/she should be referred to a sport dietitian or health care personnel for further evaluation and consultation. However, some gymnasts need to lose weight or change body composition. Therefore, recommendations published by Sundgot-Borgen and Garthe (2011) for healthy changes in body composition or weight are helpful. These are listed below and are specifically adjusted for gymnasts.

Recommendations for weight loss interventions in gymnasts

The body composition goal should be based on objective measurements of body composition. Prior to weight loss intervention, energy and nutrient status should be assessed. Furthermore, questions related to weight history and weight goal, menstrual history and status for females, dietary habits, and feelings about body image, body weight, and food should be included. If a history of disordered eating/eating disorders is present, a more intense and longer follow-up is suggested. Measurements of body composition should be done in private and the results should be explained and discussed with the athlete. The weight loss period should be done during off-season to avoid interference with competitions and sport-specific training loads.
• A 4-day or a 7-day diet record, objective measurements on body mass and fat mass and a blood test should be performed. If the gymnast has a history of amenorrhea or other indicators of low

bone mineral density (BMD), an objective measure of BMD is warranted (e.g., DXA). If a blood test indicates any specific micronutrient needs (e.g., iron, vitamin B12, and vitamin D), these vitamins should be provided and biochemical changes monitored during the period. Multivitamin, mineral, and omega-3 fatty acid supplements may be provided during the weight loss period to assure sufficient micronutrient and essential fatty acid intake.
• The gymnast should consume sufficient energy to avoid menstrual irregularities and aim for a gradual weight loss corresponding to ~0.5 kg per week. To induce a weight loss of 0.5 kg per week an energy deficit similar to ~500 kcal per day is needed, but there are individual differences. This can be achieved by reduced EI, increased energy expenditure through cardiovascular conditioning, or a combination of the two.
• A sport dietician who understands the demands of the four disciplines of Olympic gymnastics should plan nutritionally adequate eating strategies tailored to the individual. Throughout this process, the role of overall good nutrition practices in optimizing performance should be emphasized. The plan should contain at least 3–5 g kg^{-1} of carbohydrate, between 1.4 and 2 g kg^{-1} of protein per day (depending on the athlete's body composition goals), and provide between 15 and 20% of fat calories (of total EI). The focus should be on foods with low energy content but high nutrient density from a variety of sources, ingested at frequent intervals to support RMR and prolonged satiety, and prevent early fatigue during training. Post-exercise, recovery nutrition should be emphasized through timely (within 30 minutes) ingestion of carbohydrate and protein-containing foods. Foods high in whey protein, such as a flavored milk beverage to optimize muscle repair and recovery may also be recommended. Dairy products are also optimal due to their calcium content. Depending on the athlete and the situation, a well-timed recovery meal within 30 minutes post-exercise may be all that is needed, excluding the immediate recovery strategy in an attempt to reduce extra calories.
• It is important that the weight loss/change in body composition does not compromise gymnastic performance. For most, that means not to lose lean

bone mass during weight loss. If that is the case, strength training should be included during the weight loss period. A moderate energy restriction combined with strength training has been shown to alleviate the negative consequences on lean body mass and performance (Garthe *et al.*, 2011). Further, increasing protein intake can also prevent lean body mass.
• After weight loss, body fat percentage should not be lower than 5 for males and 12 for females. It is important to evaluate each gymnast using her own genetic predisposition relative to body fat and weight. Some gymnasts may tolerate a lower percent body fat at no consequence, whereas others may not do as well, meaning they may develop hormonal imbalances and consequential health and performance issues.
• Changes in body composition should be monitored on a regular basis, and athletes should be followed for at least two additional months after the weight or percent body fat goal has been reached just in case any continued or unwarranted losses or weight fluctuations occur.
• "Normal weight" gymnasts under the age of 18 years should be discouraged to lose weight.

Further research

There are a limited number of large-scale studies examining energy intake and expenditure in elite gymnasts representing all of the four Olympic disciplines. If practitioners are to tailor recommendations for weight management specific to the disciplines, more data need to be collected relative to both aspects of the energy balance equation in all four disciplines. Studies using the DLW technique should be prioritized in order to reduce the double-sided bias of dietary and PA assessment methods. More data are especially needed for male gymnasts. Large-scale prospective studies are also needed that follow cohorts of gymnasts over time, even into their retired years, to examine changes in eating and dieting behavior and associated performance and health risks. Prospective cohort studies are also suitable for examining risk and trigger factors for eating disorders among gymnasts.

Summary

It is particularly important that young gymnasts consume sufficient energy and nutrients to meet the demands of growth, training, competition, and tissue maintenance. Education and counseling regarding factors associated with optimal nutrition and body composition should be provided to both male and female gymnasts, parents, coaches, and health personnel. Circumstances that may adversely affect the gymnast's short- and long-term health include LEA, disordered eating behaviors, and eating disorders. Some gymnasts cross the line from dieting and use of pathogenic weight loss methods to serious, diagnosable eating disorders. A continuous focus on optimal EI and nutrient intake and the prevention of the female athlete triad is important for all working with young gymnasts.

References

Burke, L.M., Hawley, J.A., Wong, S.H., and Jeukendrup, A.E. (2011) Carbohydrates for training and competition. *Journal of Sports Sciences*, **29** (Suppl. 1), S17–S27.

Caine, D., Lewis, R., O'Connor, P., Howe, W., and Bass, S. (2001) Does gymnastics training inhibit growth of females?. *Clinical Journals of Sport Medicine*, **11**, 260–270.

Davison, K.K., Earnest, M.B., and Birch, L.L. (2002) Participation in aesthetic sports and girls' weight concerns at ages 5 and 7 years. *The International Journal of Eating Disorders*, **31**, 312–317.

Deutz, R.C., Benardot, D., Martin, D.E., and Cody, M.M. (2000) Relationship between energy deficits and body composition in elite female gymnasts and runners. *Medicine and Science in Sports and Exercise*, **32** (3), 659–668.

Garthe, I., Raastad, T., Refsnes, P.E., Koivisto, A., and Sundgot-Borgen, J. (2011) Effect of two different weight-loss rates on body composition and strength and power-related performance in elite athletes. *International Journal of Sport Nutrition and Exercise Metabolism*, **21**, 97–104.

Hill, R.J. and Davies, P.S. (2001) The validity of self-reported energy intake as determined using the doubly labelled water technique. *The British Journal of Nutrition*, **85** (4), 415–430.

Jonnalagadda, S.S., Bernadot, D., and Nelson, M. (1998) Energy and nutrient intakes of the United States National Women's Artistic Gymnastics Team. *International Journal of Sport Nutrition*, **8** (4), 331–344.

Economos, C.D., Bortz, S.S., and Nilson, M.E. (1993) Nutritional practices of elite athletes. Practical recommendations. *Sports Medicine*, **16**, 381–399.

Michopoulou, E., Avloniti, A., Kambas, A., Leontsini, D., Michalopoulou, M., Tournis, S., and Fatouros, I.G. (2011) Elite premenarcheal rhythmic gymnasts demonstrate energy and dietary intake deficiencies during periods of intense training. *Pediatric Exercise Science*, **23** (4), 560–572.

Manore, M.M., Kam, L.C., and Loucks, A.B. (2007) The female athlete triad: components, nutrition issues, and health consequences. *Journal of Sport Sciences*, **25** (Suppl. 1), S61–S71.

Moore, D.R., Robinson, M.J., Fry, J.L., Tang, J.E., Glover, E.I., Wilkinson, S.B., Prior, T., Tarnopolsky, M.A., and Phillips, S.M. (2009) Ingested protein dose response of muscle and albumin protein synthesis after resistance exercise in young men. *The American Journal of Clinical Nutrition*, **89** (1), 161–168.

Nattiv, A., Loucks, A.B., Manore, M.M., Sanborn, C.F., Sundgot-Borgen, J., and Warren, M.P. (2007) American College of Sports Medicine position stand. The female athlete triad. *Medicine and Science in Sports and Exercise*, **39**, 1867–1882.

Phillips, S.M. and Van Loon, L. (2011) Dietary protein for athletes: from requirements to optimum adaptation. *Journal of Sport Sciences*, **29** (Suppl. 1), S29–S38.

Sundgot-Borgen, J. and Garthe, I. (2011) Elite athletes in aesthetic and Olympic weight-class sports and the challenge of body weight and body compositions. *Journal of Sport Sciences*, **29** (Suppl. 1), S101–S114.

Recommended reading

Chen, J.D., Wang, J.F., Li, K.J., Zhao, Y.W., Wang, S.W., and Jiao, Y. (1989) Nutritional problems and measures in elite and amateur athletes. *The American Journal of Clinical Nutrition*, **49** (Suppl. 5), 1084–1089.

Cupisti, A., D'Alessandro, C., Castrogiovanni, S., Barale, A., and Morelli, E. (2000) Nutrition survey in elite rhythmic gymnasts. *The Journal of Sports Medicine and Physical Fitness*, **40** (4), 350–355.

D'Alessandro, C., Morelli, E., Evangelisti, I., Galetta, F., Franzoni, F., Lazzeri, D., Piazza, M., and Cupisti, A. (2007) Profiling the diet and body composition of sub-elite adolescent rhythmic gymnasts. *Pediatric Exercise Science*, **19** (2), 215-227.

Fogelholm, G.M., Koskinen, R., Laakso, J., Rankinen, T., and Ruokonen, I. (1993) Gradual and rapid weight loss: effects on nutrition and performance in male athletes. *Medicine and Science in Sports and Exercise*, **25** (3), 371–377.

Institute of Medicine (IOM), Food and Nutrition Board (1997) *Dietary Reference Intakes: Calcium, Phosphorus, Magnesium, Vitamin D, and Fluoride*. National Academy Press, Washington, DC.

Institute of Medicine (IOM), Food and Nutrition Board (1998) *Dietary Reference Intakes. Thiamin, Riboflavin, Niacin, Vitamin B-6, Folate, Vitamin B-12, Pantothenic Acid, Biotin, and Choline*. National Academy Press, Washington, DC.

Institute of Medicine (IOM), Food and Nutrition Board (2000) *Dietary Reference Intakes: Vitamin C, Vitamin E, Selenium, and Caratenoids*. National Academy Press, Washington, DC.

Kirchner, E.M., Lewis, R.D., and O'Connor, P.J. (1995) Bone mineral density and dietary intake of female college gymnasts. *Medicine and Science in Sports and Exercise*, **27** (4), 543–549.

Lovell, G. (2008) Vitamin D status of females in an elite gymnastics program. *Clinical Journal of Sport Medicine*, **18** (2), 159–161.

Manore, M.M., Meyer, N.L., and Thompson, J. (2009) *Sport Nutrition for Health and Performance*, 2nd edn. Human Kinetics, Champaign, IL.

Rodriguez, N.R., Di Marco, N.M., and Langley, S. (2009) American College of Sports Medicine position stand. Nutrition and athletic performance. *Medicine and Science in Sports and Exercise*, **41** (3), 709–731.

Sansone, R.A. and Sansone, L.A. (2010) Personality disorders as risk factors for eating disorders: clinical implications. *Nutrition in Clinical Practice*, **25**, 116–121.

Sundgot-Borgen, J. (1996) Eating disorders, energy intake, training volume and menstrual function in high-level modern rhythmic gymnastic gymnasts. *International Journal of Sport Nutrition*, **2**, 100–109.

Weimann, E., Witzel, C., Schwidergall, S., and Bohles, H.J. (2000) Peripubertal perturbations in elite gymnasts caused by sport specific training regimes and inadequate nutritional intake. *International Journal of Sports Medicine*, **21**, 210–215.

PART 3
TRAINING AND PERFORMANCE ASPECTS

Chapter 6
Biomechanics related to injury

Gert-Peter Brueggemann[1], Patria A. Hume[2]

[1]Institute of Biomechanics and Orthopaedics, German Sport University Cologne, Cologne, Germany
[2]Sport Performance Research Institute and Faculty of Health and Environmental Sciences, Auckland University of Technology, Auckland, New Zealand

Introduction

Gymnastics (Artistic, Rhythmic, Trampoline) is listed under the most spectacular Olympic sports. The artistry and the skills performed by gymnasts often appear to be close to the ultimate limits of the human body. Sometimes reported severe injuries lead to the assumption that the ultimate biomechanical and biological limits have been achieved. From a public and especially a media perspective, the risk of overuse and acute injuries may be high in gymnastics given the spectacular artistic movements, onset of training at an early age, extreme mechanical and mental loading, and the enormous training load, especially in elite gymnasts. Acute injuries during competitions appear rather seldom, but if they happen the outcome is often dramatic and severe. Technical training aids and close spotting by coaches often defuse the risk of injury during training.

The rate of acute and overuse injuries of US college women gymnastics related to the number of participants is relatively high in practice and competition compared to other sports (Hootman *et al.*, 2007); the same scenario was reported for children's and youth sports (Caine *et al.*, 2006), but the injury rate is moderate in relation to the number of activity hours. For example, preparatory work

in gymnastics training such as warm-up, flexibility exercises, ballet, and physical conditioning, is more or less free of the risk of acute overload and related injuries and often takes more than a third of total training hours. Coaches, gymnasts, and physical trainers need to have a general understanding of mechanical loading throughout gymnastics and the response of biological tissues from short- and long-term perspectives to ensure injury risk can be minimized. Therefore, the major topic of this chapter is to give the reader a functional approach to the mechanical stimulus and response processes on both body segment and tissue levels (macroscopic and microscopic).

Notably, the sources of knowledge on mechanical loading in all three disciplines of gymnastics-male and female Artistic Gymnastics, Rhythmic Gymnastics, and Trampoline- are very limited. Few experimental data and reliable quantitative information on tissue loading are available and the majority of reported findings are limited to ground reaction forces or contact force to the apparatus (e.g., pommel horse, rings, parallel and horizontal bars, and asymmetric bars). Especially in Rhythmic Gymnastics and Trampoline, data on potentially heavy loaded musculoskeletal structures are rare. The research of movement techniques is more or less descriptive in nature even if there are some exceptions especially in airborne movements and long swings on horizontal and asymmetric bars and rings. In order to present comparable data of mechanical loading during gymnastics this chapter focuses on quantitative information derived from similar models and

Gymnastics, First Edition. Edited by Dennis J. Caine, Keith Russell and Liesbeth Lim. © 2013 International Olympic Committee. Published 2013 by John Wiley & Sons, Ltd.

collected with the same measuring technologies. Most data presented in this chapter arise from our own data collection of elite and subelite gymnasts during training, laboratory, and competitive sessions. Some reports of tissue response in young and also former gymnasts, mostly from Artistic and Rhythmic Gymnastics, can be derived from the literature. Unfortunately, these data are rarely related to the individual loading history of the athletes. Therefore, in addition to the retrospective data of tissue reaction to general loading in gymnastics, this chapter also presents data of tissue response of gymnasts arising from a 3-year survey of elite female gymnasts (Brueggemann, 2005).

The chapter generally approaches the objective of how biomechanics and mechanical loading in gymnastics is related to acute injuries or to overuse and to biological tissue response.

Estimates of mechanical loading in gymnastics will be derived from gymnastics skills, elements, techniques, and technical training aids. Critical tissue limits and the related mechanical loading will be critically evaluated. The long-term response to gymnastics-related mechanical loading of spinal biological structures and on peripheral joints will also be reviewed. Finally, an appropriate injury prevention model will be derived from the load-response perspective.

A tissue response model related to gymnastics

Recently, there has been an upswing and a strong concentration of difficulties in the routines of male and female gymnasts both in Artistic Gymnastics and Trampoline. A similar trend can be reported for Rhythmic Gymnastics. The rate of the development of more difficult elements is increasing. An increase in skill difficulty is mainly a result of changes to the Code of Points rules. In addition to rule changes, the development of materials and apparatus, the increased knowledge of training the athletes, and probably an increased impact from scientific knowledge has influenced this rapid development.

An increase in skill difficulty corresponds to the demand for higher mechanical energy achieved. The higher mechanical energy for an element allows, for example, a higher flight and improves the flight time for the execution of the more difficult skills. With an improved flight time the tuck body configuration in an airborne skill can be replaced by a straight body configuration that increases the assessment and the difficulty defined by the Code of Points. A higher angular momentum is the prerequisite for more somersaults and/or twists. Higher amounts of mechanical energy for the most attractive flights are related to higher energy when landing from the flight and increased biomechanical requirements for the biological structures involved.

The higher demand on energy generation is related to a higher mechanical loading of the biological structures responsible for the force production, the force transmission to the skeleton, and finally the force transfer to the physical abutment at the contact area to the ground, the trampoline, or in Artistic Gymnastics to the apparatus. The higher mechanical energy for the skills is related to higher linear and rotational velocities of the entire body and its body segments, which increase the stress of the biological systems for balance and motion control. In general, biological structures and systems have the potential for functional and morphological adaptation. An increasing number of failures of the biological system of male and female gymnasts or trampoline athletes, and the increasing frequency of mistakes during the routines in competition as well as in training, indicate the structural and functional limits of both the musculoskeletal and the motion and balance control systems or the neuromuscular systems is being approached (Knoll *et al.*, 2000).

A tissue loading response model will elucidate the relation between the mechanical loading as an input signal and the biological reaction as the related output (the biological or morphological and functional response) (see Figure 6.1).

In Artistic Gymnastics, mechanical load acts on the biological response matrix in a single or a multiple series over seconds, hours, days, weeks, and years. The mechanical exercise stimulus (MES) is characterized by the loading amplitude, the

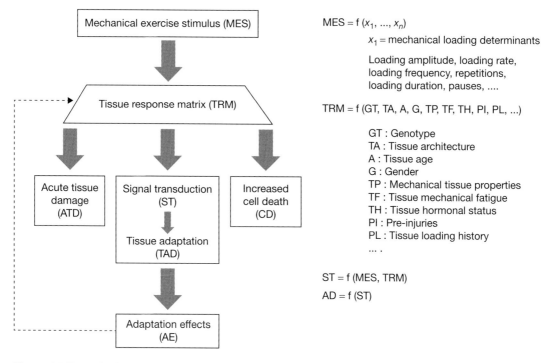

Figure 6.1 Tissue loading response model.

loading rate, the frequency and the duration of loading, and also by the pauses between the loading sequences. The biological tissue response matrix (TRM) is determined by the genotype, the tissue architecture, the tissue age, gender, pre-injuries, mechanical tissue properties, the tissue fatigue, the hormonal tissue status, and other factors. Due to the early onset of training in gymnastics and therefore the increased mechanical loading at an early age, the tissue is extremely sensitive to overuse in young gymnasts. During growth spurts the potential of tissue to withstand load bearing is temporarily decreased, which makes an appropriate load management most difficult in gymnastics.

If the MES is excessive, such loading has the potential for acute morphological and physical tissue damage (ATD), which means an acute failure of the tissue involved. If the MES is within the limits of the response matrix potential, the mechanical stimulus results in a signal transduction (ST) at the cellular level or—if the loading stimulus is not appropriate in terms of amplitude, frequency, or even direction—in an increased cell death (CD)

within the tissue under mechanical load. Assuming that the input signal to the response matrix is appropriate in terms of amplitude, direction, frequency, and intensity, ST will increase the cellular activation, which leads to tissue adaptation (TAD) on the cellular level as well as of the extracellular matrix. This is of relevance because the extracellular matrix defines and determines the mechanical properties of the tissue and is strongly related to mechanical strength of the given tissue. From this basis one can derive that tissue strength adaptation (TAD) is a function of the mechanical stimulus (MES), the response matrix (TRM), and the ST process. TAD is the source of tissue matrix change and therefore of tissue strengthening.

Tissue strength enhancement is the major concern in the physical preparation of the young gymnast allowing the tissue to withstand the extreme forces and torques in modern gymnastics. The key factor for minimizing the risk of long-term overuse is the appropriate loading of the biological structures guaranteeing TAD and strengthening. Consequently, prerequisites of load management in gymnastics' training are a sound knowledge of mechanical loading in gymnastics (MES) and a profound background of the TRM, which determines the tissue's critical strength limits. The weakness of the model is the limited knowledge of the individual characteristics of the determinants of the response matrix.

Acute and overuse tissue failure in gymnastics

ATD in Artistic and Trampoline Gymnastics results from falls on the ground, on the mats, and on the apparatus (trampoline, horizontal bars, asymmetric and parallel bars). Catastrophic injuries from direct falls with severe consequences to the spinal cord are infrequent. However, according to reports from the US National Center for Catastrophic Sports Injuries, the occurrence of this type of injury appears to be high in comparison to other sports. Acute injuries from direct falls affect the biological structures of feet, the ankle and the knee joints, the spine, the thoracic cage, and the elbows, wrists, and fingers. The mechanical energy applied to these biological structures at the collision instantaneously exceeds the actual tissue strength limits and leads to failure.

The main concern in gymnastics is overuse injury or overuse tissue failure, which is the result of frequent mechanical stimuli close to the ultimate tissue strength limits. In comparison to other sports, overuse injury rates in elite gymnastics and especially in artistic gymnasts are relatively high (Froehner, 2000). The foot, ankle, and knee joints and the spine are the most commonly injured locations. In male gymnastics the shoulder and the wrist are also ranked high in the injury frequency tables.

Studies of risk of injuries in gymnastics typically represent a broad range of performance levels, age groups, training systems, and related mechanical loading. Few retrospective studies on former elite athletes report chronic injuries and especially spinal radiological deformities of elite gymnasts (Pollaehne, 1991). Other retrospective studies (e.g., Tertti *et al.*, 1990) did not identify any major differences in early tissue degeneration between gymnasts and nongymnasts. However, many of the retrospective studies do not demonstrate results from top or elite subjects but those from subelite or recreational athletes. Froehner (2000) reported deformities and disorders of the spinal structures and the peripheral joints of 42 female and 27 male former top German gymnasts (all participated in Olympic Games, World Championships, or European Championships) 8.9 (±5.2) years after retirement from competitive Artistic Gymnastics.

Close to 10 years after their career, more than 90% of the male and female former gymnasts suffered from moderate or severe disorders of the spine, 40% of knee and ankle joints, and more than 30% of the male gymnasts of shoulders, elbows, and wrists. Severe discomfort of the spine was demonstrated in 57% of the female gymnasts (21% cervical spine, 17% thoracic spine, 52% lumbar spine) and in 58% of the male gymnasts (23% cervical spine, 19% thoracic spine, 50% lumbar spine). In 32 female former elite gymnasts Froehner (2000) identified structural changes and deformities in 42 vertebrae of the thoracic spine and in 21 vertebrae of the lumbar spine, which gives an average of two affected vertebrae per gymnast. The numbers for the male gymnasts are even higher (58 thoracic, 21 lumbar) with 3.76 affected vertebrae per gymnast. The highest frequency of structural changes of the former athletes is found in the thoracic-lumbar junction.

Spinal loading above the critical limits in regard to loading amplitude, loading rate, frequency, and duration resulting in deformation and structural changes might appear in Artistic Gymnastics especially in the thoracic-lumbar junction and more in female gymnastics in the lumbar region. Repeated hyperextension of the lumbar spine mainly in female Artistic and Rhythmic Gymnastics is assumed to pose a major risk to the lumbar spine and especially the pars interarticularis. However, a 3-year survey of elite German female gymnasts (Brueggemann & Krahl, 2000) ($n = 135$; age: 12–21 years) reports a frequency of slip instability (spondylolysis, retrolisthesis, pseudolisthesis) in 15 of 135 (11%) individuals, which is in the range of the normal population. A spondylolythesis was identified in 2.9% of the examined gymnasts. This frequency does not differ from that of a nonathletic population. The difference of these findings to earlier reports could be related to changes in the nature and type of the mechanical loading in female gymnastics. The repeated trunk flexion when landing from various heights or during take-off from the spring floor or the springboard may create compression forces sufficient to damage the anterior aspect of the vertebral endplate in the thoracic-lumbar region and disrupt further growth at this side.

Froehner's unique data demonstrate the knee and the ankle joint at second highest risk. From the 42 former female gymnasts 28% suffered from ankle joint disorders and 24% from knee-related discomfort. Among male athletes the knee showed 27% disorders and the ankle joint 15%. Upper extremities disorders were more common in the male subjects than in the female gymnasts. This can be explained by the different events and apparatus in male and female gymnastics. The females perform on three (floor exercise, balance beam, vault) of four disciplines that are intuitively prone to load the lower extremities, while the male gymnasts have only two (floor exercise, vault) of six apparatus. The total loading time of the lower extremity and the number of lower extremity loading repetitions are definitively higher in female than in male Artistic Gymnastics. Loading frequency and total loading time appear in combination with the loading amplitude as key determinants of the MES in Artistic Gymnastics.

Mechanical loading of biological structures in gymnastics

Measurement of mechanical loading

Two principal approaches are applied to study mechanical tissue load in gymnastics and other sports: (1) direct measurements and (2) indirect methods. While the direct techniques use sensors and transducers based on different technical principles and provide data describing variables directly connected to mechanical tissue loading, the indirect methods provide a compromise of mathematical models allowing a calculation or an estimation of loading-related variables on or within a biological tissue. Direct measurements are extremely seldom in gymnastics (exceptions are direct tendon force measurements in gymnastic like jumping and hopping) due to ethical and technical restrictions. The latter do not allow unhindered or nonrestricted movements for the gymnast, which is a prerequisite to approach realistic loading data. The modeling techniques applied to gymnastics used multibody models with an inverse dynamic approach and distribution models, which distribute the resultant joint moments and forces to load carrying structures and allow an estimate of mechanical load transmitted to specific tissue (bones and articular cartilage, intervertebral discs, muscle-tendon units, ligaments). Due to the fact that the mathematical models used for estimations of mechanical tissue loading have more unknowns than equations these approaches are underdetermined. Additional assumptions (e.g., tissue material properties, joint surface areas, and lever arms of ligament or tendons) must be taken into account and static optimization has often been used to minimize the solution space. It is obvious that the numerical solution is strongly related to the cost function used to solve the problem. Therefore, model outcomes have to be interpreted carefully and results of different models cannot be (quantitatively) directly compared. The data presented in this chapter are all derived from the same model and therefore comparable. The kinematic model input data are from three-dimensional (3D) motion analyses, while the kinetic data are taken from direct measurements of reaction forces on the ground (ground reaction forces) or on the apparatus (rings, horizontal bar, asymmetric bars, pommel horse, vaulting table, balance beam).

The measurement of the optic fiber transducer, which was also applied in gymnastics hopping and jumping and implanted in the Achilles and Patellar tendons (Brueggemann *et al.*, 2000), is based on modulation of light intensity by mechanical modification of the geometric properties of the plastic fiber that is inserted into the tendon. The structures of optical fibers used in animal and human experiments consist of two layered cylinders of polymers with small diameters. When the fiber is bent or compressed the light can be reduced linearly with pressure. The fiber can be inserted into the tendon or ligament with help of a hollow needle that is first passed through the tendon or ligament. The sterile optic fiber is then passed through the needle. The needle is removed and the fiber remains in situ. Both ends of the fiber are then attached to the transmitter–receiver unit. The calibration usually gives a good linear relationship between external force and optic fiber signal.

The direct methods are invasive or are often restricted to static positioning of the subject and have therefore limited application to dynamic movements and especially high-impact physical activities in gymnastics. In Artistic Gymnastics direct measurements are infrequent, whereas model-based estimations allow a first insight view into tissue loading and at least a relative comparison of loading within the spectrum of skills. Notably, the model-based quantities are conservative estimations by nature due to the chosen cost function. The real mechanical tissue loading will be even higher than the model-based estimates.

Mechanical exercise stimulus in gymnastics

As mentioned above, an increase in gymnastics skill difficulty is associated with the demand for higher mechanical energy. The further increase of mechanical energy results in higher mechanical stress on and in the biological structures. This increasing mechanical loading impacts primarily (a) the most distal joints of the kinematic chain with the hands/elbows/shoulders or the lower extremities (feet, ankle, and knee joints) and (b) the spinal structures. Due to the increased frequency of loading and the more frequent loading schedule one has to consider not only the ultimate tissue tolerances but also the modification of tissue tolerance limits in repeated loading regimes.

Spinal loading

The major and most dramatic clinical and radiological findings in gymnastics concern the thoracic-lumbar junction and the lumbar spine. There is controversy in the discussion about which skill or drill in gymnastics produces the highest loading

in regard to the thoracic-lumbar spine. One point discussed as a cause for the growth disturbances in the ring apophysis was the fast changes between flexion and extension of the thoracic-lumbar junction during the swings on the rings and horizontal bar. Some authors considered the damage at the ring apophyses in gymnasts as a flexion trauma and speculated that this could be caused by incorrect landing. This controversy led to the inclusion of gymnastic landings and long swings combined with dynamic flexion and extension of the thoracic-lumbar spine in the data acquisition to quantify spinal loading. The compressive forces at Th12/L1 in gymnastic landings are significantly higher than, for example, in running and showed the highest amplitudes compression forces of all the studied skills. Landing from a dismount (from the rings, horizontal bar, asymmetric bars) results in net compression forces to L5/S1 and therefore to the intervertebral disc of more than 11.6 times bodyweight (average force) in the first 50 milliseconds of ground contact with peak forces up to 20 times bodyweight. These resultant force data are calculated by the distribution model based on ground reaction force measurements and 3D kinematic data. Shear force to the disc at L5/S1 is estimated at 3.5 times body weight. These numbers give a compressive force to the segment L5/S1 (and the disc) for a 65 kg gymnast while landing from a dismount of at least 7500 N and a shear load to the L5/S1 disc and the pars interarticularis of >2000 N.

The few cadaver studies of young specimens loaded in a physiological environment (e.g., Genaidy et al., 1993) documented maximum compressive strength for young male adults of <8000 N and ultimate shear force tolerance of a lumbar motion segment of <3000 N. About the same loading amplitude with a little low loading rate was calculated for the motion segments of the lumbar-thoracic junction. These numbers indicate that landing in gymnastics gives tissue mechanical loading values close to the critical tissue tolerances. Vertebral deformities and growth disturbance of the anterior column of vertebrae at lumbar-thoracic junction shown (Froehner, 2000) can be explained by increased CD due to excessive loading and the related disturbed TAD. This mechanism is of major concern during growth and the higher vulnerability of the musculoskeletal system of the young gymnasts.

As expected, the compression forces increase significantly with increasing kinetic energy at touchdown and therefore with the height of the flight prior to landing. The shear forces are more or less constant with increasing height of the flight. When landing from a somersault the gymnast has to manage the linear and the angular momentum from the flight. This is related to an increased forward lean and trunk flexion. The resultant compression and shear forces at Th12/L5 gain 130–150%. Initial energy at touchdown, body position at landing, and body's angular momentum prior to landing determine the compression and shear force at the thoracic-lumbar junction and the lumbar portion of the spine in gymnastic landings.

The use of the supplementary mats demonstrates the impact of technical aids to control maximum compression and shear forces when landing from a dismount. Compressive forces during landing can be reduced to 80% by thin supplementary layers on top of the landing mats or the spring floor. Landing from a vault with a horizontal momentum close to the vertical momentum can be assumed to be related with similar or even higher spinal loading than in landing from an apparatus dismount. During the take-off from the spring floor or the springboard spinal loading appears to be lower than for landing from a flight. Maximum compression forces at L5/S1 level are estimated at 6.5–8.5 times body weight and maximum shear loading at 3.0–3.5 times body weight. This brings the take-offs on second place in the spinal loading listing. On third place of the spinal loading list rank the jumps, landings, and artistic skills on the balance beam. The cumulative spinal loading from training on the balance beam should not be underestimated given the extensive time spent and the high frequency of skills and repetitions on this apparatus.

The giant swings (e.g., in the scooped technique) on the horizontal bar and asymmetric bars, prior to dismount and flight elements with regrasp are expected as high loading demands for the spine. Compression and shear forces were calculated over the entire skills. The data demonstrate that the spinal loading is a compressive type loading during the whole drill. Muscle forces are higher than the inertial forces and compression and shear forces are counterintuitively low in comparison to the above presented activities. The long swings on rings, horizontal bar, and asymmetric bars show only moderate spinal loading. Even scooped giant swings and flight elements with regrasp are related to maximum lumbar-thoracic junction compression load of <4.5 times body weight and shear forces of <3.0 times body weight. Notably, these values represent valid and successfully performed trials. No data are available from failed movements. Health problems due to swings and giants should be explained by different overloading mechanisms rather than compression and shear loading to vertebrae and discs. Hyperextension with a high tensile strain on the anterior vertebral ligament and high tensile stress on the insertion to the vertebra may explain tissue failure.

Foot and ankle loading

The Achilles tendon is paradoxically the strongest tendon of the human body and it is frequently affected by acute and overuse injuries in gymnastics. Using cine phase-contrast magnetic resonance imaging (MRI), it was recently demonstrated that the free Achilles tendon strain is clearly higher than that of the aponeurosis (Finni *et al.*, 2003). This observation suggests that the free Achilles tendon is more compliant than the aponeurosis, which gives the free tendon the higher potential to store elastic energy. At the same time the more compliant free tendon is at a higher risk for injury. In single-leg jumping, peak tendon tensile stress up to 11 MPa have been measured in vivo using buckle transducer or optic fiber techniques. Figure 6.2 demonstrates the Achilles tendon force measured with the optic fiber device in a drop jump take-off for a forward somersault from an elastic gymnastic spring floor. Maximum load is in the mid-stance that corresponds with the peak ground reaction force. Achilles tendon force reaches a maximum tensile force of >5000 N. The loading rate is 100 kNs^{-1}, which is high in relation to single-leg jumping measures.

Achilles tendon loading during jumping on elastic surfaces is characterized by high tensile tendon force, high loading rates, and therefore

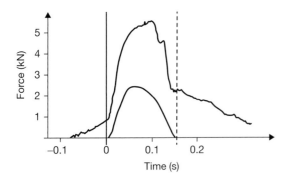

Figure 6.2 Achilles tendon force (black) and vertical ground reaction force (gray) of a drop jump take-off for a forward somersault from an elastic gymnastic spring floor. The vertical solid line gives the first contact of the feet with the ground; the dashed line indicates the last contact with the ground.

high strain rates. In general, the mid-substance of the tendon has the potential to withstand such mechanical loading as long as the entire tendon is homogeneously loaded. Differences in medial and lateral forces in cadaver Achilles tendon have been observed when separate muscles of the triceps surae were loaded. The alignment of the calcaneus plays an important role in asymmetric Achilles tendon strain. It was demonstrated in an in vitro experiment that a 7.5° calcaneal eversion leads to an increase of tensile strain at the medial column of the Achilles tendon of more than 75%. A 15° eversion is related to a 100% increase of medial strain. In addition to mediolateral axial strain differences, an intratendinous shear strain results and may cause sliding between tissue layers parallel to the acting forces. Asymmetric strain and shear strain between tissue layers should be discussed as a possible mechanism of Achilles tendon local tissue overuse, damage, and failure to free tendon. This mechanism of asymmetric strain and local tissue loading is given in gymnastics take-offs for backward somersault (on floor or from the springboard in vaulting) when the calcaneus is in an everted position. This calcaneal eversion may be related to neuromuscular weakness or fatigue or to technical deficits, or even a breakdown of spring floor or springboards. Asymmetric landing offers the option of a similar local increase of strain and tissue loading. An asymmetric Achilles tendon tensile

stress and the related tensile strain in floor exercise take-offs has the potential to lead to an acute failure through tissue loading above the critical limits or tolerances. Such asymmetric loading actions are reported when gymnasts take-off for a somersault with twists and when they initiate the longitudinal axis rotation during the contact to the ground.

From the resultant plantar flexion moment at the ankle joint one can derive the net tendon and muscle forces of the Achilles tendon and the triceps surae muscle when the lever arm of the Achilles tendon is kept in mind. The highest calculated force applied to the Achilles tendon is reported for the take-off of a (double) backward somersault after a handspring backward in gymnastics at higher than 9000 N (Brueggemann, 1985), which is about 15 times body weight. The reasons for the extreme forces are the high kinetic energy of the gymnast prior to take-off, the transfer of angular momentum to linear momentum during the take-off, and a direction change of center of mass path of >45° during the 120 milliseconds ground contact. The highest reported data of Achilles tendon loading in gymnastics was published by Panzer (1987) when subjects landed on the floor after a double backward somersault. The maximum resultant force at the Achilles tendon was estimated by one of the subjects at 25,000 N. The take-offs after a round-off or a handspring backward are related to high forces to the Achilles tendon. In jumping and some landing tasks in gymnastics the peak tendon forces are clearly approaching the ultimate strength limits of the tissue. Due to the fact that tendinous tissue has the capacity to adapt to a long term and well-organized training and adaptation, it allows the tissue to withstand such extreme loads.

The increased demands in floor exercise and tumbling with take-offs immediately after landing from a jump amplify the risk of asymmetric loading of the Achilles tendon, the foot and the stabilizing ligaments. Direct combinations of landings from a twisted somersault even scale up the risk of acute failure as well as of overuse.

Mechanical load to the heel (calcaneus) comes from the Achilles tendon and from external forces when landing on the heel. The poor landing from a forward somersault on the hard surface of the beam in female gymnastics should be related to shear loading to the calcaneus and the development of calcaneal apophysitis (Sever's disease).

For take-offs and landings on the hard floor in Rhythmic Gymnastics and on the balance beam in Artistic Gymnastics the resultant bone-to-bone force at the talonavicular joint was estimated at up to 8000 N. With foot deformities, abnormalities, or connective tissue weakness, the joint contact area is increased and the local intraarticular pressure rises up to 20 MPa, which might exceed the ultimate tissue functional potential and may lead to overuse injury.

Tissue response to loading in gymnastics

Response of bone and articular cartilage

Increased mechanical stimuli have been shown to improve bone integrity. The gain in bone mass might be explained to more than 50% by the loading rate. Impact activities like gymnastics produce an increase in skeletal mass, while athletes involved in low-impact activities such as swimming have low bone density (Grimston & Zernicke, 1993). A positive biological bone response in regard to an increased strength and/or bone mass might be related not only to high-strain (2000–3000 microstrain), low-frequency (1–3 Hz) events per activity unit but also to a persistent barrage of low-strain, high-frequency events (10–50 Hz), stemming from muscle contraction to retrain or maintain posture. This might explain the bone mass accumulation reported among samples of artistic gymnasts. Brief exposure to mechanical signals of high frequency and low intensity has been shown to provide a significant anabolic stimulus to bone (Ozcivici et al., 2010). Such low-intensity and high-frequency stimuli are related to muscle contraction and therefore to the active or bouncing loading in gymnastics and retaining posture and balance. Muscle contraction seems to play the outstanding role in maintaining and increasing bone mass; the mechanical signals generated by the muscle forces are the most important anabolic agents in bone. In gymnastics the combination of impact like loading in landings and

take-offs with intensive muscle contraction may explain the increased bone mass in gymnasts and the maintained bone density in former gymnasts.

Eckstein et al. (2002) reported that compared to bone and muscle, cartilage thickness was not modulated in the subjects after birth by an increase of mechanical stimulation. A recent study on cartilage volume and thickness of the patella femoral and the tibiofemoral joint compared former female gymnasts with nonathletic controls (Brueggemann et al., 2011). Neither the absolute cartilage volume or the volume normalized to standing height or body mass nor the absolute or normalized average cartilage height were increased in the athletic population relative to the controls.

Response of spinal structures

Froehner (2000) reported structural changes in the vertebrae of the thoracic spine and of the lumbar spine in former elite athletes with an average frequency of two affected vertebrae per female gymnast. The number for the male gymnasts was even higher than that of the female gymnasts. The highest frequency of structural changes of the former athletes was found in the thoracic-lumbar junction. The lumbar vertebrae of 16 female gymnasts (10–19 years of age) were compared with the vertebrae of 16 matched controls using 3D MRI reconstruction (Brueggemann & Krahl, 2000). A significant higher frequency of structural changes and morphological abnormalities were found in the gymnasts and increased in number according to age. The normalized heights of all lumbar vertebrae were lower for the gymnasts while the endplate areas were significantly greater in the gymnasts than in the controls. Due to the mechanical loading of the gymnasts the load carrying area increased while the vertebral height decreased. These data give an impressive example of how biological structures have the potential to respond to mechanical stimuli.

In order to illuminate the impact of mechanical loading to morphological changes of the spinal structures 37 female gymnasts were surveyed for a period of three consecutive years (Brueggemann, 2005). The individual spinal loading related to the most common and frequently performed tasks was derived by modeling estimates. The highest loading was shown for landings from dismounts and tumbling and from vaulting followed by take-offs on floor and vault. Spinal loading when performing on the balance beam was third and the swing elements on asymmetric bars ranked fourth. This gave a ranking of spinal loading in gymnastics per training unit and allowed an estimate of cumulated loading for the week, the months, and the entire year. All training units and competitions were documented for the 3 years and the cumulated spinal loading used to explain the development of spinal deformity and structural changes. In 23 of 37 gymnasts (62%) the structural changes of the lumbar and the thoracic vertebrae were explained by the cumulated spinal loading in the 3-year period. The remaining 38% of tissue response could be explained by tissue architecture, mechanical tissue properties, and genotype (see Figure 6.3).

It was demonstrated that tissue behavior and injury is strongly related to biomechanics of gymnastic loading. Morphology and mechanical properties of bony structures as well as of connective tissue are strongly determined by mechanical load. Articular cartilage does not have the potential to adjust its morphology to increased mechanical loading. But some recent research indicates that the material properties of cartilage (e.g., permeability) have the potential to adapt and that this specific tissue can be specialized to specific mechanical demands (Brueggemann *et al.*, 2011).

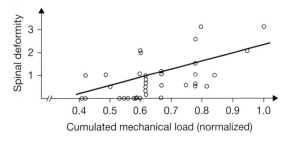

Figure 6.3 Spinal abnormalities and/or structural changes as function of cumulated mechanical spinal load of 37 elite female gymnasts in three consecutive years. Mechanical spinal load is cumulated for three consecutive years and normalized to maximum loading of the sample. Spinal deformity and/or structural changes at the lumbar region and/or the thoracic-lumbar junction are indicated as moderate (1), severe (2), or excessive (3).

Further research

This review of the gymnastics literature indicates that in the recent past biomechanics research in gymnastics was infrequent and was predominantly focused upon performance enhancement and technique optimization. Mechanical loading and especially joint and biological tissue stress and strain were not the main body of applied research to gymnastics. However, some work is available on estimates of mechanical loading in Artistic Gymnastics. Epidemiological studies of overload and related overuse injuries were retrospective and therefore solely descriptive. In addition, these studies typically represent a broad range of performance levels, age groups, training systems, and related mechanical loading. Few retrospective studies on former elite athletes report chronic injuries and especially tissue responses of elite gymnasts. A very limited number of prospective studies in elite gymnasts, considering both the cumulative MES and the tissue response, indicate the strong correlation between mechanical loading and the prevalence of overuse. Mechanical load and repetitive loading in training and competition determines at a high percentage but not completely tissue response as shown for the spinal structures. The TRM and therefore the acute tissue strength determine how the biological structure treats the mechanical stimulus.

An injury prevention model in gymnastics in general and in Artistic Gymnastics specifically has to consider the total mechanical load to the different biological structures in training and competition and the current individual strength of the biological structures involved. The current tissue capacity is highly athlete dependent and strongly related to previous loading, biological age, hormonal status, and eventually pre-injuries. This will lead to a highly individualized loading regime and a sophisticated monitoring of loading in training and competition. An elementary monitoring of the reaction forces applied to the gymnast at some given moments during training or competition may be an improvement but will not be sufficient to predict the risk of overuse injury. The numbers of repetitions, the loading amplitude, and the pauses between loading sessions should be of major importance and must be documented.

Biomechanics is strongly related to acute and overuse injuries in gymnastics. The better and more detailed knowledge of loading of different elements in gymnastics will lead to a critical review of techniques optimized for performance enhancement (e.g., hyperextension technique of handspring with 2.5 somersaults in vaulting) and to banning elements with excessive and uncontrollable loading. Examples for the latter are the recently highlighted landing on arms or neck and trunk while rolling out of somersaults in male Artistic Gymnastics.

Greater focus for injury prevention is required in the early years of gymnastics when the fundamental motor skills and the musculoskeletal system are being formed. Research has to identify and evaluate individualized loading regimes to optimize the biological adaptation process.

Future research will develop and elucidate biomarkers that allow an estimation of tissue material properties and strength of the biological structures not only for the muscle but also for bone, cartilage, and connective tissue. Such markers will permit a better control of the response to mechanical stimuli for the individual athlete. This may decrease the risk of stress-related injuries and will optimize the individual mechanical loading in training.

Finally, the strategy of supervising the individual tissue capacity will not eliminate the risk of direct falls and related injuries or overuse through extreme loading in highly evaluated movements and elements by the Code of Points. Such risks can only be reduced or partially eliminated by a critical review of the demands of Artistic, Trampoline, and Rhythmic Gymnastics, a review of the governing rules, and consequently changes in the assessment of the Code of Points, and strict bans for extremely dangerous elements.

Summary

Injuries in gymnastics are strongly related to mechanical loading. The highest mechanical demands are those to spinal structures, feet, and ankle and knee joints. In male Artistic Gymnastics

the shoulder, elbow, and wrist complete the list of highly loaded biological structures. It was shown that these structures are prone to overuse and are injured most frequently. Biological structures have the potential to respond to the mechanical stimuli as the stimulus is appropriate for the given response matrix. The TRM is defined by the tissue architecture, its mechanical properties, material fatigue, pre-injuries, and the genotype. Results from gymnastic research illustrate the potential of TAD of spinal structures, as well as of bone and cartilage in detail. An appropriate injury prevention model in gymnastics will consider the total mechanical load to the different biological structures in training and competition and the current individual strength of the biological structures involved. The current tissue capacity is highly athlete dependent and strongly related to previous loading, biological age, hormonal status, and eventually pre-injuries. This will lead to a highly individualized loading regime and a sophisticated monitoring of loading in training and competition. Future training in the high-demand sport of gymnastics may use biomarkers to estimate the tissue strength of the biological structures and to derive appropriate individual loading regimes not only for the muscle but also for bone, cartilage, and connective tissue. Such markers will permit a better control of the response to mechanical stimuli for the individual athlete. This may decrease the risk of overuse and will optimize the individual mechanical loading in training. Finally, a critical review of the demands of Artistic, Trampoline, and Rhythmic Gymnastics, and a review of the governing rules of the Code of Points and consequently changes in the assessment and the rules have the potential to decrease the risk of injuries in gymnastics.

References

Brueggemann, G.-P. (1985) Mechanical load of the Achilles tendon during rapid sport movements. In: S.M. Perren and M. Schneider (eds), *Biomechanics: Current Interdisciplinary Research*, pp. 669–674. Martinus Nijhoff, Dordrecht.

Brueggemann, G.-P. and Krahl, H. (2000) *Belastung und Risiken im weiblichen Kunstturnen (Loading and Risks in Female Artistic Gymnastics)*. Hofmann, Schorndorf.

Brueggemann, G.-P., Arampatzis, A., and Komi, P.V. (2000) Optimal stiffness and its influence on energy storage and return on elastic surfaces. In: Komi *et al.* (eds), *Proceeding Annual Congress of the European College of Sport Sciences*, Jyvaeskylae, Finland, pp. 33–34.

Brüggemann, G.-P. (2005) Biomechanical and biological limits in artistic gymnastics. In: Wang, Q. (ed.), *Proceedings of XXIII International Symposium on Biomechanics in Sports*, Beijing, China, pp. 15–24.

Brüggemann, G.-P., Brüggemann, L., Heinrich, K., Müller, M., and Niehoff, A. (2011) Biological tissue response to impact like mechanical loading. *Footwear Science*, **3**, 13–22.

Caine, D., Caine, C., and Maffulli, N. (2006) Incidence and distribution of pediatric sport-related injuries. *Clinical Journal of Sport Medicine*, **16** (6), 501–514.

Eckstein, F., Faber, S., and Muehlbauer, R. (2002) Functional adaptation of human joints to mechanical stimuli. *Osteoarthritis Cartilage*, **10**, 44–50.

Finni, T., Hodgson, J.A., Lai, A.M., Edgerton, V.R., and Sinha, S. (2003) Nonuniform strain of human soleus aponeurosis-tendon complex during submaximal voluntary contractions in vivo. *Journal of Applied Physiology*, **95**, 829–837.

Froehner, G. (2000) Retrospektive Untersuchung von Kunstturnerinnen und Kunstturnern der ehemaligen DDR (Retrospective study of female and male gymnasts of the former GDR). In: G.-P. Brueggemann and H. Krahl (eds), *Belastungen und Risiken im weiblichen Kunstturnen*, pp. 73–95. Hofmann, Schorndorf.

Grenaidy, A.M., Waly, S.M., Khali, T.M., and Hidalgo, J. (1993) Spinal compression limits for the design of manual material handling operations in the workplace. *Ergonomics*, **36**, 415–434.

Grimston, S.K. and Zernicke, R.F. (1993) Exercise related stress response to bone. *Journal of Applied Biomechanics*, **9**, 2–14.

Hootman, J.M., Dick, R., and Agel, J. (2007) Epidemiology of collegiate injury for 15 sports: summary and recommendations for injury prevention initiatives. *Journal of Athletic Training*, **42**, 311–319.

Knoll, K., Knoll, K., and Koethe, T. (2000) Grenzen der Leistungsfähigkeit des Menschen in den technisch-kompositorischen Sportarten (Limits of human performance in technical sports). *Leistungssport*, **1**, 33–38.

Ozcivici, E., Luu, Y.K., Adler, B., Quin, Y.-X., Rubin, J., Judex, S., and Rubin, C.T. (2010) Mechanical signals as anabolic agent in bone. *Nature Reviews Rheumatology*, **6**, 50–59.

Panzer, V.P. (1987) Dynamic assessment of lower extremity load characteristics during landing. Dissertation. University of Oregon.

Pollaehne, W. (1991) Ergebnisse der Wirbelsaeulen-laengsschnittauswertungen bei Hochleistungsturnern und Hochleistungsschwimmern aus radiologischer Sicht (Results of longitudinal radiological studies of elite gymnasts and swimmers). *Die Deutsche Zeitschrift für Sportmedizin*, **42**, 292–296.

Tertti, M., Paajanen, H., Kujala, U.M., Alanen, A., Salmi, T.T., and Kormano, M. (1990) Disc degeneration in young gymnasts. A magnetic resonance imaging study. *American Journal of Sports Medicine*, **18**, 206–208.

Recommended reading

Bahr, R. and Krosshaug, T. (2007) Understanding injury mechanisms: a key component of preventing injuries in sport. *British Journal of Sports Medicine*, **39**, 324–329.

Bahr, R. and Engebretsen, L. (2009) *Sports Injury Prevention. The International Olympic Committee Handbook of Sports Medicine and Science.* Wiley-Blackwell Publishers, Oxford.

Emery, C.A. (2010) Injury prevention in paediatric sport-related injuries: a scientific approach. *British Journal of Sports Medicine*, **44**, 64–69.

Kolt, G and Caine, D (2010) Gymnastics. In: D. Caine, P. Harmer, and M. Schiff (eds), *Epidemiology of Injury in Olympic Sports. Encyclopaedia of Sports Medicine*, vol. XVI, pp. 144–160. Blackwell-Wiley Publishers (England) and the International Olympic Committee (IOC) Medical Commission.

McNitt-Gray (2000) Musculoskeletal loading during landing. In: V.M. Zatsiorsky (ed.), *Biomechanics in Sport: Performance Improvement and Injury Prevention*, pp. 523–549. Volume IX of the Encyclopaedia of Sports Medicine. Blackwell Science.

Meeuwissen, W.H. (1994) Assessing causation in sport injury: a multifactorial model. *Clinical Journal of Sport Medicine*, **4**, 166–170.

Verhagen, E., and van Mechelen, W. (2010) *Sports Injury Research.* Oxford University Press, Oxford.

Chapter 7
Biomechanics: Injury mechanisms and risk factors

Patria A. Hume[1], Elizabeth J. Bradshaw[2], Gert-Peter Brueggemann[3]

[1]Sport Performance Research Institute and Faculty of Health and Environmental Sciences, Auckland University of Technology, Auckland, New Zealand
[2]School of Exercise Science, Australian Catholic University, Melbourne VIC, Australia
[3]Institute of Biomechanics and Orthopaedics, German Sport University Cologne, Cologne, Germany

Introduction

The most pressing and serious problem faced by many Olympic sports is injury. Targeted injury prevention strategies have the potential to help reduce the incidence and severity of gymnastics injuries if based upon an understanding of injury mechanisms related to biomechanical load and associated risk factors. This review focuses on the effects of mechanical loading during weight bearing/landings on gymnasts (i.e., Artistic, Rhythmic, and Trampoline). Training and performance aspects are considered to identify how high forces and decelerations, limb asymmetry and alignment, leg stiffness and joint ranges of motion, all affect risk of injury during landings.

Growing gymnasts are at increased risk of injury due to the biomechanics of their immature musculoskeletal structures. For example, muscle strength increases during growth, but it may not increase in proportion to limb inertial properties (Hawkins & Metheny, 2001). Understanding such variability in growth can be important for predicting and preventing overuse injuries to circumpubertal athletes. Overuse injuries are common when a skeletally immature athlete is exposed to high training loads, especially during periods of rapid growth (Kolt & Kirby, 1999). Growth plates are unique to young athletes and include both epiphyseal growth plates near the ends of long bones (which are mainly subjected to compression forces) and apophyseal growth plates between tendon attachments and bone shafts (which are mainly subjected to traction/tension forces). Epiphyseal growth plate injuries occur at the distal radial physis (wrist) and distal femoral physis (just above the knee), whereas Osgood–Schlatter's disease (tibial apophysitis in the lower leg, near the knee) and Sever's disease (calcaneal apophysitis in the heel) are common apophyseal growth plate injuries. Stress changes of the distal radial physis with inhibition of radial growth caused by repetitive physical loading of the limbs in female gymnasts have been reported (DiFiori *et al.*, 2006). Scoliosis (lateral curvature of the spine) is another condition thought to be exacerbated by overuse. Lower extremity injuries with a gradual onset typically include ankle impingements (from repetitive pointing of the foot), lower leg stress fractures and compartment syndromes (from the repetitive stress associated with landing), and patellofemoral knee problems (from biomechanically dysfunctional tracking movement of the patella).

Case and cross-sectional studies indicate a large number of gradual onset injuries involving the distal radius (wrist) and distal humerus (elbow), and include distal radial growth plate disorders and, primarily in females, osteochondritis dissecans of the humeral capitellum. These injuries can be severe, and are the result of compressive forces to overly stressed and immature joints. Shoulder injuries are especially common amongst male gymnasts

Gymnastics, First Edition. Edited by Dennis J. Caine, Keith Russell and Liesbeth Lim. © 2013 International Olympic Committee. Published 2013 by John Wiley & Sons, Ltd.

and are most frequently muscle strains (acute), or shoulder joint impingements (chronic) (Meeusen & Borms, 1992).

The severity of lower back problems in gymnastics is also of concern. Descriptive studies indicate that gymnastics lower back injuries tend to have a gradual onset (which may reduce the reported incidence of back problems since most injury surveillance systems record acute injuries but not overuse injuries), involving primarily advanced level gymnasts. This implicates experience and competitive level as risk factors for injury. Movements most likely to result in lower back injury are chronic repetitive flexion, and extension and rotation demanded of the spine and its associated structures during gymnastics maneuvers. High loading forces resulting from dismount and tumbling landings place the spine and lower extremities under enormous stress, especially if combined with poor landing biomechanics. The results of cross-sectional studies in the early 1990s showed a higher prevalence of spondylolysis (stress fracture) in Artistic Gymnastics than in the general population. Recent research, which is limited on spine injuries, indicates anterior spine problems.

Epidemiology studies of injury affecting gymnasts have shown that the lower limbs are most likely to sustain injuries (53% of all competition and 69% of all practice injuries) and that the majority of Women's Artistic Gymnastics competition injuries (approximately 70%) result from either landing in floor exercises or dismounts (Marshall *et al.*, 2007) (see also Chapter 10).

Biomechanics research can help identify and quantify risk factors and provide assessment of mechanisms (inciting events) resulting in these acute and overuse injuries occurring in gymnastics.

Injury mechanisms and risk factors

The mechanism of injury is the physical action or cause of injury (Bahr & Krosshaug, 2005). Examples include the strong force of muscle actions acting on bone via the tendon, compression at a joint and accumulation of damage, and repeated impact forces on bone or cartilage resulting in damage.

Exercise-induced muscle fatigue can also cause alterations in movement patterns and distribution of stress resulting in excess force transmitted to focal sites along the bone.

Mechanisms of injury are usually multifactorial. For example, biomechanical mechanisms for noncontact anterior cruciate ligament (ACL) injuries have been proposed to involve the quadriceps drawer mechanism and valgus loading, or knee abduction. Anterior tibial translation induced by a high tibiofemoral compression and tibial plateau inclination has also been proposed as a possible loading mechanism. A complete biomechanical description for ACL injury in gymnastics should quantify whole-body and knee kinematics, foot position, loading directions, magnitudes, and rates.

Frequent and/or high forces and decelerations during landings create biomechanical loads upon, and within a gymnast's body. Overuse injuries are usually caused by repetitive loading with large decelerations during landings, while acute injuries are usually caused by large forces in combination with large decelerations during landings (Beatty *et al.*, 2005). Weight-bearing impacts onto the hands and the repetitive compressive forces can lead to both acute and chronic injuries to the wrists. The biomechanical cause of injury can also be muscular in nature. The ability to develop force and power through high-velocity muscle actions is an essential component of gymnastics that influences performance but can also put the gymnast at risk of injury. For example, the mechanism of stress fractures may arise from an increase in the magnitude and frequency of the muscle action that exceeds the bone's ability to adapt, or exercise-induced muscle fatigue that causes alterations in movement pattern and distribution of stress resulting in excess force transmitted to focal sites along the bone. Injuries may be due to decreased energy absorption transfer between joints via decreased limb coordination or ineffectiveness of muscles to absorb the forces. Biomechanical factors related to noncontact ACL injury are influenced by both magnitude and timing of lower extremity energy absorption during landing (initial impact phase, terminal phase, and total landing).

Certain levels of stress and strain on the musculoskeletal system are essential in adaptation and positive enhancements to performance. Impact loading in gymnastics can increase levels of trabecular and cortical bone, therefore improving gymnasts bone mineral density. However, overload to the musculoskeletal system can lead to negative tissue damage (Brueggemann, 2010). Success in gymnastics requires gymnasts to experience high levels of biomechanical energy and loading. Genetically, gymnasts have varying stress and strain thresholds; however, due to the performance requirements, they are required to take on similar levels of biomechanical loading. Increased physical stress and strain during gymnastics can exceed the biomechanical limits of the body structures. The magnitude of forces on the gymnasts' body is approximately 4 times body weight (BW) for take-offs and 11 times BW for landings. Upper extremity forces have magnitudes of approximately 1.5 times BW for vault, 3.9 times BW for horizontal bar, 9.2 times BW for rings, 2.0 times BW for pommel horse, and 3.1 times BW for uneven bars.

Landings in sport movements can be stressful to the lower back due to increased compression and extension of the spine, especially if there is over- or underrotation. Backwards landings are more common than forward landings due to the increased preparation time available, that is, time to visually spot the landing. Therefore, because backward landings are more prevalent, there is typically more flexion of the trunk during landings than extension. Repetitive stress to the spine can result in vertebral ring apophysis inflammation. If rested and managed appropriately the injury can be resolved, but if excessive stress is continued, fractures can occur. Gymnasts can be at greater risk of developing spinal injuries if they have weak lower abdominal muscles. Gymnasts are more likely to compensate for weak abdominals by using the lumbar spine as a fulcrum or pivot point, which places greater compressive forces on the vertebrae. Excessive rotational or torsional stress can damage the small zygapophyseal (facet) joints on the vertebral arches that help link one vertebra with the next. Although only a relatively small amount of movement occurs at each joint, damage at one vertebra can result in a weak link in the spinal column "chain."

Injuries rarely occur as a result of one single risk factor, rather injuries result from a complex interaction of multiple risk factors and events (Emery, 2010). Internal and external risk factors when combined with the mechanism of injury may make a gymnast more prone to injury (see Figure 7.1). Risk factors for gymnastics' injury can include intrinsic (e.g., differences in anatomy, hormonal and neuromuscular function, musculoskeletal stiffness, muscle strength, or psychology) and extrinsic factors (e.g., equipment such as landing mat characteristics, exposure to training and competition, coaching techniques, or repetitive nature of gymnastics activities). Previous injury and a positive musculoskeletal assessment have been identified as risk factors for future injury (Caine et al., 2006) among artistic female gymnasts. Key factors that increase a gymnast's potential risk of injury are biomechanical loading, poorly designed and maintained gymnastics equipment, neuromuscular performance, reduced muscular strength, and the suboptimal technique (Brueggemann, 2010). Rules of gymnastics may also be a contributing risk factor for gymnastics injuries. Skill difficulty increases in gymnastics routines are linked to increases in biomechanical energy, which leads to higher loading and increased risk of injury.

Results of studies attempting to investigate analytical epidemiology should be viewed with caution given the design limitations present in nearly all such studies. In most cases, these studies are able to link a risk factor with injury; but this in no way suggests that the risk factor causes the injury (Meeuwisse et al., 2007). For example, taller gymnasts have been reported as more at risk of injury. This does not suggest that a particular gymnast's height caused an injury, but rather that height may be one of several contributing factors in the occurrence of an injury. It is possible that such factors as greater height, weight, and age tend to characterize older gymnasts with more years training and involvement in higher levels of training and competition.

Measurement of load

Given the high magnitude of impact load in landings, both acute and accumulative, coaches should monitor impact loads per training session, taking into consideration training quality and quantity

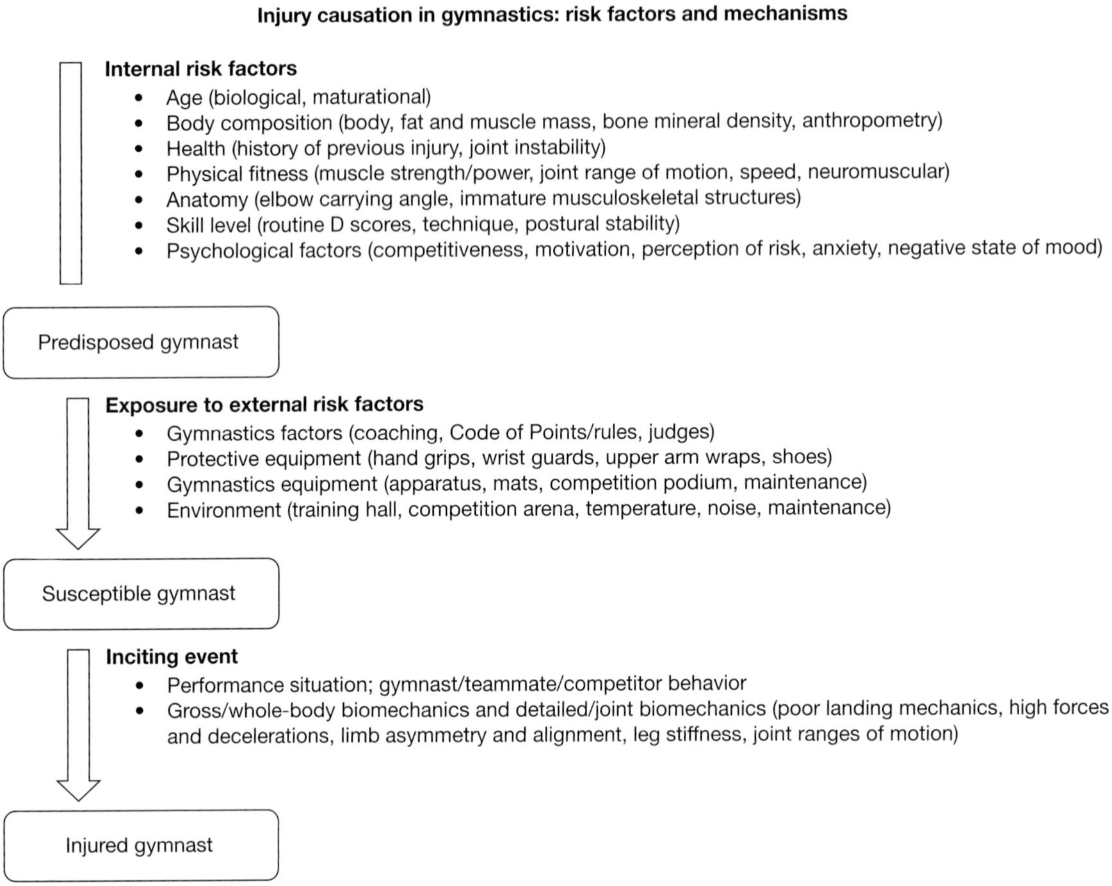

Injury causation in gymnastics: risk factors and mechanisms

Internal risk factors
- Age (biological, maturational)
- Body composition (body, fat and muscle mass, bone mineral density, anthropometry)
- Health (history of previous injury, joint instability)
- Physical fitness (muscle strength/power, joint range of motion, speed, neuromuscular)
- Anatomy (elbow carrying angle, immature musculoskeletal structures)
- Skill level (routine D scores, technique, postural stability)
- Psychological factors (competitiveness, motivation, perception of risk, anxiety, negative state of mood)

Predisposed gymnast

Exposure to external risk factors
- Gymnastics factors (coaching, Code of Points/rules, judges)
- Protective equipment (hand grips, wrist guards, upper arm wraps, shoes)
- Gymnastics equipment (apparatus, mats, competition podium, maintenance)
- Environment (training hall, competition arena, temperature, noise, maintenance)

Susceptible gymnast

Inciting event
- Performance situation; gymnast/teammate/competitor behavior
- Gross/whole-body biomechanics and detailed/joint biomechanics (poor landing mechanics, high forces and decelerations, limb asymmetry and alignment, leg stiffness, joint ranges of motion)

Injured gymnast

Figure 7.1 Internal and external risk factors when combined with the mechanism (inciting events) of injury may make a gymnast more prone to injury. (Adapted by permission from BMJ Publishing Group Ltd. Bahr & Krosshaug (2005), *British Journal of Sports Medicine*, **39**: 324–329.)

such as the control of rotation and the height from which the landings are executed. For these we need practical methods for monitoring training loads. Impact load can be measured biomechanically by the use of instrumented equipment (e.g., beat board), instrumentation on the gymnast (accelerometers), or by landings on force plates. A variety of gymnastic-specific movements have been examined in terms of impact. Pressure distribution under the sole of the foot during leaps and landings, three-dimensional analysis of arm impact during gymnastic back handsprings in children, impacts during beam and floor training in preadolescent gymnasts via video, force platform, and accelerometer (Burt *et al.*, 2007), and elbow joint forces and technique differences in

the Tsukahara vault have all been reported. Video and force analysis of six young female gymnasts showed that reaction forces at the hand during back handsprings produced large compression forces (an average of 2.37 times BW) and sizable valgus moments at the elbow (an average of 0.03 times BW) (Koh *et al.*, 1992). The combination of these forces may contribute to the occurrence of lateral compression injuries of the elbow joint such as osteochondritis dissecans of the capitellum. Correlations of measures of elbow angle and measures of reaction force showed that large elbow flexions may protect the elbow from large valgus moments.

Feedback systems via equipment instrumentation can help to monitor training loads, detect fatigue, and improve technique acquisition. However, monitoring training objectively in gymnastics, with the exception of qualitative video feedback, is not common. Some researchers have instrumented men's gymnastics apparatus such as the rings and horizontal bar; however, application to training or how they might be adapted for use with women's apparatus, remains unclear. A vault feedback system has been used to provide reliable approach velocity through to beat board contact, as well as preflight and table contact time during regular vault training of elite gymnasts. The advantage of this system was that it was designed to work as a feedback tool for coaches, with simple operation and result/data delivery via a hand-held personal digital assistant device. The system does not require a biomechanist to be present for its operation, or to analyze and interpret the data. This system has potential as an injury prevention tool by alerting a coach when the gymnast is becoming fatigued. For example, the table contact time during vaulting for female gymnasts is approximately 200 milliseconds. A 10% (20 milliseconds) increase in table contact time for an individual gymnast, depending on their task performance variability, indicates a performance decline and potential fatigue. Instrumentation of the vault table and beat board with pressure systems could potentially provide an estimate of force, or actual force could be provided via instrumentation with force plates. However, whilst instrumentation of vaulting apparatus is feasible, careful software development is needed to enable detailed information such as table contact forces to be readily and easily accessible to coaches during training.

Beatty *et al.* (2005) provided descriptive data on typical impact loads and decelerations during gymnastics training, however no insight was provided on how these measures could assist with injury prevention measures. Burt *et al.* (2007) used video analysis of training sessions along with accelerometer and force platform peak ground reaction force data to quantify the effects of participation level (international and national), apparatus (beam and floor), and training phase (precompetition and competition) on estimates of training load in gymnasts aged 7–13 years. Monitoring the quality of the training

program by counting the number of rotations and heights from which landings are executed, or measuring decelerations during impacts with accelerometers, may be a better injury prevention tool than simple quantification of training hours.

Limb asymmetry, alignment, stiffness, and joint range motion affect load

The neuromuscular control of the center of mass trajectory to control the body's momentum and angular rotation is specific to the landing task, whether landing from a height without any angular rotation, or from forward or backward somersaults (McNitt-Gray *et al.*, 2001). The amount of knee flexion has an influence on the magnitude of the impact force. A less erect landing posture through increased trunk flexion (forward lean) can encourage more knee flexion and a reduction in the landing impact forces. Either large or restricted ranges of motion are known to produce overuse injuries to the hips (Caine & Lindner, 1985) and back (Kujala *et al.*, 1997).

High-impact landings can result in undesirable movement variability that increases energy expenditure. In contrast, within- or between-joint coupling (coordination) variability may play a functional role in reducing injury through variable loading of the musculoskeletal features of the joint, providing the ability to adjust to changing environments. High coupling variability during the execution phase of a task could enable the gymnast to adjust for various intrinsic factors such as confidence and fatigue, and extrinsic factors such as competition arena temperature, which can influence their performance.

Attenuating more force on one leg amplifies the risk to gymnasts of sustaining an acute or a chronic injury, and is one of the most common means of injury in other sports (Kovacs *et al.*, 1998). Functionally symmetrical drop landings have ranged from less than 10% difference between limbs to 73% asymmetry. The ground reaction forces of two-foot landings in gymnastics are significant during training (~5 BW) and competition (~11 BW), especially if the landing is uneven (~18 BW) or if there is unusual foot placement. Landing with two feet together after high airborne skills requires tremendous stabilization and eccentric strength to prevent the knee joints from collapsing due to the high external knee joint loads. An uneven landing or unusual foot placement can result in increased dynamic valgus knee moments and increases the load on the ACL several-fold. Ideally, two-foot (toe-heel) landings should be performed with even distribution of forces between the feet that are spaced roughly shoulder width apart, with actively controlled hip, knee, and ankle dorsiflexion with the knees over the toes.

Muscles serve as the primary active stabilizers during functional loading conditions, protecting against musculoskeletal injury. Active muscle stiffness contributes to musculoskeletal behavior and is essential for the maintenance of joint stability. Musculoskeletal stiffness regulates the storage and reuse of elastic energy and is defined as the collective ability of muscles, tendons, ligament, cartilage, and bone to resist deformation from an applied force. Lower limb joint stiffness (resistance to movement) is the relationship between the deformation of the leg and the force attenuated. While some lower limb stiffness may be necessary for performance, either too much or too little stiffness may lead to injury. Too much stiffness may lead to bony injuries and ankle pathology whereas too little stiffness may lead to soft tissue injuries and knee pathology. Stiffness is well suited to quantifying the behavior of musculoskeletal components (i.e., joints, ligaments, tendons, cartilages, muscles, and bones) because it describes the resistance of a body to applied forces.

Increased lower limb musculoskeletal stiffness, as measured during self-paced repeat jump and hop tasks (15 contacts of continuous bent-knee and continuous straight-leg hops with one foot placed on each of two portable force plates), was related to an increased incidence of overuse injury in 39 adolescent female athletes involved in high-impact sports, including 17 high-level athletes (Moresi *et al.*, 2010). Screening for musculoskeletal stiffness may allow "at risk" athletes to be identified and potential athlete monitoring or intervention programs to be implemented.

Analysis of ankle stiffness measures of self-paced double-legged hopping in gymnasts has shown a potential safe zone for ankle plantarflexion stiffness. Bradshaw and Hume (2012) reported that two gymnasts from an original study by Bradshaw, who were still training 8 years later, showed increased ankle plantarflexion stiffness by 10.8 and 13.9 kN/m. Both gymnasts reported Sever's disease (calcaneal apophysitis due to overuse and repetitive microtrauma of growth plates of the calcaneus in the heel) in one or both heels and lower lumbar spine stress such as pars defect. The altered ankle stiffness of these two gymnasts in combination with the reported injuries indicates that biomechanical tests of stiffness may have potential for monitoring injury risk, especially during peak growth years.

Risk factors and injury prevention strategies to reduce biomechanical load

Injury prevention programs should place emphasis on the landing phase of gymnastics skills, as this phase seems to be critical to injury causation. Impact attenuation describes how efficiently the energy from an impact during landing is absorbed. Insufficient impact attenuation is linked to an increased injury risk as a result of overloading in tissues.

Landing techniques

Uncontrolled or repetitive landings can result in acute or overuse injuries. Therefore, there are important principles (e.g., segment alignment, attenuating forces over time, and using a large base of support) related to landings that gymnastics coaches can teach to young gymnasts. An upright trunk posture, reduced knee and hip flexion, unusual foot placement, and increased leg stiffness are potential contributing factors for injury during landings. Aiming for a "soft" (or quiet) landing means that attenuation of energy will help to reduce injury risk. Both technique and physical preparation for controlled landings should be taught at a young age, practiced often, and continued throughout athletes' participation in the sport such as described in all editions of Canadian

Level 1 coach certification manuals since 1975 and more recently in the 2009 FIG Foundation's coach education manual. Injury prevention strategies should focus on neuromuscular training and core stability programs in the off-season and preseason conditioning to enhance proper landing biomechanics.

Safety equipment

Improved gymnastics equipment, in the form of sprung floors, sprung beams, thicker landing mats, and fiberglass rails has offset the expected decrease in injury incidence by enabling the performance of increasingly complicated and risky performance routines. Poorly maintained or positioned safety equipment is implicated in some injuries such as spraining an ankle by landing between badly aligned mats.

Marshall *et al.* (2007) reported from analysis of collegiate women's gymnastics injuries over 16 years, the rate of injury in competition was more than two times higher than in practice (15.19 versus 6.07 injuries per 1000 athlete-exposures; rate ratio = 2.5, 95% confidence interval [CI] = 2.3, 2.8). A gymnast was almost six times more likely to sustain a knee internal derangement injury in competition than in practice (rate ratio = 5.7, 95% CI = 4.5, 7.3). It is understood that USA college female gymnastics represents a unique population in the world of gymnastics and these results therefore should not be generalized to other gymnastics populations. These high rates of injury during competition have led to some suggestions of increasing the thickness of landing mats used in competitions. Identification of the most important characteristics of gymnastics mat design for injury reduction has been gained from modeling impact energy absorption of surfaces and quantifying the response of gymnastic sports surfaces to dynamic loading. A seven-link wobbling mass model was used (Mills *et al.*, 2010) to investigate how changes in the material properties of a multilayer model of a gymnastics competition landing mat could minimize ground reaction forces and internal loading of a gymnast during landing. Minimal changes to the mat's stiffness (0.5%) but increased damping (272%) compared to a competition landing mat resulted in reduced peak vertical and horizontal ground reaction forces

(12%) and reduced bone bending moments (6%) in the shank and thigh compared to a matching simulation. Design of landing mats to allow better damping of forces whilst retaining landing stability should be a focus for future research.

Training conditions

There is epidemiological evidence that sudden onset injuries occur more frequently relatively early or late in training sessions or when doing familiar skills (i.e., possibly due to inattention) (Caine *et al.*, 1996). Training sessions should therefore involve more frequent apparatus changes to decrease the likelihood of a gymnast becoming inattentive. A number of studies across the gymnastics sports have reported increased injury rates for specific training periods. Coaches need to be aware of increased risk of injury when there is an increase in training intensity, increased anxiety (e.g., during periods immediately prior to competition, during competition, when learning new skills, or performing underprepared routines), increased levels of fatigue, or when there is less protection (competing without spotting and extra safety landing pads).

There is some controversy in the literature regarding the effect of skill level on injury. Caine *et al.* (2003) reported that the relative risk of injury was 1.47 times greater in the advanced versus beginning level American gymnasts. However, Kolt and Kirby (1999) reported that the rate of injuries per 1000 training hours was increased for subelite Australian gymnasts (4.11 per 1000 hours) compared with elite gymnasts (2.63 per 1000 hours). It is possible that reported injury rate differences are due to data collection differences used in the Australian and American studies. As gymnasts reach a higher level of competition, they perform more complex (and risky) maneuvers. Elite gymnasts may be more at risk of being pressured to return to full training too early after injury because of the level they are performing at, and where there are greater implications for time loss from training and competition. Those gymnasts are therefore at heightened risk of reinjury or compensatory injuries from altered biomechanics due to their incomplete rehabilitation.

Research on men's and women's gymnastics events show that most injuries occur on the floor, however, studies are required that include event-specific exposure time as the injury rate denominator. It is unclear whether the number of injuries on the floor is due to the nature of floor exercises themselves (e.g., repetitive trauma from tumbling) or because more time is spent on the floor, or a combination of the two.

Physique

Biomechanical efficiencies may be gained with particular physiques. Decreased height and weight elicit a greater ratio of strength to weight, greater stability, and a decreased moment of inertia. Body fat adds to mass without adding to power producing capability, therefore fat mass is detrimental to the gymnast. There can be increased risk of injury during periods of rapid body growth due to increased moments of inertia, increased muscle-tendon tightness, and decreased physis strength. Female artistic gymnasts who are mature and have a physique characterized as relatively tall with high lean body mass are at a greater risk for developing positive ulnar variance in the wrist (Claessens *et al.*, 1996).

Musculoskeletal dynamic screening

Incorrect biomechanics during movement patterns can increase inappropriate loading. There are a number of screening protocols that can help identify movement dysfunction or technique faults. A whole-body functional movement competency screen that challenges fundamental movement patterns of the BW squat, the BW lunge and twist, the push-up, the BW bend and pull, and the single-leg squat, has been developed for use by sport and health professionals. The coach video records the athlete performing five repetitions of each movement task from the front and side, and then rates segment movement quality for the head, shoulders, lumbar spine, hips, knees, ankles, and feet, then rates quality of balance and joint range of movement. Initial evidence has shown movement competency screen scores can predict trunk injury for male and female elite athletes, however there is no evidence yet for gymnasts. Having screening movement tasks that can help predict performance or injury will enable coaches to monitor and

prescribe exercises for gymnasts to enhance their performance and reduce their injury risk.

The importance of lower extremity dynamic malalignment in many lower extremity injuries (Willson & Davis, 2009) emphasizes the need to be able to screen gymnasts at least annually (more regularly during peak growth periods). There is an increasing body of research that is showing the use of biomechanics of functional movements to improve musculoskeletal screening. Dynamic alignment of the lower limb resulting in knee valgus may predispose the gymnast to ACL injury. Patella femoral syndrome is initiated by factors including weakness in the medial most quadriceps muscle, tightness in the lateral most quadriceps muscle, and weakness within the hip flexor, extensor, and adductor muscles. Other technologies beside video analysis may be used by biomechanists for screening. Achilles strain measures using ultrasonography during a ramped protocol with three different loads of isometric heel raises may provide a potential screening tool. Aside from profiling physical performance qualities, biomechanical (kinetic) testing has the potential to also aid in the assessment and management of the athlete's functional musculoskeletal health (rehabilitation, injury risk). Investigation is needed to determine reliable functional tests that closely mimic gymnastics movements.

Further research

Although theoretically biomechanics can be used to help prevent injury via monitoring training forces, or predicting injury risk via musculoskeletal screening and technique analysis, there have been few studies that actually provide evidence of effectiveness of injury prevention intervention strategies based on biomechanical analysis (Bradshaw & Hume, 2012). Biomechanics research on gymnastics has predominantly focused upon the high-performance participation levels, with quantitative descriptions of specific skills. Greater focus for injury prevention is required on the elementary years of gymnastics when the fundamental motor skills of jumping and landing are being formed and also on the lower to middle competitive levels that involves the bulk of participants and similar rates of injury. Key strategies that maximize technique and safety need to be identified. Biomechanics can potentially help improve gymnastics performance and reduce injury risk to provide positive participation and competition experiences.

Computer simulation forward modeling exhibits promise for influencing coaching and training practice. This is because coaches with gymnasts seeking the epitome of competition performance are always seeking to know how to push skills further, such as the number of somersaults and/or twists that can be successfully performed on floor or vault. Simulation of the aerial skiing twisting performance is a relevant example of how coaches may be assisted by modeling research in gymnastics. Knowledge of take-off velocity and technique required to accomplish a quadruple twist for gymnastics skills would allow a coach to develop a gymnast safely through skill progressions to ensure that the final technique could be achieved.

From our review of the literature we can say that monitoring training loads should help decrease the risk of injury. Small, portable, and cost-effective means of assessing biomechanical loads on gymnasts are promising. Until practical validated methods are available, it is suggested that given the high magnitude of impact load (both acute and accumulative), coaches should monitor impact loads via the number of impact landings per training session, taking into consideration the height from which the landing is made and the control of body rotation during landing. Peak growth should be identified by tracking the gymnast's peak height velocity given the biological versus chronological age differences and understanding how biological age can affect biomechanics and skill development. Prospective multifactorial risk analyses for elite gymnasts aged 10–14 years should be conducted. Studies could include assessment of strength and power and training loads, musculoskeletal stiffness and alignment, growth and development, bone health, and a nutrition profile. The effectiveness of gymnasts with a previous history of ankle sprain using an ankle brace to decrease the risk of recurrent injury should be determined. There is evidence from other sports that ankle taping is not effective after a very short period of intensive training or competition (Hume & Gerrard, 1998), therefore this issue needs to be researched in gymnasts.

Summary

Large impact forces, in combination with poor lower limb geometry during landings, in gymnastics are resulting in injuries predominantly to the lower limbs. Using functional movement screening, biomechanically instrumented equipment (e.g., beat board, rings, and bars), or instrumentation on the gymnast (e.g., accelerometers) to monitor gymnasts' motion, and equipment and techniques to help reduce biomechanical loading should be useful. Given the high magnitude of impact load, both acute and accumulative, coaches should monitor impact loads in training, considering quality and quantity such as control of rotation and heights from which landings are executed. Evidence-based injury prevention interventions should be developed for gymnastics focused on reducing biomechanical loading during landings.

References

Bahr, R. and Krosshaug, T. (2005) Understanding injury mechanisms: a key component of preventing injuries in sport. *British Journal of Sports Medicine*, **39**, 324–329.

Beatty, K.T., McIntosh, A.S., and Frechede, B.O. (2005) Measurement of impact during gymnastics skills. *British Journal of Sports Medicine*, **39**, 374.

Bradshaw, E. and Hume, P.A. (2012) Biomechanical approaches to identify and quantify injury mechanisms and risk factors in women's artistic gymnastics. *Sports Biomechanics*, **11** (3), 324–341.

Brueggemann, P. (2010) Neuromechanical load of biological tissue and injury in gymnastics. In: R. Jensen, W. Ebben, E. Petushek, C. Richter, and Roemer, K. (eds), *XXVIII International Symposium of Biomechanics in Sports 2010*. Department of Health Physical Education and Recreation, College of Professional Studies, Northern Michigan University, International Society of Biomechanics in Sports, Marquette, MI.

Burt, L., Naughton, G., and Landeo, R. (2007) Quantifying impacts during beam and floor training in pre-adolescent girls from two streams of artistic gymnastics. In: H.J. Menzel and M.H. Chagas (eds), *XXV International Symposium on Biomechanics in Sports 2007*. Federal University of the State of Minas Gerais in Belo Horizonte, International Society of Biomechanics in Sports, Ouro Preto, Brazil.

Caine, D., Knutzen, K., Howe, W., Keeler, L., Sheppard, L., Henrichs, D., and Fast, J. (2003) A three-year epidemiological study of injuries affecting young female gymnasts. *Physical Therapy in Sport*, **4**, 10–23.

Caine, D.J., Daly, R.M., Jolly, D., Hagel, B.E., and Cochrane, B. (2006) Risk factors for injury in young competitive female gymnasts. *British Journal of Sports Medicine*, **40**, 91–92.

Caine, D.J., and Lindner, K.J. (1985) Overuse injuries of growing bones: the young female gymnast at risk?. *Physician and Sports Medicine*, **13**, 51–64.

Caine, D.J., Lindner, K.J., Mandelbaum, B.R., and Sands, W.A. (1996) Gymnastics. In: D.J. Caine (ed.), *Epidemiology of Sports Injuries*. Human Kinetics Publishers, Champaign, IL.

Claessens, A.L., Lefevre, J., Beunen, G., De Smet, L., and Veer, A.M. (1996) Physique as a risk factor for ulnar variance in elite female gymnasts. *Medicine and Science in Sports and Exercise*, **28**, 560–569.

DiFiori, J., Caine, D., and Malina, R. (2006) Wrist pain, distal radial growth plate injury, and ulnar variance in the young gymnast. *American Journal of Sports Medicine*, **34**, 840–849.

Emery, C.A. (2010) Injury prevention in paediatric sport-related injuries: a scientific approach. *British Journal of Sport Medicine*, **44**, 64–69.

Hawkins, D. and Metheny, J. (2001) Overuse injuries in youth sports: biomechanical considerations. *Medicine and Science in Sports and Exercise*, **33**, 1701–1707.

Hume, P.A. and Gerrard, D.F. (1998) Effectiveness of external ankle support: bracing and taping in rugby union. *Sports Medicine*, **25**, 285–312.

Koh, T.J., Grabiner, M.D., and Weiker, G.G. (1992) Technique and ground reaction forces in the back handspring. *American Journal of Sports Medicine*, **20**, 61–66.

Kolt, G.S. and Kirby, R.J. (1999) Epidemiology of injury in elite and subelite female gymnasts: a comparison of retrospective and prospective findings. *British Journal of Sports Medicine*, **33**, 312–318.

Kovacs, R., Santha, A., Balajti, N., Martos, E., and Balogh, E. (1998) Overuse changes of distal radial epiphysis in professional gymnasts. *Hungarian Review of Sports Medicine*, **39**, 171–180.

Kujala, U.M., Taimela, S., Oksanen, A., and Salminen, J.J. (1997) Lumbar mobility and low back pain during adolescence: a longitudinal three-year follow-up study in athletes and controls. *American Journal of Sports Medicine*, **25**, 363–368.

Marshall, S.W., Covassin, T., Dick, R., Nassar, L.G., and Agel, J. (2007) Descriptive epidemiology of collegiate women's gymnastics injuries: National Collegiate Athletic Association Injury Surveillance System, 1988-1989 through 2003–2004. *Journal of Athletic Training*, **42**, 234–240.

McNitt-Gray, J.L., Hester, D.M.E., Mathiyakom, W., and Munkasy, B.A. (2001) Mechanical demand and multi-joint control during landing depend on orientation of the body segments relative to the reaction force. *Journal of Biomechanics*, **34**, 1471–1482.

Meeusen, R. and Borms, J. (1992) Gymnastic injuries. *Sports Medicine*, **13**, 337–356.

Meeuwisse, W.H., Tyreman, H., Hagel, B.E., and Emery, C.A. (2007) A dynamic model of etiology in sport injury: the recursive nature and risk of causation. *Clinical Journal of Sports Medicine*, **17**, 215–219.

Mills, C., Yeadon, M.R., and Pain, M.T.G. (2010) Modifying landing mat material properties may decrease peak contact forces but increase forefoot forces in gymnastics landings. *Sports Biomechanics*, **9**, 153–164.

Moresi, M., Bradshaw, E., Greene, D., and Naughton, G. (2010) Jump kinetics, bone health and nutrition in elite adolescent female athletes. 28th International Conference on Biomechanics in Sport, Marquette, MI.

Willson, J.D. and Davis, I.S. (2009) Lower extremity strength and mechanics during jumping in women with patellofemoral pain. *Journal of Sport Rehabilitation*, **18**, 76–90.

Recommended reading

Butler, R.J., Cowell, H.P., and McClay Davis, I. (2003) 'Lower extremity stiffness: Implications for performance and injury'. *Clinical Biomechanics*, **18**, 511–517.

Kolt, G., and Caine, D. (2010) Gymnastics. In: D. Caine, P. Harmer, and M. Schiff (eds), *Epidemiology of Injury in Olympic Sports. Encyclopaedia of Sports Medicine*. Wiley-Blackwell (England) and the International Olympic Committee (IOC) Medical Commission.

Krosshaug, T. and Verhagen, E. (2010) Investigating injury risk factors and mechanisms. In: E. Verhagen and van Mechelen (eds), *Sports Injury Research*. Oxford University Press.

Norcross, M.F., Blackburn, J.T., Goerger, B.M., and Padua, D.A. (2010) 'The association between lower extremity energy absorption and biomechanical factors related to anterior cruciate ligament injury'. *Clinical Biomechanics*, **25**, 1031–1036.

Soriano, P.P., Belloch, S.L., and Alcover, E.A. (2006) Partial implementation of the Q.F.D. methodology for the identification of the most important characteristics and features of Gymnastics mats design. *International Journal of Applied Sports Sciences*, **18**, 65–77.

Chapter 8
Gymnastics physiology

Neil Armstrong[1], N.C. Craig Sharp[2]

[1]Children's Health and Exercise Research Centre, University of Exeter, Exeter, UK
[2]Centre for Sports Medicine and Human Performance, Brunel University, Uxbridge, UK

Introduction

Gymnastics is a complex sport consisting of routines performed on different pieces of apparatus for varying periods of time and with different physiological demands. Men's Artistic Gymnastics routines range in length from ~5 seconds in the vault through ~35 seconds on the rings, pommel horse, parallel bars, and high bar to ~70 seconds on the floor. Women's Artistic Gymnastics routines vary in length from ~5 seconds in the vault, through ~45 seconds on the uneven bars to ~90 seconds on the beam and floor. Rhythmic Gymnastics routines last from ~90 seconds in individual routines to ~150 seconds in group routines. The balance between the contributions of the physiological variables underpinning gymnastics routines varies according to the length and demands of particular routines and the age, maturation, sex, and state of training of the gymnasts.

It is not unusual to see 2-year-old children in gymnasium initiation programs and training time increases with age with elite gymnasts training for ~30 hours or more each week. Approximately 80% of all gymnasts are younger than 18 years with the vast majority between 9 and 16 years of age. Most girls reach their competitive peak in their mid- to late teens whereas males tend to reach their competitive peak in their early 20s. It is therefore

Gymnastics, First Edition. Edited by Dennis J. Caine, Keith Russell and Liesbeth Lim. © 2013 International Olympic Committee. Published 2013 by John Wiley & Sons, Ltd.

apparent that to understand gymnastics physiology the principal physiological demands of different aspects of the sport must be identified and considered in the context of the gymnasts' age, growth, maturation, and sex.

Exercise metabolism and the supply of energy during gymnastics

Anaerobic metabolism

At the onset of exercise, muscle contraction is supported by the energy released during the hydrolysis of adenosine triphosphate (ATP). The intramuscular stores of ATP relative to muscle size are similar in adults and children at ~5 mmol/kg wet weight of muscle but this is insufficient to support maximal exercise for more than ~2 seconds. ATP must be resynthesized before total depletion and anaerobic resynthesis of ATP occurs almost immediately from phosphocreatine (PCr) stores in the muscles. PCr is depleted rapidly during high-intensity exercise such as gymnastics. PCr resynthesis of ATP reaches its peak within ~2 seconds and is the primary energy component during vaults. PCr stores decline rapidly and during the final few seconds of a routine on the bars or rings the contribution of PCr to ATP resynthesis is ~2% of that during the first few seconds. For high-intensity performance to be sustained beyond a few seconds ATP supply must be maintained and this is ensured, at least in the short term, by the processes of glycolysis and glycogenolysis.

Carbohydrates are stored in the muscles and in the liver as glycogen. At the onset of exercise muscle glycogen is very quickly converted to glucose-6-phosphate (G-6-P). Liver glycogen is catabolized and released into the blood as glucose where it is available to the muscle and other cells as an energy substrate. Once glucose enters the muscle it is phosphorylated to G-6-P and thereafter glycolysis and glycogenolysis follow a common pathway in the muscle sarcoplasm. Despite the number of reactions involved, the anaerobic catabolism of G-6-P to pyruvate is rapid with a time constant (τ, the time taken to achieve 63% of the change) of ~1.5 seconds. Peak production of ATP is therefore reached within ~6 seconds and the glycolytic pathway becomes the main provider of ATP within ~10 seconds of the onset of maximal exercise. At its peak, glycolysis resynthesizes ATP at about half the rate of resynthesis from PCr. During rings, pommel horse, and bar routines glycolysis is the predominant energy source.

To sustain glycolysis pyruvate is either reduced to lactate or oxidized in the muscle mitochondria through the tricarboxylic acid cycle to carbon dioxide and water. The rate of muscle lactate production during high-intensity exercise is dependent on the balance between the anaerobic and aerobic catabolism of pyruvate and therefore the availability of oxygen or the demand for power. In the muscle the accumulation of lactate is accompanied by an increasing acidosis that inhibits the activity of the key glycolytic regulatory enzyme (phosphofructokinase, PFK), interferes with the muscle contractile mechanism, and stimulates the free nerve endings in the muscle giving rise to the painful sensations that accompany fatigue from high-intensity exercise and lead to cessation of exercise. As young children rely less on anaerobic metabolism than adolescents or adults they experience these cautionary fatigue indicators less intensely and are more likely than older people to overheat or experience nausea during rigorous exercise. They therefore need careful supervision.

An increase in the glycolytic resynthesis of ATP results in a corresponding increase in lactate production by active muscle fibers. Lactate metabolism is, however, a dynamic process and while some muscle fibers produce lactate, adjacent fibers simultaneously consume it as an energy source. Nevertheless, as exercise proceeds lactate accumulates within the muscle and diffuses into the extracellular space and into the blood where it is often measured and used as an indicator of glycolytic activity. Blood lactate accumulation does not directly reflect muscle lactate production as it is a function of several processes including consumption in the muscle, rate of diffusion into the blood, and rate of removal from the blood. The interpretation of blood lactate accumulation during childhood, adolescence, and young adulthood is clouded by theoretical and methodological issues and reports of the blood lactate threshold (T_{LAC}) associated with gymnastics activities need to be interpreted cautiously.

Aerobic metabolism

The initial step of carbohydrate oxidative metabolism is the passage of pyruvate into the mitochondria, followed by conversion into acetyl CoA, and subsequent entry into the tricarboxylic acid cycle where the energy liberated during the process resynthesizes ATP. The rate at which ATP can be resynthesized aerobically in the muscle mitochondria is much slower than that of anaerobic ATP resynthesis but the capacity for energy generation is much greater and reinforced by the ability to use both free fatty acids and amino acids as substrates. Young people respond to high-intensity exercise with a faster aerobic τ than adults. In a step change from rest or low-intensity exercise to high-intensity exercise the pulmonary oxygen uptake ($p\dot{V}O_2$) τ of young people is ~20 seconds with maximal values of $p\dot{V}O_2$ being reached within ~80 seconds. During high-intensity exercise aerobic resynthesis of ATP gradually increases with time and the oxidative contribution becomes dominant in gymnastics routines longer than ~60 seconds. During vaults, pommel horse, bars, and rings routines the anaerobic supply of energy predominates but during floor exercises and Rhythmic Gymnastics routines aerobic metabolism is the principal source of energy. In addition, oxidative metabolism can use carbohydrates, free fatty acids, and amino acids as substrates and although this may be of minor importance during gymnastics competitions it is important as a glycogen-sparing mechanism during the many hours of training in which elite gymnasts engage.

Direct estimation of energy costs during gymnastics routines

Attempts have been made to directly measure the energy cost of gymnastics routines for over 50 years but technological difficulties with apparatus and flawed methodologies have limited the interpretation of the data.

Jemni (2011) described studies that required male gymnasts to perform their routines while breathing through a mouthpiece into a Douglas bag. At the end of each routine, gymnasts held their breaths until the investigators attached another bag to collect the expired air during recovery. Analysis of the respiratory gases indicated that the event with the highest energy cost was the floor followed in decreasing order by the pommel horse, rings, high bar, parallel bars, and vault. Another investigation measured the excess post-exercise oxygen consumption during the first 30 seconds following female gymnastic routines and reported floor exercises to have the highest energy cost followed by the uneven bars, the balance beam, and the vault.

In a more recent investigation into the energy cost of ball routines in Rhythmic Gymnastics, Guidetti *et al.* (2000) measured heart rate (HR) during the routines and blood lactate accumulation on completion of the routines. To facilitate the interpretation of the data the 14–16-year-old girls had their HR, $p\dot{V}O_2$, and blood lactate accumulation monitored during an incremental treadmill test to exhaustion. During the ball routine the girls' mean peak HR was 188 beats/min. The mean average HR during the whole ball routine was 177 beats/min, which corresponded to 88.2% of treadmill-determined maximum HR. In this study the ball-routine HRs were similar to the HRs at T_{LAC} on the treadmill and the post-exercise blood lactate confirmed that the girls performed their competitive routines at an intensity around their T_{LAC}. From $p\dot{V}O_2$ collected pre- and post-exercise and post-exercise blood lactate accumulation the energy cost of the routines was estimated. It was concluded that the most taxed energy system was the aerobic system.

Developmental exercise physiology underpinning gymnastics performance

The assessment and interpretation of young people's muscle strength and aerobic fitness are well documented and data on elite young athletes are readily available even though they are often difficult to interpret. The responses of young people to short-term high-intensity exercise in relation to age, growth, maturation, and sex are less clear and our understanding of gymnastics-related exercise is clouded by technical issues, including the non-specificity of current methods of assessment.

Developmental exercise metabolism

Muscle biopsy studies

For both ethical and methodological reasons, the muscle biopsy technique has rarely been used with healthy children. The few muscle biopsy studies that have been performed with children have focused on resting and post-exercise measures and have generally been restricted to small samples of boys. Nevertheless, some interesting patterns have emerged from the literature.

Muscle fiber size increases with age from birth to adolescence and in males into young adulthood. The percentage of type I fibers in the vastus lateralis decreases in healthy males over the age range 10–35 years. No clear age-related fiber distribution changes have been observed in females but this might be a methodological artefact as few data on girls and women are available. Studies comparing the muscle fiber composition of boys and girls are confounded by the small number of participants and large interindividual variations that cloud statistical analyses. However, there is a consistent trend with adolescent and young adult males exhibiting, on average, 8–15% more type I fibers in the vastus lateralis than similarly aged females in the same study.

In the 1970s, Eriksson and his colleagues (Eriksson, 1980) carried out a series of muscle biopsy studies of small samples of 11–15-year-old boys, which have influenced the interpretation of pediatric exercise metabolism for almost 40 years.

No similar data are available on girls. Muscle biopsies from the quadriceps femoris revealed resting ATP stores that were stable over the age range of 11.6–15.5 years and similar to values others had reported with adults. The concentration of ATP remained unchanged following 6 min bouts of submaximal cycle ergometer exercise but minor reductions were observed following maximal exercise.

The mean resting PCr stores of the 11-year-old boys were 14.5 mmol/kg wet weight of muscle whereas the mean resting values of the 15-year-olds were 63% higher at 23.6 mmol/kg wet weight of muscle and similar to values recorded previously in adults. The PCr concentration gradually declined following exercise sessions of increasing intensity with values of less than ~5 mmol/kg wet weight of muscle reported following maximal exercise.

Muscle glycogen concentrations at rest were reported to average 54 mmol/kg wet weight of muscle at 11 years rising to 87 mmol/kg wet weight of muscle at 15 years, which is comparable with adult values reported by others. A decrease in glycogen following exercise was observed in all age groups but the depletion was three times greater in the oldest compared to the youngest boys indicating enhanced glycogenolysis with age. The age-related increase in the glycolytic contribution to metabolism is reflected in Eriksson's studies by muscle lactate accumulation increasing by 76% from 8.8 mmol/kg wet weight of muscle at 11 years to 15.5 mmol/kg wet weight of muscle at 15 years. On the basis of an "almost significant" relationship between lactate accumulation in the muscles and testicular volume Eriksson hypothesized a maturational effect on lactate production, which remains to be proven.

Eriksson reported levels of PFK and succinic dehydrogenase (an aerobic enzyme) to be 50% lower and 20% higher, respectively, than adult values his group had observed previously. They suggested that children might have a lower glycolytic and more enhanced oxidative capacity than adults during exercise. More recent muscle biopsy analyses have been generally supportive and reported glycolytic enzyme activity to be positively correlated with age and oxidative enzyme activity to be negatively correlated with age over the age range 6–17 years, in both males and females. A consistent finding is that the ratio of glycolytic to oxidative enzyme activity is higher in adults than in adolescents and children, indicating a relatively greater potential for anaerobic exercise in adults.

Magnetic resonance spectroscopy studies

Magnetic resonance spectroscopy (^{31}P-MRS) provides in real time a window through which muscle can be interrogated during exercise. ^{31}P-MRS studies are constrained by exercising within a narrow tunnel and the need to synchronize the acquisition of data with the rate of muscle contraction. There is a leap of faith in the extrapolation of exercise data from a specific muscle group, normally the quadriceps, using laboratory technology to the whole-body activity of a gymnastics routine, but ^{31}P-MRS studies have provided new insights into the physiology underpinning young people's performance.

^{31}P-MRS allows the monitoring of ATP, PCr, and inorganic phosphate (Pi) spectra during exercise. During an incremental exercise test to exhaustion, Pi increases with a corresponding decline in PCr. The expression of muscle Pi/PCr against power output therefore provides an index of mitochondrial function. In other words, a muscle with a greater oxidative capacity will require a lower change in Pi/PCr for a given increment of power output. An incremental exercise test to exhaustion results in nonlinear changes in the ratio Pi/PCr plotted against power output. As power output increases an initial shallow slope is followed by a steeper slope and the transition point is known as the intracellular threshold ($IT_{Pi/PCr}$). The $IT_{Pi/PCr}$ is analogous to other metabolic thresholds such as the T_{LAC}.

During exercise at and below the $IT_{Pi/PCr}$ the cellular energetic state is similar in children and adults and between sexes. During exercise above the $IT_{Pi/PCr}$ adults display a steeper Pi/PCr slope than children, which is also the case for girls compared with boys.

The results of incremental exercise studies have been supported by those from ^{31}P-MRS kinetics studies in which the PCr kinetic response to a step change in exercise intensity has been monitored. The similar PCr kinetics of children and adults at the onset of exercise below the $IT_{Pi/PCr}$ indicate a comparable capacity for oxidative metabolism during low-intensity exercise. The PCr kinetic response to the onset of exercise above the $IT_{Pi/PCr}$ shows boys to have a significantly faster PCr kinetic response to high-intensity exercise than men.

These findings are supported further by studies that have monitored the resynthesis of PCr during recovery from maximal exercise and reported boys to have a faster PCr τ during recovery than men. The lesser accumulation of Pi and fall in PCr during exercise above T_{LAC} is consistent with an enhanced recruitment of type I muscle fibers in children compared to adults and in boys compared to girls. This indicates a reduced mitochondrial oxidative capacity with age.

Pulmonary oxygen uptake kinetics studies

An understanding of $p\dot{V}O_2$ kinetics is important for all sports that require step changes in exercise intensity (e.g., changes of pace in gymnastics routines). It is technically difficult to measure the $p\dot{V}O_2$ kinetics response during gymnastics activities and there are no data available on young people. In the laboratory $p\dot{V}O_2$ kinetics are studied by the use of a step transition where a period of low-intensity exercise, such as pedaling a cycle ergometer without a resistance, is followed by a sudden increase in exercise intensity to a predetermined level.

At the onset of exercise there is an almost immediate increase in $p\dot{V}O_2$ measured at the mouth. This cardiodynamic phase (phase I), which lasts ~15 seconds is independent of $\dot{V}O_2$ at the muscle ($m\dot{V}O_2$) and is associated with an increase in cardiac output that occurs prior to the arrival at the lungs of venous blood from the exercising muscles. Phase I is followed by an exponential increase in $p\dot{V}O_2$ (phase II or primary phase) that drives $p\dot{V}O_2$ to a steady state during exercise below the T_{LAC}. Phase II $p\dot{V}O_2$ kinetics are described by their τ and it has been demonstrated that they reflect within ~10% the kinetics of $m\dot{V}O_2$ and therefore provide a noninvasive window into muscle metabolism.

During phases I and II, ATP resynthesis cannot be supported fully by oxidative phosphorylation and the additional energy requirements are met from muscle oxygen stores, PCr, and glycolysis. During exercise below the T_{LAC} children reach a steady state in $p\dot{V}O_2$ within ~100 seconds, but

during exercise above the T_{LAC} the overall oxygen cost of exercise increases over time. A slow component of $p\dot{V}O_2$ is superimposed upon the primary component and the achievement of a steady state is delayed by ~600–900 seconds. The mechanisms underlying the $p\dot{V}O_2$ slow component remain speculative but appear to be a function of muscle fiber distribution, motor unit recruitment, and the matching of oxygen delivery to active muscles.

Children have faster $p\dot{V}O_2$ kinetics responses than adults during the transition to exercise both above and below their T_{LAC}. During the transition to exercise above the T_{LAC} girls are characterized by slower phase II $p\dot{V}O_2$ kinetics than boys. This greater aerobic contribution to ATP resynthesis in children compared to adults and, during high-intensity exercise, boys compared to girls suggests an enhanced oxidative capacity, which might be due to greater oxygen delivery or better oxygen utilization by the myocyte or both. Muscle blood flow and therefore oxygen delivery during exercise has been reported to decrease with age in boys aged 12–16 years. Peak $\dot{V}O_2$, which is primarily dependent on oxygen delivery, is not related to $p\dot{V}O_2$ kinetics during youth and there is no compelling evidence to suggest that increased delivery of oxygen influences the τ of children's $p\dot{V}O_2$ kinetics. Faster phase II $p\dot{V}O_2$ kinetics therefore reflect an enhanced capacity for oxygen utilization by the mitochondria, which might be partially explained by an enhanced aerobic enzyme profile and/or reduced creatine concentration (as inferred from muscle PCr stores).

Girls have a greater relative $p\dot{V}O_2$ slow component compared to boys and in both sexes the $p\dot{V}O_2$ slow component increases with age. The increase with age is likely to be related to changes in muscle fiber recruitment patterns and the data are consistent with children having a higher percentage of type I muscle fibers than adults and in accord with boys having a higher percentage of type I fibers than similarly aged girls.

Aerobic fitness

Floor routines and Rhythmic Gymnastics are predominantly dependent on aerobic fitness. The best single measure of young people's aerobic fitness is

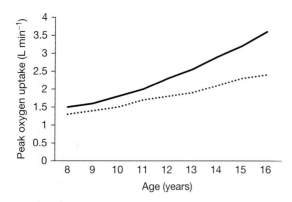

Figure 8.1 Peak oxygen uptake in relation to age and sex. Boys, solid line; girls, dotted line.

peak V̇O₂, the highest rate at which oxygen can be consumed during exercise. In the laboratory peak V̇O₂ is normally determined on a treadmill or a cycle ergometer and as there is no well-established ergometer with which to specifically assess gymnasts' peak V̇O₂ laboratory data must be interpreted with caution.

As illustrated in Figure 8.1, treadmill-determined boys' peak V̇O₂ (L/min) shows a linear increase with chronological age and girls' data demonstrate a similar but less consistent trend with some studies indicating a tendency to level-off at about 14 years of age. From 8 to 16 years peak V̇O₂ increases by ~150% and ~80% in boys and girls, respectively, with the sex difference rising to ~35% by age 16. The physiological explanation for sex differences in peak V̇O₂ during childhood is complex but the balance of evidence suggests that, although there are no sex differences in maximal HR or arterial-venous oxygen difference, maximal stroke index is higher in boys than in girls and therefore boys deliver more oxygen to the muscles. During adolescence boys' greater muscle mass is the dominant influence in enhancing peak V̇O₂ and in late adolescence this is reinforced by boys' higher concentration of blood hemoglobin.

The peak V̇O₂ of the arms is important in several gymnastics activities. Peak V̇O₂ determined using an arm ergometer is only about two-thirds that of the peak V̇O₂ of the legs but it presents the same underlying trends during youth.

Peak V̇O₂ is strongly correlated with body mass and this is conventionally controlled for

by simply dividing peak V̇O₂ (mL/min) by body mass (kg) and expressing it as the simple ratio mL/kg/min. When peak V̇O₂ is expressed in this manner a different picture emerges with boys' peak V̇O₂ remaining essentially unchanged from 8 to 18 years at ~48 mL/kg/min while girls' values decline from ~45 to 35 mL/kg/min over the same age range. Boys demonstrate higher mass-related peak V̇O₂ than girls throughout childhood with the sex difference being reinforced by the greater accumulation of body fat by girls during puberty.

The conventional use of mass-related (ratio) values has clouded understanding of peak V̇O₂ during growth and maturation. With body mass appropriately controlled for by using allometry, boys' peak V̇O₂ has been shown to increase through childhood and adolescence into young adulthood. Girls' peak V̇O₂ increases at least into puberty and possibly into young adulthood. Longitudinal studies have clearly demonstrated that maturation is associated with increases in peak V̇O₂ above those explained by body size, body composition, and chronological age. Furthermore, ratio scaling "over scales" (i.e., favors light children and penalizes heavy children) and as gymnasts consistently present body masses below the 50th percentile it is futile to use ratio scaling to compare the aerobic fitness of young gymnasts with athletes from other sports.

Several authors (summarized by Jemni, 2011) have concluded that mass-related peak V̇O₂ is not directly related to performance parameters in gymnastics and that it is therefore unnecessary to enhance gymnasts' peak V̇O₂ but a recent study of elite rhythmic gymnasts has demonstrated the importance of aerobic fitness when interpreted correctly. Douda *et al.* (2008) analyzed the physiological and anthropometric predictors of rhythmic gymnasts' performance, which was defined from the total ranking score of each athlete in a national competition. A multiple regression analysis of elite and nonelite gymnasts separately revealed that 92.5% of the variations in elite gymnasts' performance was explained by peak V̇O₂ (58.9%), arm span (12%), mid-thigh circumference (13.1%), and body mass (8.5%). High peak V̇O₂ (L/min) was the first predictor of performance. As expected, mass-related peak

$\dot{V}O_2$ (mL/kg/min) was not well correlated with performance score.

Blood lactate accumulation

Blood lactate accumulation must be interpreted with caution and should not be assumed to reflect a direct relationship with muscle lactate production. Nevertheless, when interpreted appropriately blood lactate accumulation acts as a useful measure of submaximal aerobic fitness that can be used to monitor improvements in muscle oxidative capacity with training in the absence of changes in peak $\dot{V}O_2$. Post-exercise blood lactate can be used to indicate effort during short-term high-intensity exercise and to estimate the anaerobic contribution to exercise.

At the onset of a progressive, incremental exercise test to exhaustion there are minimal changes in blood lactate accumulation. It is not unusual for blood lactate to initially increase and then fall back to near-resting levels due to the interplay between type I and type II muscle fiber recruitment. As exercise progresses, blood lactate accumulation increases and reaches an inflection point where it begins to increase more rapidly with a subsequent steep rise until exhaustion. The point at which blood lactate increases nonlinearly in response to an increase in exercise intensity is defined as the T_{LAC} that serves as a measure of submaximal aerobic fitness.

To avoid blood sampling some authors have used the ventilation threshold (i.e., the point during incremental exercise where ventilation increases disproportionally with the increase in $p\dot{V}O_2$) to estimate the T_{LAC}. With some exercise protocols a clear inflection point is not always discernible and to circumvent this fixed blood lactate reference values have been used to estimate submaximal aerobic fitness. These reference values are not recommended for use with gymnasts as they are not equivalent to the T_{LAC}. Fixed reference values and T_{LAC} vary both within an individual and independently with age and possibly maturation. A lactate reference value (e.g., 2.5 or 4 mmol/L) might be above or below the individual's T_{LAC} and not comparable with the relative performance of another gymnast.

Data on blood lactate accumulation during youth are equivocal but a consistent finding is that young people accumulate less blood lactate than adults during both maximal and submaximal exercise. Lower exercise-induced blood lactate accumulation in children than in adults might reflect faster removal from the blood, and/or a smaller muscle mass with a higher percentage of type I fibers combined with a facilitated aerobic metabolism rather than lower muscle lactate production. There is no conclusive evidence of significant sex differences in performance at fixed submaximal blood lactate levels during childhood and adolescence.

Blood lactate accumulation during gymnastics exercises has been reported but confusion with steady state and nonsteady state exercise models of blood lactate confound analyses and interpretation. Direct comparisons (and averages) of gymnasts' blood lactate accumulation following routines of different duration and intensity and using predominantly different muscle groups (e.g., floor versus rings versus pommel horse) have been reported and summarized by Jemni (2011) but add nothing of significance to the literature.

Short-term high-intensity exercise

Vaults, pommel horse, and bars routines are predominantly supported by anaerobic metabolism. During the vaults the main source of energy comes directly from the breakdown of ATP and PCr in the muscle with a small contribution from glycolyis and a minute contribution from aerobic metabolism. The pommel horse and bar routines are primarily supported through glycolysis following an initial contribution from high-energy phosphates with the aerobic contribution increasing with the length of the routine.

The direct examination of muscular energetics during short-term high-intensity exercise is complex and research has focused on tests that assess leg power output during maximal exercise. A plethora of tests involving jumping, running, and cycling has been developed but none are specific to gymnastics performance. All performance tests have flaws but data generated during growth

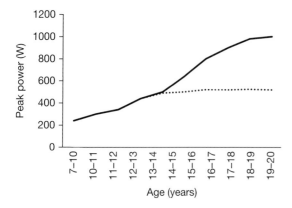

Figure 8.2 Peak power output in relation to age and sex. Boys, solid line; girls, dotted line.

and maturation are generally consistent. The Wingate anaerobic test (WAnT) that allows the determination of cycling peak power (CPP), usually over a 1-, 3-, or 5-second period and cycling mean power over the 30-second test period has emerged as the most popular test of leg power. Data from variants of this test have mapped out the development of leg peak power output during growth and maturation. Arm peak power can be determined in the same manner with either alternate or simultaneous arm exercise and the sparse data available suggest that arm power output follows the same profile but tends to be ~60% of leg power.

As illustrated in Figure 8.2, cross-sectional data show that in both boys and girls there is an almost linear increase in CPP from age 7 years until ~13 years when, in boys but not girls, a second and steeper linear increase in CPP through to young adulthood is observed. The indistinguishable difference in CPP between boys and girls until age 13 years is confounded by the paucity of studies simultaneously considering chronological age and stage of maturation of the participants. By young adulthood the sex difference in CPP is ~50%. Longitudinal data have emphasized the sex difference in CPP in relation to growth and maturation by showing that 12-year-old girls and boys, respectively, generate ~60% and ~45% of the CPP they achieve at 17 years of age (Armstrong *et al.*, 2001; Armstrong & Welsman, 2001). Over the age range 12–17 years, CPP increased by 121% in boys

and 66% in girls whereas increases in peak $\dot{V}O_2$ were somewhat less at 70% and 50% for boys and girls, respectively.

Sustained or repeated use of the glycolytic energy pathway during bouts of high-intensity exercise inevitably leads to an increase in acidity, an accumulation of lactate in the muscle, and symptoms of muscle fatigue that are more marked during the use of smaller muscle groups such as the arms. The ability to perform without imperfection despite being under "metabolic stress" is particularly important in gymnastics but during a well-organized gymnastics competition with appropriate rest periods, or preferably low-intensity activity recovery periods between events, this should not be a major problem with suitably trained gymnasts. However, during training when anaerobic-type activities are likely to be repeated several times with limited rest-recovery periods coaches must be aware of the build-up of metabolic by-products that will cause deterioration in performance and risk of injury during complex movements.

With gymnasts undertaking training for ~30 hours per week and including frequent bouts of high-intensity exercise coaches also need to consider long-term glycogen depletion. It is, however, well documented that young people recover faster than adults following high-intensity exercise. This might be explained by children and adolescents having enhanced oxidative capacity, faster PCr resynthesis, better acid–base regulation, and lower production and/or more efficient removal of metabolic by-products. It has also been suggested that young people's faster recovery from exercise might simply be a direct consequence of their limited capacity to generate power from anaerobic sources compared to adults.

Muscle strength

Muscle strength underpins the successful performance of most gymnastics routines, particularly those on apparatus, thus coaches require a clear understanding of the development of strength during growth and maturation.

The maximal force that can be generated by skeletal muscle is primarily a function of muscle cross-sectional area but there is compelling evidence that during late adolescence a higher percentage of motor units can be voluntarily activated than during childhood.

Muscle mass increases from early childhood reaching a peak during late adolescence or young adulthood. In addition, changes in muscle pennation during adolescence positively influence the expression of strength. The percentage of type II fibers increases and attains adult values during young adulthood. There are no published data on the relationship between muscle fiber distribution and the expression of voluntary strength in young people but type IIA and type IIX fibers in adults' quadriceps have been shown to have, respectively, 3 and 10 times greater shortening velocity than type I fibers. If this is also the case in adolescents it confers a huge advantage to mature boys in sports such as gymnastics that demand both strength and high power output.

From ~7 years of age boys have a larger absolute and relative (to body mass) amount of muscle compared to girls. Girls' muscle mass increases from ~40 to 45% of body mass between 5 and 13 years and then declines in relation to body mass, but not absolutely, due to body fat accumulation during adolescence. Boys' percentage muscle mass increases from ~42 to 54% of body mass from childhood to young adulthood with a marked spurt during adolescence. Peak muscle growth velocity occurs several months later than peak height velocity (PHV) and peak muscle strength growth velocity occurs ~1.0–1.5 years after PHV. Earlier maturing male gymnasts are therefore strongly advantaged over later maturers during this window as the benefits of enhanced muscle strength become apparent in late adolescence. It is, however, young adulthood before male peak strength is achieved.

In boys, muscle strength increases linearly with chronological age from early childhood until ~13–14 years of age when there is a marked increase in strength through the pubertal years, followed by a slower increase into the early-, mid-, or even late 20s. Girls experience an almost linear increase in strength with age until ~14–15 years with no clear evidence of an adolescent spurt. Sex-related differences in strength have been reported in children as young as 3 years of age but differences are small prior to puberty and there is a considerable overlap of male and female scores. As girls tend to enter puberty ~2 years ahead of boys it is not unusual for 10–11-year-old girls to be stronger than similar aged boys. The prepubertal strength difference is, however, greatly magnified during late adolescence by which time very few girls outscore boys on strength measures. The sex-related difference is more marked in the upper extremity and the trunk than in the lower extremity, even after adjusting for body size differences.

Correlations between measures of muscle strength from different muscle actions and/or muscle groups are generally quite low. Nevertheless, regardless of muscle action and whether individual strength or composite strength scores from several muscle groups are examined data describing the development of strength during growth and maturation are consistent and are illustrated using grip strength data in Figure 8.3.

Changes in body shape during puberty advantage earlier maturing boys over later maturing boys. For example, during puberty, as well as an increase in muscle strength, boys experience an increase in limb length and a marked spurt in shoulder breadth. Small differences in shoulder breadth can result in large differences in upper trunk muscle mass and the greater leverage of longer arms enhances the expression of strength.

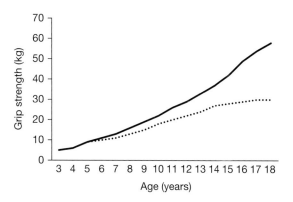

Figure 8.3 Grip strength in relation to age and sex. Boys, solid line; girls, dotted line.

Physiological principles underlying gymnastics training

Endurance training

Endurance training consists of a structured exercise program that is sustained for a sufficient length of time and at sufficient intensity and frequency to induce an improvement in aerobic fitness. As demonstrated in previous sections, aerobic fitness is a vital component of gymnastics performance and is particularly important during floor and Rhythmic Gymnastics routines.

It is well established that training at an intensity at or slightly above the T_{LAC} produces a rightward shift in the blood lactate response in relation to exercise intensity or percentage peak $\dot{V}O_2$ (see Figure 8.4). Changes in the T_{LAC} might be a function of either a reduced rate of muscle lactate production or an enhanced removal of lactate from the blood or a combination of both. Muscle lactate production might be diminished by an increased ability to resynthesize ATP aerobically following training and therefore a lower reliance on glycolysis.

Peak $\dot{V}O_2$ is the only component of aerobic fitness on which there are sufficient data to examine dose-response effects of endurance training during youth. Genetic influences on the responsiveness of peak $\dot{V}O_2$ to endurance training are not well understood but it appears that there is a continuum from high responders to nonresponders. Assuming that gymnasts in training are not nonresponders the evidence is overwhelming that peak $\dot{V}O_2$ can be

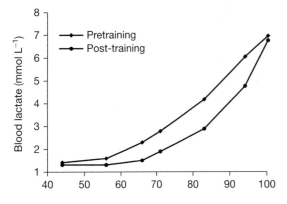

Figure 8.4 Blood lactate response to exercise pre- and post-training.

enhanced with training during both childhood and adolescence. It has been hypothesized that there is a "maturational threshold" below which the effects of training will be minimal but recent research has demonstrated that this is clearly not the case. Early studies suggesting that prepubertal children do not respond to training or that girls are less receptive than boys to training are confounded by programs using less than optimum intensity exercise.

In order to induce significant changes in peak $\dot{V}O_2$ the relative intensity of the exercise needs to be higher than that which has been shown to be effective with adults. The optimum intensity lies within the HR range 85–90% of maximum (i.e., 170–180 beats/min). There are no age, maturation, or sex effects on the magnitude of changes in peak $\dot{V}O_2$ during youth, although training-induced changes tend to be less than those expected with adults. Following an appropriate 12-week training program using large muscle groups, three to four sessions per week, for 40 minutes per session, an improvement in peak $\dot{V}O_2$ of ~10% would be expected. The improvement in peak $\dot{V}O_2$ is largely due to enhanced oxygen delivery to the muscles through an increase in maximum stroke volume.

High-intensity and resistance training

Initial studies of resistance training suggested that it was hazardous with children but recent research has demonstrated that appropriately supervised resistance training is not more likely to induce injury than participation in other sporting activities. Similarly, although several early studies of high-intensity training and resistance training failed to demonstrate significant changes in either muscle power output or muscle strength during youth, the positive effects of both modes of training have now been well documented. Following high-intensity and/or resistance training prepubertal children normally experience similar (or greater) relative gains in muscle strength and/or power output than adolescents and adults but smaller absolute gains. There are no, or only small, sex-related differences in responses to resistance training among prepubertal and early pubertal children although absolute muscle strength and power output increases are likely to be more pronounced in boys during late adolescence and young adulthood.

The mechanisms underlying training-induced changes in muscle strength vary with age, maturation, and possibly sex. It is difficult to quantify the relative contribution of muscle hypertrophy and neurological adaptations such as enhanced neural drive, increased motor unit recruitment and synchronization, and reduced central nervous system inhibition during youth. However, in prepubertal children strength gains can be principally attributed to neurological adaptations with muscle hypertrophy, the dominant influence in late adolescence, particularly in boys.

Resistance training programs during youth are probably best included as part of an overall gymnastics general fitness program with no more than two or three sessions per week, on nonconsecutive days, devoted to them. Training loads on weight machines can be quantified in terms of the individual's repetition maximum (RM) and with children it is best to begin with relatively low resistances, perhaps 12–15 RM and gradually progress to greater resistances and fewer repetitions in accord with the gymnast's growth and maturation. Muscle strength improvements of 10–40% have been demonstrated in young children following 12-week resistance training programs.

Overtraining or the unexplained underperformance syndrome

Gymnasts training for ~30 hours per week over several years might find themselves victims of a syndrome loosely termed overtraining but perhaps more accurately viewed as the unexplained underperformance syndrome (UPS) (Budget *et al.,* 2000). UPS occurs where high-intensity training, frequent competition, and non-sport-specific stressors combine to negatively affect the young gymnast. In addition to long lasting (i.e., longer than 2 weeks) decrements in performance, the signs and symptoms of UPS include some or all of the following: increased fatigue and perception of effort during training, unusually "heavy" or sore muscles, sleep disturbances, loss of appetite, mood disturbances, and upper respiratory tract infections. During episodes of UPS, the young gymnast might experience some or all of the following: decreased interest in training and competition, increased frustration

with lack of improvement with training, decreased self-confidence, inability to concentrate, short temper, depression, increased conflicts with family, coach, and friends, and elevated levels of stress.

There are few data on the prevalence of this syndrome in elite young athletes but recent surveys suggest that aspects of UPS have been experienced by ~30% of elite young athletes with a higher prevalence in individual sports, such as gymnastics, than team sports and in girls than boys.

Very high training loads and intense, frequent competitions provide the primary underlying cause of UPS in elite young athletes but it is likely that the problem is even more multidimensional. For example, the anxiety caused by striving to meet the expectations of coaches and parents, the loss of autonomy in lifestyle planning through devotion to a single goal, and stress from other pressures such as trying to cope with both school and training/competition demands are some of the most common contributors to UPS during childhood and adolescence.

Though there are some promising research leads, there are no specific diagnostic tests, and initially a possible underlying illness must be eliminated. UPS as a condition is not treated so much as managed over 4–12 weeks. This involves modest levels of aerobic exercise, possibly cross-training, vital for morale as well as physical benefits, together with moderate (i.e., quantitatively and qualitatively) skill work. Massage by qualified sports masseurs, hydrotherapy, and counseled relaxation sessions may also be beneficial, and monitoring body fat is important, as weight may stay constant during the relative lay-off, but muscle mass may decrease and fat mass increase. Weekly psychological questionnaires may be useful to monitor progress but must be used sensitively so as not to induce more stress. Full training and competition should be introduced as a gradual progression, with attention being paid to rest periods and days, and incremental levels of competition.

Further research

^{31}P-MRS and breath-by-breath $p\dot{V}O_2$ kinetics studies have untapped potential. Data collection, analysis, and modeling techniques using these new technologies are now well established and the recent introduction of experimental models such as "priming exercise," "work to work transitions," and "manipulations of pedal rates" provide intriguing theoretical avenues for future research into muscle metabolism during growth and maturation (Armstrong & Barker, 2012). However, the confident application of data from laboratory investigations of muscle metabolism founded on constrained exercise patterns to a comprehensive understanding of the specific metabolic pathways underpinning complex gymnastics performances awaits the development of appropriate technology and exercise models.

Gymnastics movement patterns are extremely difficult to replicate in the laboratory during the monitoring of physiological functions. Current test batteries used to assess and interpret the fitness of gymnasts lack the specificity required for confident extrapolation to gymnastics performances and require further research and development (Breivik, 2007). Laboratory assessment of peak $\dot{V}O_2$, p$\dot{V}O_2$ kinetics, peak power output, and muscle strength and interpretation in relation to age, growth, maturation, and sex are well documented. But, specific data on gymnasts are sparse and await the development of appropriate ergometers and unobtrusive techniques of physiological data collection during gymnastics performances.

Dose-response data on aerobic training and resistance training during youth are readily available although data from high-intensity exercise training are less secure. Further research is necessary to interpret the specific effects of gymnastics training on both general aerobic fitness and the local muscle fitness required for gymnastic routines. Well-designed and rigorously executed training programs reported in the literature are limited to ~12 weeks in duration. There are no secure longitudinal data on the specific and/or general physiological effects of intensive training, for 20–30 hours per week, from childhood through adolescence and into young adulthood. Similarly, there are no data on the interaction between long-term aerobic and resistance training programs during stages of growth and maturation. The incidence, causes, symptoms, and treatment of UPS in young gymnasts require further investigation.

Summary

Gymnastics performances are supported by overlapping energy systems and the relative contribution of these systems is dependent on exercise intensity and duration in relation to age, growth, maturation, and sex. Vaults are heavily reliant on ATP resynthesis from PCr. The predominant energy sources during routines on the rings, pommel horse, beam, and bars are also anaerobic but with ATP resynthesis from glycolysis rapidly assuming the primary role as the contribution from PCr breakdown declines over the first few seconds. Aerobic resynthesis of ATP is the primary energy source during floor routines and Rhythmic Gymnastics although both PCr breakdown and glycolysis make a significant contribution to the energy demand.

Although data from specific gymnastics tests are lacking, laboratory data are consistent and clearly show age-, growth-, maturation-, and sex-related changes in anaerobic and aerobic performance that are asynchronous. During adolescence and into young adulthood both sexes experience a more marked increase in the ability to perform exercises supported by anaerobic metabolism than those supported by aerobic metabolism. Muscle strength increases with age in an almost linear manner until the mid-teens when boys, but not girls, experience a marked spurt in both muscle mass and muscle strength. Girls' strength tends to level-off from ~16 years of age but boys' strength continues to increase into young adulthood.

In the absence of dietary disorders and energy imbalance there is no evidence to indicate that exercise training during youth has adverse effects on growth and maturation. Aerobic fitness, muscle power output, and muscle strength are important components of gymnastics performance and all can be enhanced with training during both childhood and adolescence.

Significant numbers of elite young athletes on long-term intensive training and competition programs suffer from the UPS. The problem is due to a cluster of effects related to the duo of prolonged very hard training and frequent competition. Coaches and parents need to be aware of the symptoms, recognize the problem, and be ready to address sympathetically and manage sensitively the causes of the malaise.

Gymnasts' responses to exercise and training are dependent upon age, genetics, growth, maturation, and sex. Individual biological clocks run at their own rate and to interpret the performance and progress of gymnasts coaches require an understanding of developmental exercise physiology and the ability to apply physiological concepts to gymnastics training programs and long-term performance planning.

References

Armstrong, N. and Barker, A.R. (2012) New insights into paediatric exercise metabolism. *Journal of Sport and Health Science*, **1**, 18–26.

Armstrong, N., Welsman, J.R., Chia, M. (2001) Short-term power output in relation to growth and maturation. *British Journal of Sports Medicine*, **35**, 118–125.

Armstrong, N., Welsman, J.R. (2001) Peak oxygen uptake in relation to growth and maturation. *European Journal of Applied Physiology*, **28**, 259–265.

Breivik, S.L. (2007) Artistic gymnastics. In: E.M. Winter, A.M. Jones, R.C.R. Davison, P.D. Bromley, and T.H. Mercer (eds), *Sport and Exercise Physiology Testing*, pp. 220–224. Routledge, Oxford.

Budget, R., Newsholme, E., Lehmann, M., and Sharp, N.C.C. (2000) Redefining the overtraining syndrome as the unexplained underperformance syndrome. *British Journal of Sports Medicine*, **34**, 67–68.

Douda, H.T., Toubekis, A.G., Avloniti, A.A., and Tokmakidis, S.P. (2008) Physiological and anthropometric determinants of rhythmic gymnastics performance. *International Journal of Sports Physiology and Performance*, **3**, 41–54.

Eriksson, B.O. (1980) Muscle metabolism in children – a review. *Acta Paediatrica Scandinavia*, **283** (Suppl.), 20–28.

Guidetti, L., Baldari, C., Capranica, L., Persichini, C., and Figura, F. (2000) Energy cost and energy sources of ball routine in rhythmic gymnasts. *International Journal of Sports Medicine*, **21**, 205–209.

Jemni, M. (2011) Physiology for gymnastics. In: M. Jemni (ed.), *The Science of Gymnastics*, pp. 1–21. Routledge, Oxford.

Recommended reading

Armstrong, N. (ed.) (2007) *Paediatric Exercise Physiology*. Churchill Livingstone, Edinburgh.

Armstrong, N. and McManus, A. M. (eds) (2011) *The Elite Young Athlete*. Karger, Basle.

Armstrong, N. and Van Mechelen, W. (eds) (2008) *Paediatric Exercise Science and Medicine*, 2nd edn. Oxford University Press, Oxford.

Bar-Or, O. and Rowland, TW. (2004) *Pediatric Exercise Medicine*. Human Kinetics, Champaign, IL.

Hebestreit, H. and Bar-Or, O. (eds) (2008) *The Young Athlete*. Blackwell Publishing Ltd, Oxford.

Rowland, TW. (2005) *Children's Exercise Physiology*. Human Kinetics, Champaign, IL.

Chapter 9
Gymnastics psychology

Thomas Heinen[1,2], Pia M. Vinken[3,4], Konstantinos Velentzas[5]

[1]Institute of Sport Science, University of Hildesheim, Hildesheim, Germany
[2]Federation Internationale de Gymnastique (FIG), Lausanne, Switzerland
[3]Institute for Sport Teaching Skills, German Sport University Cologne, Cologne, Germany
[4]Institute of Sport Science, Leibniz University, Hanover, Germany
[5]Department of Sport Science, Bielefeld University, Bielefield, Germany

Introduction

A typical competition situation in gymnastics reveals a great diversity in behaviors. While the gymnast prepares for the upcoming routine, the coach may give some final instructions to him/her. Another group of gymnasts could be relaxing or preparing themselves in the gymnast's area. Judges are estimating the quality of the presented routines. Spectators watch the performing gymnasts and applaud when appropriate. The different behaviors may result from a variety of influencing factors. For example, the behavior of the spectators and the judges predominantly rely on the performance of the gymnasts. The behavior of the relaxing gymnasts may rely on their current arousal level. The behavior of the coach relies on previous observations of the performance of his/her gymnast(s), and the preparation of a particular gymnast may rely on further factors, such as observation of previous routine, current arousal level, current confidence level, and so forth. The preparation itself may in turn influence the gymnasts' behavior in the upcoming routine.

The diverse behaviors in gymnastics are thought to be goal-directed and intentionally driven (Hackfort, 2006). They result from the dynamic interplay of a person acting in a particular environment with regard to specific task demands (see Figure 9.1). In gymnastics, the task is predominantly defined by the competitive rules, the boundary conditions of the gymnastics apparatus, together with biomechanical and functional constraints related to an appropriate movement technique. Task demands may vary from performance to performance, and gymnasts have to adapt their performance to different settings or to apparatuses from different manufacturers. Being able to vary skill performance according to such influences is an important characteristic of elite gymnasts. Regarding the acting person, physiological factors as well as psychological factors are thought to influence performance. While, for instance, personality traits of the gymnast may only change in the long run, there are other factors such as psychological states that may change in the short run depending on the current situation. The environment comprises physical factors and social factors such as social support, peer groups, or norms that can have a strong influence on the gymnast.

Keeping the factors just described in mind, the first and foremost goal in gymnastics psychology is to optimize the person–environment relationship with regard to a given task in order to enable a gymnast to optimize his/her behavior to best suit a given situation. It is thus essential to organize a person–task–environment fit for the attainment of peak performance (Schack & Hackfort, 2007). Optimizing the environment by using, for instance, a vaulting table from a different manufacturer does not necessarily lead to

Gymnastics, First Edition. Edited by Dennis J. Caine, Keith Russell and Liesbeth Lim. © 2013 International Olympic Committee. Published 2013 by John Wiley & Sons, Ltd.

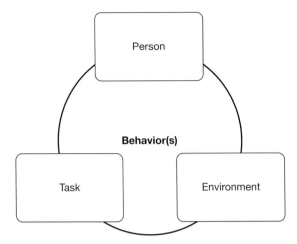

Figure 9.1 Observable behaviors in gymnastics are the results of person acting in a particular environment with regard to specific task demands. The execution and the effects of the diverse actions produce feedback for the acting person. The environment and the task may influence each other as well as the person. A person–task–environment fit is a precondition for the optimization of actions and thus for the optimization of complex behaviors in a particular situation (e.g., competition).

significant changes in observable performance in the short run, but the gymnast may have a better "feeling" of the performed vaults. This, however, could be a precondition for significant changes in observable behavior. In order to optimize the person–environment relationship with regard to a given task one fundamental step would be to equip the gymnast with skills that may support this. Nevertheless, influences hampering a person–task–environment fit may contribute to the development of certain problems (Schack & Hackfort, 2007).

In the following sections we will at first summarize psychological influences and performance-related challenges in high-performance gymnastics with regard to the acting person, the environment, and the task. Afterwards, we will derive psychological intervention methods that have proven to be advantageous for gymnasts to optimize the person–task–environment fit, and that can easily be applied in gymnastics training. Finally, we will pose several questions that still need to be answered with regard to gymnastics psychology.

Psychological influences and performance-related demands in high-performance gymnastics

Person: gymnasts' personality traits and psychological states

Physiological and psychological factors are thought to influence gymnasts' behavior and thus their performance. Two categories of psychological factors can be distinguished. The first category comprises enduring personality traits that may serve as templates for assimilating and accommodating environmental stimuli. The second category deals with psychological responses in particular situations, called states. For example, to be anxious in a wide variety of situations is a personality trait, whereas the actual manifestation of anxiety prior to performing a complex skill the first time without coach assistance is situation-specific and thus more a state rather than a trait.

Empirical evidence indicates that differences in athletes' personality traits covary with factors such as type of sport, skill level, competition level, gender, and cultural background. Personality alone is thus a rather weak predictor of gymnasts' behavior and performance in a wide variety of situations. Therefore, it is noted that information about gymnasts' personality, plus information about the situation, plus information about the interaction of gymnasts' personality with the situation better predict a gymnasts' performance than a personality or a situation analysis alone (Vanden Auweele *et al.*, 2001).

Using such a multidimensional and interactional approach, sport psychologists attempt to characterize a psychological profile for elite gymnasts in which selected psychological characteristics are identified that covary with gymnasts' expertise. Compared to their less-skilled counterparts or as compared to novices, elite gymnasts are thought to have a high degree of self-confidence, are less anxious, are mentally tough, have a clear focus on the task, view difficult situations as challenging, are intrinsically motivated, attribute failures more to external events, and are strongly committed to gymnastics. In contrast, aspects such as low self-confidence, a high degree of anxiety, focus on distractions, perceiving difficult situations as being over-challenging, being extrinsically motivated, or attributing failures to oneself are usually associated with poor gymnastics performance (Spink, 1990). It is thus the right mixture of perceptions, cognitions, emotions, and behaviors that influences the pathway to performance. Despite the mentioned differences between elite gymnasts and less-skilled counterparts it should be kept in mind that the contribution of psychological characteristics (traits/states) explains only approximately 30% of athletes' behavioral variance.

Seen in the long run, psychological factors in combination with the gymnasts' physiological state, the environment, and the task play important roles in differentiating between elite gymnasts and less-skilled gymnasts. Several authors agree that the systematic use of psychological skills and strategies may support optimizing psychological states in the short run and may in turn lead to changes in personality traits in the long run. These skills and strategies should be learned and continually practiced, as well as integrated into gymnasts' physical preparation, and refined if necessary so that a gymnast is able to perform to his/her maximum potential. The systematic application of psychological skills and strategies should support the balance between psychological and environmental factors, thus facilitating learning und stabilizing performance.

It can be summed up, first, that there are several personality traits and psychological states that seem to be more beneficial to a gymnast's performance, development, and mental health than others, and second, that continually practicing psychological skills and strategies may influence psychological states in the short run. These changes in psychological states may in turn lead to changes in personality traits in the long run, leading to enhancements in personality development.

Environment: coach's behavior related to gymnasts' development

From a psychological point of view, the environment is comprised of the various social factors incorporating social support, peer groups, or norms, and thus has a potential influence on the gymnast. Elite gymnasts compete and train in a physical, social, psychological, and organizational environment that can have both facilitative and debilitative effects upon the achievement of ideal performance states, and a lot of elite gymnasts have modified their lifestyle for the sake of their training. Furthermore, one should acknowledge that the active or passive presence of other people can have direct or indirect influences on the gymnast. Although gymnastics can be seen as an individual sport, gymnasts spend most of their time with their training groups, so that peer pressure and other interindividual phenomena occur as a consequence. Family as well as other team members could strengthen or weaken gymnasts' performance by the way they interact with each other. One of the most influencing environmental factors is without question the coach and thus we will focus on this factor in the next few paragraphs.

It is argued that good coaches are able to develop gymnasts to their personal best. However, coaches' work is a multidimensional and also a highly dynamic process. Coaches not only organize and manage training but also support and interact with the gymnasts before, during, and after competition. Coaches furthermore deal with aspects such as parental influences, spectators, or gymnasts' personal concerns, as well as represent the sport of gymnastics, and fulfill expectations of committees, federations, and others. Given this diversity in coaching demands, early research centered on the personality traits of coaches and it was believed that great coaches were born not made. Since then, however, research has evolved to support the notion of a situation-specific leadership whilst highlighting the interaction between the personality of the coach (leader), the situation, and factors such as characteristics of the followers, which are likely to influence coaches' behavior (Horn, 2008).

In a multidimensional approach of leadership, consequences in both gymnasts' performance and satisfaction evolve as a result of the interaction of three components of coaches' behavior: (1) required behavior, (2) preferred behavior, and (3) actual behavior. Required behaviors are those that conform to the established norms in gymnastics. For example, national team coaches are expected to behave in a certain manner in the presence of their gymnasts. Preferred behaviors are those behaviors of a coach that are preferred by the gymnasts. Members of a league team could prefer that their coach also has an eye on the social part of the sport activity. Actual behaviors are those behaviors that the coach exhibits in a particular situation. Empirical evidence highlights that the congruence between the three components is a significant predictor of gymnasts' satisfaction and performance (Cox, 2007). In other words: gymnasts are likely to perform better and they are more satisfied when actual and required behaviors are in line with the gymnasts' preferred coach behavior.

Required behaviors of gymnastics coaches predominantly differ as a function of coaching level, whereas preferred coaching behaviors predominantly differ depending on gymnasts' gender and age. Actual coaching behaviors such as establishing a high level of trust with gymnasts, being aware of gymnasts' individual (psychological and social) needs, making fair and comprehensible decisions, setting realistic expectations for each individual, or remaining calm under pressure are only some examples that are thought to have a strong influence on gymnasts' performance, independent of preferred and required behaviors. One aspect that integrates most of the aforementioned characteristics is the compatibility between coach and gymnast. Compatible coach–gymnasts dyads are characterized by effective and open communication and the presence of rewarding behavior for effort and performance in a two-sided free interaction. Both sides feel respect for each other and appreciate the other's role.

It may sound that the aforementioned attributes are impossible to adopt for a coach in the multidimensional and complex setting of gymnastics. However, we feel that as it is a hard piece of work for a young gymnast to acquire the diverse gymnastics skills, it may also be a hard piece of work for a young coach to acquire the diverse attributes and characteristics that may support gymnasts to perform to their personal best. Taken together, effective coaching depends on the coaches' qualities, the chosen leadership behavior or style, the athletes' qualities, and the given situational factors. This can lead to positive personality development (including psychological well-being) for the gymnasts in the long run as well as prevention or clarification of emerging problems in the short run.

Task: acquiring, controlling, and losing gymnastics skills

When a gymnast leaves the springboard to perform, for example, a Yurchenko vault, his/her actions look quite fluid and easy but they are in reality quite complex. Information from different sensory systems needs to be integrated in order to perform a complex skill in a precise and safe manner. The higher the expertise level of a gymnast, the more likely he/she will regulate his/her actions directly based on environmental information, and motor actions are strongly contingent upon the acquired sensory input. However, given the complexity and dynamic character of gymnastics skills, performance may differ from training to competition, and environmental influences may lead to changes in psychological states, thus influencing task execution in different situations.

Dramatic changes in psychological states are thought to be a potential precondition for movement errors and (in the worst case) for injuries. They are also thought to be preconditions for a phenomenon implying that skills appear to be suddenly lost by a gymnast (Day et al., 2006). When suffering from such a "lost-skill syndrome," gymnasts find themselves unable to perform a skill that was previously performed in an automatic manner. Such a loss of skill often results from a singular situation in which the gymnast performed a complex skill and lost spatial orientation during skill performance, sometimes leading to a serious fall. This loss of skill can have significant consequences. For instance, most gymnasts show a strong stress response when trying to perform a "lost" skill, which usually leads to a complete avoidance of skill execution or breakdown in motor control. This stress response often comprises perceptual and attentional changes, heightened levels of cognitive and somatic anxiety, perceived loss of control, and negative self-talk. Some gymnasts are still able to initiate an intended skill. However, during skill execution they often find themselves performing a different skill than the one that was intended (e.g., somersault with one and a half twist instead of somersault with two and a half twist). Finally, the loss of a skill often transfers to skills with a similar movement structure. In sum, a loss of skill could imply a career-destroying potential for a gymnast, since this phenomenon seems to be very resistant to change.

Taken together, dramatic changes in psychological states are thought to be a potential precondition for a loss of skill, which can have negative consequences for a gymnast. Even if the causes of lost-skill syndrome are still not fully understood, a systematic implementation of psychological interventions in gymnastics training could not only be one fruitful way to prevent a loss of skill but also to equip a developing gymnast with skills that may support him/her in attaining peak performance.

Psychological interventions in gymnastics

In this section methods for optimizing gymnasts' performance on a systematic basis will be discussed. It was already highlighted that elite gymnasts possess certain (psychological) characteristics that make it possible for them to experience unprecedented success. Empirical evidence highlights that psychological intervention programs are effective in developing and enhancing psychological skills, and thus are effective in enhancing gymnasts' performance. Furthermore, several psychological models and theories have been formulated to clarify the guidelines for an optimized psychological preparation, and to evaluate the development of psychological skills (Gardner & Moore, 2004).

From the current research it is also apparent that there are not necessarily linear relationships between the use of specific psychological methods and the development or change in specific psychological skills. Therefore, using psychological methods in gymnastics training is not trivial. It may seem obvious that imagery training (as a psychological method) influences imagery skill when practiced regularly. However, imagery training may also lead to changes in aspects such as self-confidence and anxiety. In light of this, coaches should be able to

provide their gymnasts with a base of psychological support. In order to assist gymnasts in reaching peak performance and taking into account the complexity of task, environmental/social demands, characteristics of the gymnast, as well as interactions between the three entities, it becomes obvious that the application of specific psychological methods can be a decisive factor, making the difference between success and failure in a competitive context. Gymnastics coaches are thus advised to apply state-of-the-art knowledge on psychological methods in a person-centered approach when working with gymnasts of all ages. Seen in the long run, we argue that such an approach is most effective if the gymnast is able to personalize and claim ownership of specific methods in such a way that they become useful strategies for him/her. In the next paragraph we will characterize three strategic approaches for training and competition as well as important psychological methods to be integrated in gymnastics training.

Strategies for training and competition

The general purpose of using psychological methods is to put oneself in an optimally aroused, confident, and focused state immediately before as well as during routine execution. This aim, however, implies that the used methods have been developed in gymnastics training on a systematic basis leading to the intended changes in arousal, confidence, or focus. Imagine, for instance, a gymnast who is going to perform his high bar routine in a world championship competition. He is the last competitor and knows that he would be able to make it to the first place if he performs the routine without any major errors. What can he do to cope with this situation? Or, extending the question, what could have been done in his training, prior to this competitive situation? From the current research and from the authors' own experiences as sport psychologist, it is proposed that the aforementioned questions can be addressed by means of the following three intertwined descriptions (Cox, 2007).

First, coaches are encouraged to develop training and competition plans together with their gymnasts. These plans should comprise the individual goals, the steps and behaviors necessary to reach these goals, as well as the steps that should be taken in case of emerging problems. Using training diaries is only one way of implementing this strategy. Gymnasts' individual goals should be evaluated in a systematic way relative to the individual development of the gymnast (e.g., by using competitive simulation), and refined if necessary and/or appropriate.

Second, coaches may integrate general psychological skills training programs into gymnasts' physical training on a regular basis. These programs should aim at teaching gymnasts different psychological methods to optimize different psychological skills. Such training programs usually consist of several sessions. Each session can address different psychological methods and psychological skills, such as relaxation techniques (e.g., awareness of abdominal breathing), self-talk techniques (e.g., using positive self-talk to cope with fear), focusing (e.g., shifting focus from narrow to broad), or imagery techniques (e.g., shifting imagery perspective from internal to external). When applying such a program, the gymnast should be given time to explore which psychological methods are more appropriate for him/her in affecting specific psychological skills. While using autogenic training for controlling arousal level may satisfy one gymnast, another gymnast may prefer to use progressive muscular relaxation. From the authors' own experience it is beneficial to begin integrating such a program in gymnastics groups at ages 11–13 for two 30-minute sessions per week over a time period of 6–7 months.

Third, while the previous step is of high importance in advancing young gymnasts to apply psychological techniques in daily training and in competition, most sport psychologists would argue that psychological methods are most effective if they are adapted individually to each gymnasts' strengths and weaknesses. It is likely that different gymnasts will exhibit different profiles relative to their psychological skills. At first, it may therefore be beneficial to assess the gymnasts' psychological strengths and weaknesses and use this as a starting point to equip the gymnast with further psychological methods or to improve the application of already known methods. At this step it is

recommended to consult a professional sport psychologist. Afterwards, selected psychological methods should be integrated into individual programs that comprise a particular, yet individual, collection of psychological methods that best suit the gymnasts' needs. These methods can have different functions and they can be applied during training, in order to regulate psychological states or to facilitate skill acquisition. In the following paragraphs we will characterize some of the most important psychological methods in gymnastics and describe how they can be incorporated into an individual program for an upcoming vault performance.

Psychological methods integrated into gymnastics routines

When the gymnast prepares his-/herself and walks towards the starting point on the run-up track, he/she could use particular coping methods (e.g., self-talk or abdominal breathing) to balance his/her arousal level as well as to create an atmosphere of self-confidence. Afterwards, the gymnast could use a short imaging period during which he/she imagines several key points/phases of the intended vault as well as a successful outcome. When he/she is signaled to vault, the attention could be focused on a relevant external (e.g., springboard or vaulting table) or internal cue (thought). This shift in attention leads to the execution of the vault. As the vault is executed, the gymnast stays calm. If possible he/she can use visual spotting for spatial orientation during the vault. After finishing the vault, the gymnast could apply a strategy to clear the mind for the next apparatus. Critical analysis should be saved for the next training session. Additionally, during breaks, he/she could engage a conversation with the teammates or listen to relaxing music while imaging a restful scene.

To be effective, the aforementioned methods and strategies must be practiced systematically. Their temporal length should be consistent from trial to trial, and its execution should occur at a consistent time relative to the execution of the vault. Since psychological methods can be very individual in nature, the reader should try to understand the following paragraphs as modules that can be used to prepare specific mental skills for individual gymnasts.

The first module refers to methods the gymnast could use to cope with a particular (stressful) situation. In gymnastics, coping predominantly refers to expending effort to master, minimize, or tolerate stress, which is likely to occur immediately prior to the execution of a gymnastics routine, and which can recur on each apparatus during a competition. Coping can focus on the stress-causing problem itself (problem-focused coping) or on the accompanying emotions (emotion-focused coping) when under stress. The gymnast can furthermore actively engage the problem or the emotion (approach coping) or try to avoid the current problem or the emotion (avoidance coping). There are several factors influencing the effectiveness of different coping strategies. First, it is thought, that females benefit more from the use of emotion-focused coping than males do. They also report to benefit more from social support to cope with stressful situations. Knowing the coping preferences of individual gymnasts is an important precondition for psychological interventions. Second, coping strategies that match the stressor are most effective. A problem-focused coping strategy should be more effective in dealing with cognitive anxiety as compared to an emotion-focused strategy. This may, however, differ from gymnast to gymnast. Therefore, it is also necessary to know the psychological responses of a stressed gymnast. Third, approach and avoidance coping are both beneficial in the short run, but only approach coping (problem- and emotion-focused strategy) is effective in the long run. Coping strategies are usually integrated in gymnastics training with either a somatic focus (e.g., deep abdominal breathing), or a cognitive focus (e.g., self-talk). Abdominal breathing or self-talk can easily be applied in almost every environmental setting or competitive situation when needed. Further, the combination of abdominal breathing and self-talk (or imagery, see below) as autogenic training or progressive relaxation can, for instance, be applied prior to a competition or after an exhausting training session.

The second module comprises the use of imagery as a psychological method. Imagery as a process implies using all senses to create or recreate an experience in the mind. In gymnastics, imagery may be used for motivational or cognitive purposes. Imagery is thought to be an effective technique for practicing as well as adjusting technical and tactical elements of the routines (in the short run and in the long run) as well as a technique to prevent injury by reducing the number of repetitions practiced. These could include mentally simulating competitive environments, as well as building self-confidence and focus. The relationship between imagery use and performance in gymnastics seems to be affected by several factors such as the content of imagery, the skill level of the gymnast, the imagery ability of the gymnast, the perspective and sensory focus used during imagery, and the amount and duration of imagery use during training (Weinberg, 2008).

For imagery to be effective, first, the content of imagery needs to be adapted to each individual gymnast depending on his/her current setting and goals. A young gymnast may be more receptive to using metaphorical images such as imaging being a fast running panther, whereas a more experienced gymnast may be more receptive to imaging certain technical details of gymnastics skills. Second, a certain amount of skill is necessary, and thus, experienced gymnasts will potentially benefit to a larger degree from imagery. Good imagery ability is another significant predictor of the effectiveness of imagery. When working with gymnasts, coaches will find that some gymnasts are able to imagine gymnastics skills vividly with a lot of detail and a high degree of controllability whereas other gymnasts have difficulties imaging even simple situations and skills from their sport. Third, while imagery can be used from different perspectives (internal, external) and focused on different senses (e.g., visual, kinesthetic, or auditory), empirical evidence suggests that a kinesthetic focus is superior for the acquisition and optimization of motor skills. However, experienced gymnasts often report to have specific preferences in imagery perspective and sensory modality, and it may be advisable to assess gymnasts' preference in each individual case.

A third module comprises visual spotting as a psychological method to be used during skill performance. When a gymnast intentionally fixates his/her gaze, for example, to a particular reference point in the environment (e.g., end of the balance beam during a standing scale), this is what is called visual spotting. It is assumed that fixating the gaze to environmental reference points during skill execution enables the gymnast to optimize visual information pickup for spatial orientation. Empirical evidence suggests that gymnasts use visual spotting in the performance of gymnastics skills, and that there exist relationships between visual spotting and movement kinematics, thus arguing for the functional role of spotting in the optimization of skill execution (Heinen, 2011). Visual spotting helps the gymnast to engage a more external focus of attention, which usually leads to a more fluid and precise movement execution even in stressful situations. It is therefore suggested that spotting techniques should be integrated in gymnastics training on a systematic and regular basis. It should, however, be acknowledged that gaze during visual spotting should be first and foremost directed to the invariant properties of the environment, or the specific apparatus, that the gymnast will find in different gyms or when performing on an apparatus from a different manufacturer. This may help the gymnast to stabilize skill execution even if he/she engages in a stressful situation or has to deal with problems such as lost-skill syndrome or alike.

To sum up, it is stated that the discussed psychological methods can be thought of as a set of tools that a gymnast could use to optimize his/her psychological states and in turn to optimize subjective and objective performance. From the authors' point of view the discussed modules are highly effective when integrated in gymnastics training. However, there may be other psychological intervention strategies that could prove to be effective for individual gymnasts. To be effective, the methods should be practiced in a systematic and regular manner, and they should be integrated with physical training in such a way that the gymnast is able to personalize and claim ownership of the methods for his/her individual needs.

Further research

Elite gymnasts not only possess specific psychological states but also regulate complex skills more precisely than their less-skilled counterparts.

However, dramatic changes in psychological states are thought to be a potential precondition for movement errors, injuries, or even for a loss of skill. Further research should try to better understand these. Experienced gymnasts are far from being "machines" that produce the same pattern of movement in every trial. Even if this might look so at first sight, biomechanical analyses usually reveal that there will always remain some trial-to-trial variability, and the question would be which (psychological) factors influence this variability and when does this variability support and when does it hamper performance. Such questions can only be addressed when trying to integrate fields such as psychology, movement science, and biomechanics. Such an integrative approach implies specific methods such as measuring gaze behavior, and movement behavior (kinematics and muscular activation) during complex skill performance. An additional line of research should focus on evaluating different intervention strategies in case of a manifested lost-skill syndrome.

Taking into account the development of new media and new technologies such as virtual reality devices, or augmented reality devices, it could be one interesting way in gymnastics psychology to research the potential and usability of such devices in psychological interventions. Finally, and taking into account recent trends in fields such as neuroscience or psychophysiology, it could be interesting to see to what degree psychophysiological or neurophysiological intervention strategies (e.g., transcranial magnetic stimulation or galvanic vestibular stimulation) could support psychological training, physical training, or both in high-performance gymnastics.

The relationship between psychological characteristics and gymnasts' performance may covary with other factors such as gender, age, cultural background, and so on. Therefore, investigating these relationships could be one fruitful way for further research. This could also help to address questions related to talent identification and talent selection in gymnastics. It could potentially reveal alternative explanations for the development of serious problems in gymnastics, such as eating disorders, drug abuse, injury, burn out, or drop out. It would additionally be interesting to broaden such research to gymnasts with particular expertise on a particular apparatus and to compare their psychological profile to all-around gymnasts or to specialists on other apparatus. This could address the question why gymnasts develop particular preferences for an apparatus while others do not.

There is a variety of influences in the environment and it would be fruitful for further research to assess the short-term effects of influences from factors such as coaches, spectators, judges, or other gymnasts' behavior on gymnasts' psychological states, as well as long-term effects of factors such as parents, peers, or other gymnasts from the same club or same team on gymnasts' (personality) development. While one would agree that social support could be important in the personality development of a gymnast, the effects of rather "pushy" or "ignorant" parents, highly competitive training regimes, or situations like gymnasts living far away from home, on gymnasts' personality development are less clear, and should be studied more.

Summary

The diverse behaviors in gymnastics result from the interplay of person acting in a particular environment with regard to specific tasks. A person–task–environment fit is a significant precondition for gymnasts' optimization of actions in a particular situation (e.g., competition) and thus for the attainment of peak performance. There are several personality traits and psychological states that seem to be related to gymnasts' performance, development, and mental health. Psychological methods can be thought of as a set of tools that a gymnast could use to optimize his/her psychological states and in turn to optimize performance. To be effective, the methods should be practiced in a systematic and regular manner, and they should be integrated with physical training in such a way that the gymnast is able to personalize and claim ownership of the methods for his/her individual needs. Continually practicing psychological methods and strategies may influence psychological states in the short run. These changes in psychological states may in turn lead to changes in personality traits in the long run, leading to

enhancements in personality development, which should be considered positive in nature. However, the relationship between the configuration of psychological characteristics and gymnasts' performance may covary with other factors such as gender, age, cultural background, and so on. Gymnastics coaches are advised to apply state-of-the-art knowledge on psychological methods in a person-centered approach when working with gymnasts of all ages. Effective coaching is characterized by an open communication and the presence of coaches' rewarding behavior for gymnasts' effort and performance. The coach and the gymnasts feel respect for one another and appreciate each other's roles.

References

Cox, R.H. (2007) *Sport Psychology. Concepts and Applications*. McGraw-Hill, New York.

Day, M.C., Thatcher, J., Greenlees, I., and Woods, B. (2006) The causes of psychological responses to lost move syndrome in national level trampolinists. *Journal of Applied Sport Psychology*, **18**, 151–166.

Gardner, F. and Moore, Z. (2004) The multi-level classification system for sport psychology (MCS-SP). *The Sport Psychologist*, **18**, 89–109.

Hackfort, D. (2006) A conceptual framework and fundamental issues for investigating the development of peak performance in sports. In: D. Hackfort and G. Tenenbaum (eds), *Essential Processes for Attaining Peak Performance*, pp. 10–25. Meyer & Meyer Sport, Oxford.

Heinen, T. (2011) Evidence for the spotting hypothesis in gymnasts. *Motor Control*, **15**, 267–284.

Horn, T.S. (2008) Coaching effectiveness in the sport domain. In: T.S. Horn (eds), *Advances in Sport Psychology*, 3rd edn, pp. 239–267. Human Kinetics, Champaign, IL.

Schack, T. and Hackfort, D. (2007) An action theory approach to applied sport psychology. In: G. Tenenbaum and R.C. Eklund (eds), *Handbook of Sport Psychology*, 3rd edn, pp. 332–351. John Wiley & Sons, Inc., New York.

Spink, K.S. (1990) Psychological characteristics of male gymnasts: differences between competitive levels. *Journal of Sports Sciences*, **8**, 149–157.

Vanden Auweele, Y., Nys, K., Rzewnicki, R., and Van Mele, V. (2001) Personality and the athlete. In: R.N. Singer, H.A. Hausenblas, and C. Janelle (eds), *Handbook of Sport Psychology*, 2nd edn, pp. 239–268. John Wiley & Sons, Inc., New York.

Weinberg, R. (2008) Does imagery work? Effects in performance and mental skills. *Journal of Imagery Research in Sport and Physical Activity*, **3** (1), Article 1.

Recommended reading

Arkaev, L.I. and Suchilin, N.G. (2004) *How to create champions. The Theory and Methodology of Training Top-Class Gymnasts.* Meyer & Meyer Sport, Oxford.

Chase, M.A., Magyar, M., and Drake, B. M. (2005) Fear of injury in gymnastics: self-efficacy and psychological strategies to keep on tumbling. *Journal of Sports Sciences,* **23** (5), 465–475.

Cottyn, J., De Clerq, D., Pannier, J.L., Crombez, G., and Lenoir, M. (2006) The measurement of competitive anxiety during balance beam performance in gymnasts. *Journal of Sports Sciences,* **24** (2), 157–164.

Fournier, J.F., Calmels, C., Durand-Bush, N., and Salmela, J.H. (2005) Effects of a season-long PST program on gymnastic performance and on psychological skill development. *International Journal of Sport and Exercise Psychology,* **3**, 59–77.

Grandjean, B.D., Taylor, P.A., and Weiner, J. (2002) Confidence, concentration, and competitive performance of elite athletes: a natural experiment in Olympic gymnastics. *Journal of Sport and Exercise Psychology,* **24**, 320–327.

Heinen, T., Vinken, P. M., and Fink, H. (2011) The effects of directing the learner's gaze on skill acquisition in gymnastics. *Athletic Insight,* **3** (2), 165–181.

Jemni, M. (ed.) (2011) *The Science of Gymnastics.* Routledge, Oxon.

Krane, V. and Williams, J.M. (2006) Psychological characteristics of peak performance. In: J.M. Williams (ed.) *Applied Sport Psychology: Personal Growth to Peak Performance,* 5th edn, pp. 207–227. McGraw-Hill, New York.

Schack, T. and Bar-Eli, M. (2007) Psychological factors in technical preparation. In: B. Blumenstein, R. Lidor, and G. Tenenbaum (eds) *Psychology of Sport Training,* 2nd edn, pp. 62–103. Meyer & Meyer Sport, Oxford.

PART 4
SPORT MEDICINE ASPECTS

Chapter 10
Epidemiology of injury in gymnastics

Dennis Caine[1], Marita L. Harringe[2]

[1]College of Education and Human Development, University of North Dakota, Grand Forks, ND, USA
[2]Stockholm Sports Trauma Research Center and Care Sciences and Society, Karolinska Institutet, Stockholm, Sweden

Introduction

Current day Olympic Games include Men's and Women's Artistic Gymnastics, Rhythmic Gymnastics, and Trampoline Gymnastics. Gymnastics is a sport that is well known for intense training and relatively young age of participants. Like many sports that involve children and adolescents, gymnastics has experienced increased participation in recent years, with changes most pronounced following the excitement and media attention associated with the Olympics. Elite female and male artistic gymnasts may initiate training for their sport as early as ages six and nine, respectively, with peak performance being 10 or more years away. Published studies on Artistic Gymnastics report weekly hours of preparation ranging from 7 to 36 hours among females and from 10 to 33 hours among males, depending on competitive level. Top-level gymnasts typically train twice each day, 5–6 days per week and up to 12 months of the year.

Extraordinary levels of athleticism and biomechanical loading during training and competition are associated with this trend toward earlier and increased competition. The difficulty and range of skills that have come to characterize the sport have changed considerably over the years. Every 4 years, for example, rule changes are made in accordance with the Federation International de Gymnastique (FIG) Code of Points, essentially increasing the required levels of difficulty with each revision. The increased participation in gymnastics is encouraging because physical activity clearly provides many health-related benefits to those who participate. However, increased involvement and difficulty of skills practiced at an early age and continued through the years of growth, with the intense training required, strongly suggest the possibility of increased risk of injury. It is perhaps not surprising that concern has been raised regarding the incidence rate, severity, and long-term effects of injury sustained in competitive gymnastics. Most competitive gymnasts, particularly those who progress to elite levels of training and competition, typically do not pass through their gymnastics careers without incurring injury.

The purpose of this chapter is to provide information on the epidemiology of gymnastics injury as reported in the literature. Several systematic reviews of the epidemiology of injury in men's and women's gymnastics have been published since 2000 (Caine & Nassar, 2005; Kolt & Caine, 2010; DiFiori & Caine, 2012). Consistent with the purpose of the IOC Handbook series, the intent of this manuscript is to draw on these previous reviews with the purpose of capturing generally accepted principles and information and avoiding lengthy discussion of controversial findings. To update the overall picture, however, relevant material published since the most recent reviews will also be covered.

The main focus of the chapter, as determined by the available published research literature, will be

Gymnastics, First Edition. Edited by Dennis J. Caine, Keith Russell and Liesbeth Lim. © 2013 International Olympic Committee. Published 2013 by John Wiley & Sons, Ltd.

on competitive Men's and Women's Artistic Gymnastics. There have been only a few injury studies arising from competitive Rhythmic and Trampoline Gymnastics. Studies of Trampoline Gymnastics largely predate the inclusion of this sport at the Olympic level (1998) and are limited primarily to case series of recreational injuries. The literature on gymnastics injuries comes mainly in the form of observational epidemiological studies (e.g., prospective, retrospective, and cross-sectional), including studies that have investigated the relationship between injury and risk factors. Study designs such as case series, case reports, and anecdotal reports are also common in the gymnastics injury literature. However, the majority of emphasis in this chapter will be on information arising from observational epidemiological studies as they provide more generally accepted information on the incidence, distribution, and determinants of injury.

Gymnastic injury research limitations

Much of the existing literature on injury in gymnastics deals with females, with only a few studies addressing male gymnasts. In reviewing the existing literature, several methodological limitations arise as summarized below (Kolt & Caine, 2010):

• Diversity of study populations with respect to age, type of gymnastics, competitive level, apparatus, event, and type of training environment.
• Study duration is relatively short in most studies. With differences in injury incidence between training and competition, comparing different periods of an annual performance and training cycle is difficult and can be seen as problematic.
• Frequent use of self-report questionnaires that may not capture accurate details of the diagnosis and exact nature of injury.
• In the absence of detailed injury records retrospectively collected data are susceptible to gymnast and coach recall bias and tend to miss the more minor injuries, thereby resulting in lower overall injury rates.
• Variability in injury definition across studies thus resulting in different approaches to "counting" injuries.
• Nonrandom selection resulting in the possibility that those gymnastic programs most concerned with injury will be overrepresented in the published literature.
• Paucity of studies on gymnasts from outside of North America. With different training methods across countries, findings from one country may not be readily generalized to other countries.
• The popularity, participation, and financial support for the sport may vary internationally.
• With significant changes in gymnastics training (including increased difficulty of skills being performed), equipment, and rules over the years, comparing results from different periods of time should be done with caution.
• Many of the studies that investigated risk factors did not account for the multifactorial nature of injury risk.

It is important for the reader to consider the generally accepted principles arising from the gymnastics injury research in light of these limitations.

The epidemiological approach

Participants in gymnastics and everyone who works with them, whether they are parents, sports medicine personnel, sports governing bodies, or coaches, need to know answers to important questions such as: What is the risk of injury and does the risk vary relative to type or level of gymnastics? When and where are injuries most likely to occur? What is the outcome of injury? Are some factors associated with an increased risk of injury? These are all questions that need to be answered through scientific investigation. Providing this information is an important objective of epidemiological research related to Olympic gymnastics.

Injury epidemiology is the study of the distribution and determinants of varying rates of injuries in human populations for the purpose of identifying and implementing measures to prevent their development and spread. A model outlining the epidemiologic approach to sports injury prevention was first proposed by Willem van Mechelen *et al.* (1992) and involves a "sequence of prevention" (Figure 10.1). In the first step, research establishes the extent of injury. This involves quantifying injury occurrence (*how much*) with respect to *who* is affected

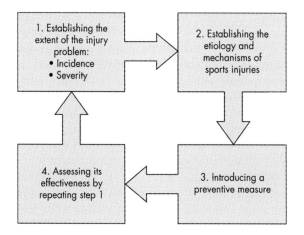

Figure 10.1 Four-step sequence of injury prevention research. (Source: Van Mechelen W., Hlobil H., Kemper J.C.G. (1992) Springer Healthcare © Adis Data Information BV 2012. All rights reserved.)

by injury, *where* and *when* injuries occur, and *what* is their outcome. The study of the distribution of varying rates of injuries (i.e., who, where, when, what) is referred to as descriptive epidemiology. In the second step, research explores the causes and implications of injury, the *why* and *how* of injury. Third,

research creates a prevention strategy to reduce the injury burden. In the fourth step, research evaluates the effectiveness of the implemented prevention strategy by reexamining the extent of injury. The study of the determinants of an exhibited distribution of varying rates of injuries (i.e., why and how) and the identification and implementation of preventive strategies is referred to as analytical epidemiology. The focus in this chapter will be on the first two steps of this sequence. A focus on steps three and four will be provided in Chapter 14.

Descriptive epidemiology

Descriptive epidemiology is by far the most common type of epidemiologic research that has been published in the gymnastics injury literature. A diagram illustrating important aspects of the descriptive epidemiology of sports-related injuries is shown in Figure 10.2 (Caine *et al.*, 2006). These components are discussed below with the purpose of highlighting their various contributions to understanding the incidence and distribution of injury in gymnastics.

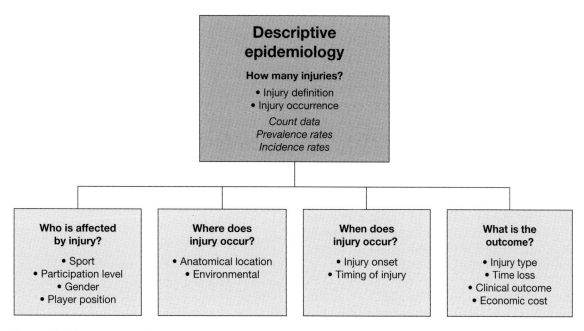

Figure 10.2 Descriptive epidemiology of sports injuries. (Source: Caine *et al.* (2006)).

How many injuries?

In descriptive epidemiology the researcher attempts to quantify the occurrence of injury. The most basic measure of injury occurrence is a simple count of injured persons. In order to investigate the rate and distribution of injuries it is necessary to know the size of the source population from which the injured individuals were derived, or the population-at-risk. The two most commonly reported rates in the sports injury literature are incidence and prevalence. Prevalence rates pertain to the total number of cases, new or old, that exist in a population at risk at a specific period of time. Prevalence rates published in the gymnastics injury literature typically include rates for specific conditions such as wrist pain and/or radiologic abnormalities of the thoracic-lumbar spine among gymnasts.

The two types of injury incidence most commonly reported in the gymnastics injury literature are clinical incidence and incidence rates. Clinical incidence refers to the number of incident injuries divided by the total number of athletes at risk and usually multiplied by some *k* value (e.g., 100). In the gymnastics injury literature these rates have most often been presented as injuries per 100 gymnasts. Prior to 1990, clinical incidence was widely reported in the gymnastics injury literature. However, clinical incidence does not account for potential variance in exposure of participants to risk for injury (Knowles *et al.*, 2006). For example, an injured gymnast who is not training in all parts of practice is not at the same risk of sustaining injury as an uninjured gymnast. Incidence rate refers to the number of incident injuries divided by the total time-at-risk and usually multiplied by some *k* value (e.g., 1000). It is the preferred measure of incidence in research studies because it can accommodate variations in exposure time of individual athletes. Different units of time-at-risk, varying in precision, have been used to calculate incidence rates in the gymnastics literature. These include reporting the number of injuries per *k* athlete exposures (an athlete exposure or AE is defined as one gymnast participating in one practice or competition in which there is the possibility of sustaining an athletic injury), per *k* time exposures (one time exposure is typically defined as one gymnast participating in

1 hour of activity in which there is the possibility of sustaining an athletic injury), or per *k* element exposures (one element exposure is defined as one gymnast participating in one element of activity in which there is the possibility of sustaining a gymnastics injury, e.g., during a vault). Most recent studies on gymnastics injuries report injury rates per *k* time exposures (e.g., 1000 hours), although there are difficulties associated with this approach, especially with regards to determining time spent competing (O'Kane *et al.*, 2011). Rates expressed per *k* gymnast exposures have been reported by the National Collegiate Athletic Association injury surveillance system (NCAA ISS) (Marshall *et al.*, 2007). Although attractive in terms of ease of data collection, this approach lacks precision in terms of actual time exposed. A difficulty that may arise in comparing incidence rates from different studies relates to the injury definition employed. A review of the gymnastics injury epidemiology literature reveals that few common operational definitions exist for injury. Definitions include such criteria as presence of a new symptom or complaint, decreased function of a body part or decreased athletic performance, cessation of practice or competition activities, and consultation with medical or training personnel. Defining injury in gymnastics is problematic due to the tendency for gymnasts to train "around" injuries. For example, a gymnast with an ankle injury may continue training on the uneven bars providing she avoids the dismount. Clearly, if injury is defined differently across studies, a meaningful comparison of injury rates is compromised due to different criteria for determining numerator values. Notably, several sports including soccer (football), rugby union, and thoroughbred horse racing have recently published methodological consensus statements that identify definitions and methodology to ensure consistency and comparability of results in studies examining injury in their sports.

Who is injured?

As might be expected, injury rates are most often categorized according to the way in which gymnastics participants are organized for sports (e.g., artistic, rhythmic, or trampoline) or level of sport (e.g., recreational, high school, club college, or international).

Given the variance in injury definitions across studies, perhaps the most reliable within- or across-sport comparisons arise from those studies that use a common, exposure-based injury definition and surveillance protocol and where certified athletic trainers or other health professionals record the injury data. Examples include research reports arising from the NCAA ISS and the RIO™ (Reporting Information Online). For example, the NCAA ISS reported a 15-year average of intercollegiate injuries (Hootman et al., 2007). Women's gymnastics had the second highest rate of competition injuries among women's intercollegiate sports, preceded by women's soccer. In practice, women's gymnastics ranked highest among women's sports followed by soccer. Unfortunately, there is presently no organized ISS to track and monitor injuries occurring in club gymnastics or at gymnastics schools, which is where most competitive gymnasts train and compete.

Comparison of injury rates across reported studies is difficult given that most authors have not taken into account the exposure to injury risk, but rather reported injury rates per season. Those who did calculate exposure-based overall injury rates reported rates ranging from 0.5 injuries per 1000 hours of participation to 5.3 injuries per 1000 hours of participation for female club gymnasts (Kolt & Caine, 2010; DiFiori & Caine, 2012), which is relatively high and similar to injury rates sustained by girls in sports such as soccer and basketball (Caine et al., 2006). Unfortunately, there are no overall (practice and competition combined) exposure-based injury rates reported for male gymnasts.

There is also a dearth of injury data for participants in Rhythmic and Trampoline Gymnastics. Cupisti et al. (2007) carried out an 8-month prospective study with 70 club-level rhythmic gymnasts aged 13–19 years. They reported 49 significant injuries over the study period, equating to a rate of 1.08 injuries per 1000 hours of training. Whilst Trampoline Gymnastics is a relatively new discipline to the Olympic gymnastics family (since 1998), only one study has reported on the epidemiology of injuries in this sport (Grapton et al., 2012). Based on data gathered by the French Federation of Gymnastics (FFG) over a 5-year period, 226 injuries were incurred in conjunction with trampoline training and competition.

Where does the injury occur?

The "where" of injury distribution involves the anatomical as well as the environmental or situational location (see Figure 10.2). Anatomical locations include body region of injury (e.g., upper extremity) as well as specific body parts (e.g., shoulder or ankle). Identification of commonly injured anatomical locations alerts sports medicine personnel to injury sites in need of special attention during preparticipation musculoskeletal assessment and important "targets" for preventive measures.

Environmental locations provide information on where the injury occurred. Environmental locations reported in the gymnastics injury literature include whether the injury occurred in competition or training; and apparatus used or event, such as balance beam or parallel bars in gymnastics. Information on high-risk injury locations and settings provides important "targets" for further study and preventive measures.

Anatomical location

The lower extremity is the most commonly injured body region for both club-level gymnasts and for high school and college female gymnasts (35.9–70.2% of all injuries) (Kolt & Caine, 2010; O'Kane et al., 2011; DiFiori & Caine, 2012). This finding is not surprising given the repetitive dismounts practiced on the various pieces of gymnastics apparatus. The next most frequently injured region is the upper extremity (7.7–36.0% of all injuries), followed by the trunk and spine (0–43.6% of all injuries), and the head (up to 8.8% of all injuries). A more specific look at these body regions highlights that injuries to the knee are the most common, followed by those to the ankle and the lower back.

The distribution by anatomical location has also been reported in studies of male artistic gymnasts (Kolt & Caine, 2010; DiFiori & Caine, 2012). Similar to that for female gymnasts, the lower extremity was the most injured region (32.8–72.2% of all injuries) in most studies followed by the upper limb (12.5–53.4%) and trunk and spine (7.9–31.3% of all injuries). However, male gymnasts tend to experience a greater proportion of injuries affecting specific upper extremity locations (e.g., shoulder or wrist) than female gymnasts, likely reflecting the skills practiced and apparatus used in men's gymnastics.

Data on anatomical location of injury is limited for Rhythmic Gymnastics. Cupisti *et al.* (2004) reported a 10.5% prevalence of low back pain among rhythmic gymnasts compared with 26.0% of matched controls (nongymnasts). In a later study, Cupisti *et al.* (2007) investigated 70 club-level rhythmic gymnasts over an 8-month period. The most common anatomical sites for injury were the foot (38.3%), knee and lower leg (19.1%), and back (17.0%).

Among competitive trampoline gymnasts the most commonly affected injury sites in one study (Grapton *et al.*, 2012) were the lower limb (49.1%), followed by the spine (32.3%), and upper limb (18.6%). The most frequently injured body parts were knee (19.9%), followed by the lower back (16.8%) and ankle (15.5%).

Environmental location

Not unlike competitive swimming, gymnastics is a sport characterized by long hours of training and repetition and very few hours spent in competition. It is not unusual for some gymnasts, despite training up to 36 hours per week, to participate in only 5–10 competitions per year. It is not unexpected, therefore, that a greater proportion of injuries is associated with training. Several studies of female gymnasts report that 71.0–96.6% of all injuries occur in practice and 3.4–21% in competition (Kolt & Caine, 2010; O'Kane *et al.*, 2011). However, when exposure is accounted for the rate of injury is two to three times greater in competition. For example, collegiate female gymnasts were six times more likely to sustain a knee internal derangement and almost three times more likely to sustain an ankle ligament sprain in competition than in practice (Marshall *et al.*, 2007). Gymnasts are much more likely to participate at a greater intensity in competition than in practice, thus increasing the risk of sustaining an injury. Also, in gymnastics when routines are performed in practice, an effort is made to ensure that the training environment is as safe as possible by performing the routine in smaller pieces, using protective mats

and harnesses, and spotting by coaches to a degree not possible in competition (O'Kane *et al.*, 2011). Other factors possibly contributing to higher competition injury rates include higher pressure to perform, travel, and the different equipment and environment inherent in traveling to a competition (O'Kane *et al.*, 2011). Given the higher rate of injury during competition, an increased focus and analysis of risk factors and preventive measures associated with competition injuries is required.

No studies of injury in Rhythmic or Trampoline Gymnastics have examined injury data in relation to whether injury occurred during training or competition.

With gymnasts participating in a wide variety of events or apparatus (six for men, four for women, and many other nonapparatus training drills), it is important to understand where the greatest risk of injury lies. However, it is difficult to fully understand the relationship between gymnastic event and injury because most research reports a percentage distribution of injury by event, and therefore does not account for time exposed. It is likely that the incidence rate of injury would be greatest during floor routines in Artistic Gymnastics due to the high frequency of dismounts and landings. However, this hypothesis awaits confirmation from exposure-based research.

In Men's Artistic Gymnastics and Rhythmic and Trampoline Gymnastics, exposure-based data in relation to event are not available in the published literature.

When does injury occur?

As Figure 10.2 indicates, the next characteristic of injury distribution is the when of injury occurrence. Time factors are typically expressed in terms of injury onset and timing of injury.

Injury onset

There are two broad categories of injury onset that differ markedly in etiology. Overuse injuries are more subtle and develop gradually over time. They are the result of repetitive microtrauma to the tendons, bones, and joints. Common examples include growth plate injuries, patellar tendinosis, and medial tibial stress syndrome. Injuries that occur suddenly are often termed acute or sudden impact injuries and are usually the result of a single, traumatic event. Common examples include wrist fractures, ankle sprains, and shoulder dislocations. An injury history may actually involve both categories of injury onset, such as when an acute injury is superimposed on a chronic mechanism. However, this third injury category is not often distinguished in the epidemiologic literature on gymnastics injuries. Most studies in the gymnastics injury literature do not distinguish between acute and overuse injuries. However, this is an important oversight since risk factors for overuse and acute injuries may differ. Determination of activity or apparatus at the time of injury should be limited to acute injuries (O'Kane et al., 2011). The importance of identifying injury onset is also important given the growing evidence of overuse problems in gymnastics, particularly among child and adolescent gymnasts.

In gymnastics, where a high number of training hours are required for high-level performance, and where a number of high-risk skills are performed, it is expected that both overuse and acute injuries will occur. Studies reporting injury onset for female gymnasts indicate a range of 21.9–55.8% for overuse and 44.2–82.3% for acute injuries (Kolt & Caine, 2010; O'Kane et al., 2011). O'Kane et al. (2011) reported incidence rates of 1.8 and 1.3 injuries per 1000 hours for overuse and acute injuries, respectively.

Studies of male gymnasts also show a greater proportion of sudden versus gradual onset injuries (Kolt & Caine, 2010). The proportion of overuse versus acute injuries may vary according to anatomical location and competitive level with advanced-level gymnasts showing a higher proportion of overuse injuries in some studies.

The main injury study in Rhythmic Gymnastics to date (Cupisti et al., 2007) did not report the onset of injury as overuse or acute.

Timing of injury

Examples of timing of injury include time into practice, time of day, and time of season when injury occurs. It stands to reason that if rates are higher during a particular time, then efforts to better understand the risk factors for increased incidence are in order. For example, if the proportion or incidence rate of injuries is shown to be greater during the latter part of a training session or competition, or when the gymnast has been on an apparatus for an extended period of time, then fatigue and possible loss of concentration could be considered as possible contributing factors.

When examining timing of injury, both timing within a practice session and timing during a year-long season are important. Several studies have reported that the early part of a training session or competition is a period where a relatively high frequency of injury occurred (Kolt & Caine, 2010) suggesting insufficient warm-up.

Several studies have also followed the time into the season for injury occurrence in women's gymnastics. These findings indicate that injury rates can increase following periods of decreased training, during periods of practice of competitive routines, during weeks just prior to and during competition, and during competitive seasons (Kolt & Caine, 2010).

What is the outcome of injury?

As Figure 10.2 indicates, the next characteristic of injury distribution is injury outcome related to severity, or the "what" of injury occurrence. Injury severity can span a broad spectrum from abrasions to fractures, to those injuries that result in severe permanent functional disability (i.e., direct catastrophic injury). In the epidemiologic literature on sports injuries, injury severity is typically indicated by one or more of the following: injury type, time loss, need for medical treatment, and residual symptoms. Assessment in each of these areas is important to describe the extent of the injury problem. It may be, for example, that injury incidence is similar in two sports; however, the severity of injury may vary considerably between these sports.

Injury type

Identification of common injury types is important because it alerts sports medicine personnel to injury types in need of special attention and it directs researchers in identifying and testing related risk factors and preventive measures. Most gymnastics injury studies report injury types in general terms such as contusion or fracture, with few specifics on type of fracture, grade of injury, and so forth. Injury types are generally reported as percentage values. However, it would be preferable to report incidence rates for specific injury types, for example, anterior cruciate ligament (ACL) injuries, to better facilitate the analysis of risk factors and preventive measures.

Injury types in gymnastics have been categorized differently across studies, making comparison difficult. For example, some studies combine lower leg and ankle injuries, while others separate these injury types. A recent review of injury types in gymnastics (Kolt & Caine, 2010) indicates that sprains (15.9–43.6%) are the most common type of injury followed by strains (6.4–31.8%). Typically caused by inversion ankle injuries, ankle ligament sprains are the most common acute injuries in gymnastics (DiFiori & Caine, 2012). Other types of injuries that are common include contusions, fractures, and inflammatory conditions.

Although pain may not necessarily result in time loss and/or injury, pain among gymnasts is problematic and may affect performance. Many gymnasts continue training and competing with pain. For example, Caine and Nassar (2005) reported that injuries or conditions treated at the 2002–2004 USA Gymnastics National Women's Artistic Championships ranged from 27.6 to 80% of the junior and from 62.5 to 70% of senior gymnasts. Next to sprains (27.4%), the most common treatments were for overuse conditions (17.8%) and nonspecific pain (14.4%). Similarly, Harringe *et al.* (2004) noted that half of the team gymnasts (58%) in their study competed despite having symptoms from an injury on the day of competition.

Wrist pain is common among gymnasts of both sexes who train and compete at advanced skill levels. Prevalence estimates of wrist pain among these participants range from 46 to 79% (DiFiori & Caine, 2012). Chronic wrist pain in young gymnasts does not appear to be a transient phenomenon and may result in stress-related injury (e.g., stress changes to the distal radial physis). Prevalence studies also indicate that low back pain may

be common among artistic gymnasts; however, these data arise from cross-sectional studies published more than 20 years ago (Caine *et al.*, 1996). Radiological findings indicate the potential damaging effects of excessive mechanical loading on the immature spine of gymnasts including damage to the pars interarticularis resulting in spondylolyis or spondylolisthesis, discogenic pathology, and vertebral endplate abnormalities (Caine *et al.*, 1996). However, several researchers have suggested that anterior column spine problems, such as anterior vertebral endplate fractures, are becoming more common than posterior column spine problems (Caine & Nassar, 2005; Marshall *et al.*, 2007).

In prior literature, the frequency of head injuries and concussion is quite low, ranging from 0 to 0.7% among female artistic gymnasts (Caine & Nassar, 2005), and 2.3% of practice injuries and 2.6% of competition injuries among collegiate female gymnasts (Marshall *et al.*, 2007). However, in the most recent study published on Women's Artistic Gymnastics injuries (O'Kane *et al.*, 2011), the percentage of gymnasts reporting head injury was 8.8%, and a history of concussion ranged from 15.6 to 30.2% depending on the definition of concussion.

The data on injury types for male gymnasts are scanty, but indicate a similar distribution to that experienced by female artistic gymnasts.

For Rhythmic Gymnastics, only one study has reported injury type (Cupisti *et al.*, 2007). They found that, of the 46 injuries recorded, 26.1% were strains, 15.2% sprains, 17.4% contusions, 6.5% fractures, 2.2% dislocations, and 32.6% were classified as other. Injury types among competitive Trampoline Gymnastics (Grapton *et al.*, 2012) are mainly ligament sprains (44.2%) affecting the lower limb, followed by bone (31.9%) and muscular injuries (18.6%). The most frequently injured body parts were knee (19.9%), followed by the lower back (16.8%) and ankle (15.5%).

Time loss

A useful measure of injury severity used in the literature on gymnastics injuries is the duration of restriction from athletic performance subsequent to injury. Understanding the time lost to training or competition as a result of injury is important for coaches, sports medicine personnel, and participants. Not only does it provide an indication of the severity of injury, but also the impact that the injury has on overall training and competition programs. Most studies reporting time loss use days lost from practice or competition as a measure of injury severity. These time loss data are often categorized by time periods (e.g., 7 or less days) indicating degree of severity. Although the use of days lost from participation may be among the more precise representations of injury severity in the literature, this approach is not without problems. For example, subjective factors, such as personal motivation, peer influence, or coaching staff reluctance/encouragement, may determine if and when gymnasts return to practice or competition. Accessibility to a health care professional and location of injury may also impact decision of when to return to gymnastics. As noted previously, it is not uncommon for gymnasts to participate at competitions with chronic injury problems (Harringe et al., 2004; Caine & Nassar, 2005).

Gymnastics is a sport characterized by very little total time loss from full participation. That is, in the presence of most injuries, participants can continue to train in a modified manner or on apparatus or skills that do not impact on the injured body part. In many cases this is important as a method to maintain skill and fitness levels. Although most gymnastics injuries are relatively minor in terms of time loss, there is some research that indicates that particularly advanced level gymnasts may spend a substantial portion of their training at less that full practice (Kolt & Caine, 2010). For example, over 16 years, 39% of all women's intercollegiate competition injuries and 32% of all training injuries resulted in a time loss of 10 or more days (Marshall et al., 2007).

For competitive rhythmic gymnasts, Cupisti et al. (2007) found that for each injury sustained, 4.1 training sessions were missed and 32 were modified.

Need for medical treatment

There are few data published that provide an insight into the number of gymnasts who seek medical attention for injury and the cost of this treatment. As mentioned above, 27.6–80% of the junior and from 62.5 to 70% of senior gymnasts, respectively, were treated for pain or injury at the USA National Women's Artistic Championships between 2002 and 2004 (Caine & Nassar, 2005). During a 1-year injury surveillance of advanced club-level female gymnasts, 36 of 50 gymnasts consulted with a physician for 59 injuries (Caine et al., 1989).

Clinical outcome

Clinical outcome of injury includes such factors as recurrent injury, nonparticipation, and residual effects. An unfortunate outcome of many injuries, at all levels of sport, is recurrent injury. Gymnastics is a sport where participants experience recurrent injuries for several reasons including premature return to activity, inadequate rehabilitation, and underestimation of the severity of the primary injury. A gymnast with previous injury who returns to participation may be characterized by a changed injury risk profile, particularly if the original injury has not been properly rehabilitated. In studies of competitive female artistic gymnasts between 24.5 and 32.3% of all injuries were reinjuries (Kolt & Caine, 2010). No recent published data are available on rates of recurrent injury, nor are there any data available for male artistic gymnasts.

Another important but infrequently researched aspect of injury outcome relates to the frequency of season- or career-ending injuries (i.e., nonparticipation). An important question to address is how many gymnasts drop out of their sport, either temporarily or permanently due to injury. Data on season-ending injuries have been provided in only a few studies of young gymnasts. The types of injuries that were involved in decisions to drop out included ACL rupture, osteochondritis dissecans of the elbow, knee meniscus lesions (although these are now more easily managed with arthroscopic treatment), navicular stress fracture, chronic rotator cuff conditions, and injuries to the low back. Other studies that have examined the relationship between injury and dropping out of sport found that between 16.3 and 52.4% of those who dropped out of club-level gymnastics had an injury at the time of withdrawing from the sport (Kolt & Caine, 2010). Although this may suggest that injury played a role in the withdrawal, there are several other factors (e.g., age, transition to other sports, or loss of motivation or interest) that could have influenced this decision. Notably, O'Kane *et al.* (2011) reported that a little more than half of the gymnasts in their study played other sports.

Perhaps the most important question one can ask related to injury severity concerns residual or long-term effects of injury. Although engaging in physical activity has many health benefits, there is also risk of injury that may have long-term consequences on the musculoskeletal system resulting in reduced levels of physical activity or medical treatment. If residual symptoms are slight, they may cause the gymnast to modify his or her level of training. In some cases, however, functional limitations resulting from injury may preclude further participation in gymnastics or, following participation, result in reduced levels of activity secondary to residue from injury. For example, a link between acute knee or ankle injury and osteoarthritis is likely. Several studies found no differences between former gymnasts and control groups (nongymnasts) in back pain, but reported a higher prevalence in radiological changes (e.g., degenerative changes) in the gymnastic groups (Kolt & Caine, 2010).

In extreme cases, such as catastrophic injury, serious physical damage may result in permanent, severe functional disability such as quadriplegia. There is concern in gymnastics regarding catastrophic injury given the "high-risk" skills being trained and competed. The limited data on catastrophic injuries in gymnastics arise from case reports and series from the United Kingdom, China, the United States, Japan, and Germany (Kolt & Caine, 2010) and include those injuries suffered in Trampoline Gymnastics. Data arising from the National Center for Catastrophic Sports Injury Research (http://www.unc.edu/depts/nccsi/; accessed on February 22, 2013), which has tracked catastrophic injuries in high school and college settings since 1982, indicate a total of 20 direct catastrophic injuries that occurred among high school ($n = 13$) and college ($n = 7$) gymnasts during 1982–2011. Catastrophic injury rates (per 100,000 participants) were relatively high in gymnastics compared to other sports. In contrast, data arising from multiple cohort studies of club-level

and recreational gymnasts indicate no catastrophic injuries (Kolt & Caine, 2010).

The Cupisti *et al.* (2007) study of Rhythmic Gymnastics did not identify any catastrophic injuries.

Analytical epidemiology

Analysis of gymnastics injury risk factors has produced a number of significant injury predictors—including such factors as age, competition, periods of rapid growth, previous injury, and stressful life events—which have shown consistent results across multiple studies. However, much of the analytical literature suffers from one or more of the following limitations: injury definitions and methods of injury data collection that are extremely variable, incidence rates based on clinical incidence rather than incidence rates (i.e., rates based on hours or sessions of exposure) are often used to distinguish high-risk athletes, failure to account for the different categories of injury onset, and inappropriate analyses for detecting multifactorial risks. As a result, much of the risk factor research should be viewed as initial work in the important search for injury predictors and that may provide interesting variables for manipulation in other study designs.

Injury risk factors

For injury intervention and rehabilitation programs to be effective, an in-depth knowledge of injury risk factors is paramount. This is particularly so given that gymnastics is a sport with relatively high injury rates. Risk factors may be classified as intrinsic or extrinsic. Intrinsic factors are individual biological and psychosocial characteristics predisposing a person to the outcome of injury such as previous injury, strength, or life stress. Extrinsic (or enabling) risk factors are factors that have an impact on the gymnast "from without" and include such factors as coach's qualifications, training time, and level of competition. Intrinsic and extrinsic risk factors may interact to increase the risk of injury.

Risk factors can also be divided into modifiable and nonmodifiable factors. Modifiable risk factors refer to those that can be altered by injury prevention strategies to reduce injury rates. Although non-modifiable risk factors such as gender or age may be important considerations in many studies of injury prediction and should be accounted for in statistical analyses, it is above all important to study factors that are potentially modifiable. What complicates the identification and quantification of risks is that causality associated with injury is both extremely complex and dynamic in nature. Willem Meeuwisse *et al.* (2007) proposed a dynamic recursive model that accommodates a multifactorial assessment of causation in athletic injuries and emphasizes the fact that adaptations occur within the context of repeated participation in sport (both in the presence and absence of injury) that alter risk and affect etiology in a dynamic, recursive fashion (see Figure 10.3). In this model, intrinsic factors are viewed as factors that predispose the athlete to react in a specific manner to an injury situation. However, what is important to understand is that intrinsic factors are not constant and may change in response to injury or to absence

of injury (i.e., adaptive changes such as increased intrinsic strength).

Once the athlete is predisposed, extrinsic or "enabling" factors such as faulty equipment or coaching behavior may facilitate manifestation of injury. According to the dynamic recursive model extrinsic risk factors, like intrinsic risk factors, are also subject to change in the context of repeated participation in sport. For example, rule changes or equipment may result in risk modification, thus changing susceptibility to injury.

Intrinsic factors

Some studies showed that body size (height and weight), age, and body fat were all greater in injured or high-injury-risk gymnasts (Kolt & Caine, 2010; DiFiori & Caine, 2012). However, it is possible in these studies that factors such as greater height and weight characterize older gymnasts who are competing at higher levels of competition. Some research also indicates that a rapid period

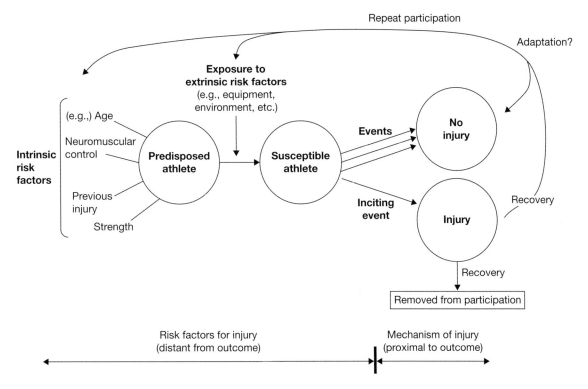

Figure 10.3 Recursive model of etiology of sport injury. (Source: Meeuwisse *et al.* (2007)).

of growth and previous injury are associated with increased risk of injury (Kolt & Caine, 2010; DiFiori & Caine, 2012). An interesting but underresearched area of injury risk in gymnastics is the role that psychosocial factors play. Increased levels of life stress were associated with the number of and severity of injury in some research (Kolt & Caine, 2010; DiFiori & Caine, 2012). The retrospective nature of some of these studies, however, means that the direction of the relationship between life stress and injury cannot be accurately determined.

Extrinsic factors

There is some evidence that advanced club-level gymnasts are at increased risk of injury compared to their beginning level counterparts, especially in competition, and that intercollegiate competition injury rates were higher in those competing in higher level versus lower level divisions (Kolt & Caine, 2010). One would expect injury rates to increase with higher levels of competition because advanced-level gymnasts have more years training since competitive initiation and the technical difficulty of the skills they perform is also greater (Caine *et al.*, 1996).

Inciting events

Very few studies provide information on the action or activity leading to injury in gymnastics. Existing research indicates that a majority of injuries occur during landings in floor exercise or when dismounting from other apparatus. Contact with floor, mat, or equipment is also related to injuries in practice and competition (Kolt & Caine, 2010; O'Kane *et al.*, 2011). In women's intercollegiate gymnastics the majority of competition injuries (70.7%) resulted from other contact, primarily during landings. This category was also the leading mechanism for practice injuries (Marshall *et al.*, 2007).

Further research

Although we have learned a great deal from epidemiological studies of injury affecting gymnasts, there remain many unanswered questions and areas of needed research. We list below what we feel to be the most important areas for further research:

• Above all, this overview of the gymnastics injury literature underscores the need to establish national and international ISS's designed to provide current and reliable data on injury trends in boys and girls club-level gymnastics.

• An international guideline with respect to grading of different levels of gymnastics would provide a possibility to compare studies at international levels.

• There is a pressing need for a FIG consensus statement that identifies injury definitions and research methodology to ensure consistency and comparability of results in epidemiological studies examining injury in gymnastics.

• Further work on injury in relation to exposure time data is required. To date, only a few studies have looked at injury in light of the amount of time gymnasts actually spend in preparation and competition.

• With significant changes in gymnastics over the past 10–15 years (including equipment changes and rule changes), injury data on current day gymnasts are required. In this regard, nationally organized injury surveillance programs are needed.

• Research on injury in male gymnasts is clearly lacking and needs attention. This should specifically include descriptive and analytic risk factor studies.

• Research on injury in Rhythmic Gymnastics is also clearly lacking and needs attention. With very different physical demands in Artistic Gymnastics, relying on generalization of findings across disciplines is not advised. Both descriptive and risk factor studies are required.

• There is a paucity of research specifically on Trampoline Gymnastics. As this discipline becomes more popular, research findings will be required to help guide training and injury prevention and rehabilitation. Future research on Trampoline Gymnastics should include descriptive and risk factor studies.

• Further research is required on the cost and extent of surgery procedures required, which relate to gymnastics injury as well as the residual effects of injuries later in life. With many gymnastics injuries being long-term or chronic in nature, it is important to ascertain the longer term effects of such events.

• More accurate research on risk factors of injury in gymnastics is needed. This research should be done prospectively and should encompass modifiable risk factors that could be developed into injury prevention strategies. Risk factors of particular interest include injury history, pain history, coaching qualifications, periods of rapid growth, and psychosocial factors.

• As most of the research to date has relied on self-report of injury, medical evaluation of injury is required to more accurately categorize and diagnose injuries.

• As many as one-third of all injuries sustained by gymnasts may be recurrent injuries signaling the need for improved rehabilitation prior to return to training.

It is important to emphasize that it is only through concerted collaborative efforts that optimal results can be achieved. The research team should include the coach, athletic trainer, physician, and epidemiologist who interact in a very dynamic and fluid manner.

Summary

Much of the existing epidemiologic literature on injury in gymnastics deals with female artistic gymnasts, with only a few cohort studies addressing male gymnasts, rhythmic gymnasts, and trampoline gymnasts. Comparison of results across studies was compromised due to methodological limitations, and the absence of national and international ISS's. Nonetheless, the following generalizations arise from the extant literature on the epidemiology of injury in Artistic Gymnastics:

• Injury rates among artistic gymnasts are relatively high compared to those reported for other sports.

• The most commonly injured body region for both male and female gymnasts is the lower extremity likely reflecting the high proportion of injuries associated with landings and dismounts. In particular, the knee, ankle, and lower back are the most commonly injured anatomical locations.

• Although there tends to be a greater proportion of acute injuries, overuse injuries appear to be increasingly common at advanced levels of training and competition.

• The findings of some studies indicate that the frequency of injury is relatively high during the early part of training and competition suggesting insufficient warm-up.

• Studies also indicate increased injury rates following periods of decreased training, during periods of practice of competitive routines, during weeks just prior to and during competition, and during competitive seasons.

• Although most injuries are relatively minor in gymnastics, the severity of injury appears to be high among advanced level gymnasts.

• Catastrophic injuries appear to be an infrequent occurrence in gymnastics; however, the clinical incidence at the collegiate level appears to be relatively high compared to other sports.

• Preliminary analysis of risk factors suggests that the following may be associated with increased risk of injury among gymnasts: periods of rapid growth, history of previous injury, excessive life stress, and advanced levels of training and competition.

Given the life-changing impact injury can have on gymnasts, both in the short- and long-term, the current paucity of well-designed epidemiological studies of all forms of Olympic gymnastics injuries is disturbing. The importance of establishing denominator-based injury surveillance in obtaining an accurate picture of injury risk and severity and as a basis for testing risk factors cannot be overemphasized. We feel that there is an ethical imperative for gymnastics governing bodies, both nationally and internationally, to provide incentive and guidance for epidemiological research in all forms of Olympic gymnastics.

References

Caine, D., Caine, C., and Maffulli, N. (2006) Incidence and distribution of pediatric sport-related injuries. *Clinical Journal of Sport Medicine*, **16** (6), 501–514.

Caine, D., Cochrane, B., Caine, C., and Zemper, E. (1989) An epidemiologic investigation of injuries affecting young competitive female gymnasts. *The American Journal of Sports Medicine*, **17**, 811–820.

Caine, D. and Nassar, L. (2005) Gymnastics injuries. In: *Epidemiology of Pediatric Sports Injuries. Part 1. Individual Sports*, vol. 48, pp. 17–58. Karger Publishers, Basel, Switzerland.

Cupisti, A., D'Alessandro, C., Evangelisti, I., Piazza, M., Galetta, F., and Morelli, E. (2004) Low back pain in competitive rhythmic gymnasts. *Journal of Sports Medicine and Physical Fitness*, **44**, 49–53.

Cupisti, A., D'Alessandro, C., Evangelisti, I., Unbri, C., Rossi, M., Galetta, F., Panicucci, E., Lopes Pegna, S., and Piazza, M. (2007) Injury survey in competitive sub-elite rhythmic gymnasts: results from a prospective controlled study. *Journal of Sports Medicine and Physical Fitness*, **47**, 203–207.

DiFiori, J.P. and Caine, D.J. (2012) Gymnastics. In: F.G. O'Conner, D.J. Casa, B.A. Davis, P. St Pierre, R.E. Sallis, and R.P. Wilder (eds), *ACSM's Sports Medicine: Comprehensive Review*, pp. 649–656. McGraw-Hill Publishers.

Grapton, X., Lion, A., Gauchard, G.C., Barrault, D., and Perrin, P.P. (2012) Specific injuries induced by the practice of trampoline, tumbling and acrobatic gymnastics. Knee surgery, sports traumatology and arthroscopy. doi: 10.1007/s00167-012-1982-x.

Harringe, M.L., Lindblad, S., and Werner, S. (2004) Do team gymnasts compete in spite of symptoms from an injury? *British Journal of Sports Medicine*, **38**, 398–401.

Hootman, J.M., Dick, R., and Agel, J. (2007) Epidemiology of collegiate injury for 15 sports: summary and recommendations for injury prevention initiatives. *Journal of Athletic Training*, **42**, 311–319.

Knowles, S.B., Marshall, S.W., and Guskiewicz, K.M. (2006) Issues in estimating risks and rates in sports injury research. *Journal of Athletic Training*, **41**, 207–215.

Kolt, G. and Caine, D. (2010) Gymnastics. In: D. Caine, P. Harmer, and M. Schiff (eds), *Epidemiology of Injury in Olympic Sports*. International Olympic Committee, vol. XVI, pp. 144–160. Wiley-Blackwell, Oxford.

Marshall, S.W., Covassin, T. and Dick, R. (2007) Descriptive epidemiology of collegiate women's gymnastics injuries: National Collegiate Athletic Association Injury Surveillance System, 1988–1989 through 2003–2004. *Journal of Athletic Training*, **42**, 234–240.

Meeuwisse, W., Tyreman, H., Hagel, B., and Emery, C. (2007) A dynamic, recursive model of etiology in sport injury: the recursive nature of risk and causation. *Clinical Journal of Sport Medicine*, **17**, 215–219.

O'Kane, J., Levy, M.R., Pietila, K., Caine, D., and Schiff, M.A. (2011) Survey of injuries in Seattle area level 4–10 gymnastics clubs. *Clinical Journal of Sport Medicine*, **21**, 486–92.

van Mechelen, W., Hlobil, H., and Kemper, H.C. (1992) Incidence, severity, aetiology and prevention of sports injuries. A review of concepts. *Sports Medicine*, **14**, 82–99.

Recommended reading

Bahr, R. and Engebretsen, L. (2009) *Sports Injury Prevention. The International Olympic Committee Handbook of Sports Medicine and Science*, Wiley-Blackwell Publishers, Oxford.

Caine, D. (2003) Injury epidemiology. In: W. Sands, D. Caine, and J. Borms (eds), *Scientific Aspects of Women's Gymnastics. Sports Science and Medicine Series*, vol. 45. Basel Karger Publishers, Switzerland.

Caine, D., Lindner, K., Mandelbaum, B., and Sands, W. (1996) Gymnastics. In: C. Caine, D. Caine, and K. Lindner (eds), *Epidemiology of Sports Injuries*, pp. 213–246. Human Kinetics, Champaign, IL .

Emery, C.A. (2010) Injury prevention in paediatric sport-related injuries: a scientific approach. *British Journal of Sports Medicine*, **44**, 64–69.

Mueller, F. and Cantu, R. (2011) National Center for Catastrophic Sports Injury Research. 29th Annual Report Fall 1982 – Spring 2011. URL http://www.unc.edu/depts/nccsi/2011Allsport.pdf [accessed on February 22, 2013].

Rivera, FP., Cummings, P., Koepsell, T.D., Grossman, D.C., and Maier, R.V. (eds) (2001) *Injury Control: A Guide to Research and Program Evaluation*. Cambridge University Press, Cambridge.

Verhagen, E. and van Mechelen, W. (2010) *Sports Injury Research*. Oxford University Press, Oxford.

Chapter 11
Treatment and rehabilitation of common upper extremity injuries

Stephen Aldridge[1,2], W. Jaap Willems[3]

[1]Royal Victoria Infirmary *and* Newcastle University, Newcastle Upon Tyne, UK
[2]British Gymnastics, Newport, UK
[3]Onze Lieve Vrouwe Gasthuis/de Lairesse Kliniek, Amsterdam, The Netherlands

Introduction

Gymnasts have complex and unique functional demands of their upper limbs. Few other activities have similar requirements. Not only do apparatus, such as beam, pommel horse, and parallel bars, require that the full body weight is supported by the arms, but furthermore the gymnast lands repetitively on the hands, and takes off again whilst tumbling, and on vault and floor. These activities put enormous strain through a limb, which is not normally required to undertake these forces. The arm is also required to maintain extreme strength for activities on the rings, without losing any of the flexibility without which many activities for gymnasts would be impossible, such as swinging on the high, uneven or parallel bars. To complicate things further these activities are all honed during the gymnasts growing years, before skeletal maturity, when damage to growth plates can occur. All of these factors together leave gymnasts at risk of developing upper limb problems. Problems, which are minor for most people, can be debilitating for gymnasts. This requires that medical personnel understand the rigors of the sport, and that despite normal examination there may be an underlying cause of functional impediment for high-level performance. Also, gymnasts may have

a range of movement outside normal levels with marked increased laxity, which is normal for them, and does not imply a pathological instability.

Gymnastic injuries can be defined as acute or as chronic. Acute injuries are sustained at a specific event, such as fractures and dislocations, more than 40% of which affect the upper limb (Singh *et al.*, 2008). Chronic injuries are longstanding and develop either through overuse, or as a consequence of an acute injury, such as shoulder instability or osteochondral defects.

Acute injuries

Fractures

Fractures are a common injury, which can frequently be treated with good results without needing operations. It is beyond the scope of this book to describe the best treatment for individual fractures, but the principle of treatment of all fractures is the same:

- Reduction into an acceptable position.
- Immobilization by plaster, internal fixation (plate, screws, or nails), or external fixation (rare in the upper limb).
- Rehabilitation.

In general terms, displaced fractures, open fractures, unstable fractures, and those with vascular injuries require surgery to avoid long-term functional deficits. There may be an argument made for surgery to allow earlier return to activities, and this

Gymnastics, First Edition. Edited by Dennis J. Caine, Keith Russell and Liesbeth Lim. © 2013 International Olympic Committee. Published 2013 by John Wiley & Sons, Ltd.

may be more common in elite gymnasts to allow continued training. This is a relative indication for surgery, and needs in-depth discussion with an orthopedic surgeon to make a good judgment, as there are risks to operating, which may delay return to training.

As a sport, gymnastics puts the body at risk from fractures due to falls from height, and twisting injuries, but the wrist and forearm are at risk from accidents with the dowel grip of the wrist guards on bars, which can lock causing a hyperflexion injury of the wrist, which can result in fracture and extensor tendon rupture. This should be avoided with proper fitting and maintenance.

Fractures occurring to the hand and fingers are common, and the treatment whether surgical or nonoperative needs to allow early mobilization of the fingers to avoid long-term stiffness and tethering of the tendons.

Most forearm and clavicle fractures take 4–6 weeks to heal, and humeral fractures double this time. It is important to maintain core stability and lower limb conditioning during this time, and, if allowed, to maintain range of motion (ROM) of other joints of the chain, to prepare for return to training.

Dislocations

The most common dislocations of the upper limb are of the acromioclavicular joint (ACJ), shoulder, and the elbow. All typically occur after a fall. The diagnosis is often obvious due to the deformity, pain, and inability to move the affected part.

ACJ dislocations (also known as shoulder separations) occur after a fall onto the point of the shoulder (Figure 11.1). Dislocations are graded by the severity of the stabilizing structures affected. Treatment of low-grade injuries (with minimal soft tissue injury) consists of rest and rehabilitation, the duration of which depends on severity, and the return to sport is guided by loss of local tenderness and a pain-free range of movement. Extreme dislocations with incarceration of the clavicle in surrounding tissues require surgical correction, but there is controversy about requirement for surgery for completely displaced disruptions, which are not incarcerated.

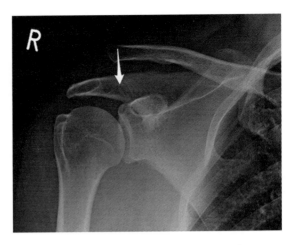

Figure 11.1 Plain radiograph of acromioclavicular joint (ACJ) dislocation. The white arrow denotes the position the lateral clavicle ought to line up with against the acromion.

Glenohumeral joint dislocation is a common sports injury, which occurs most frequently from indirect trauma with the shoulder forced into abduction and external rotation, causing an anterior dislocation. It can however occur as a direct injury by landing on the humeral head, and in any direction. The initial treatment requires reduction of the dislocation as quickly as possible by a competently trained practitioner. Ideally, a prereduction radiograph should be taken to exclude any associated fracture, and the limb should be examined for any neurovascular injury, particularly to exclude an axillary nerve injury. Once the shoulder is reduced it should be immobilized in a sling for 3–4 weeks following a rehabilitation program, progressing from initial isometric cuff strengthening whilst immobilized to external rotation and active movement, avoiding abduction and external rotation for 6 weeks. Young athletes have a high recurrence rate after dislocation and often suffer with instability symptoms. As a result, arthroscopy and stabilization should be considered following a dislocation to reduce these risks from 60% recurrence rate to 5% at 2 years (Brophy & Marx, 2009). Consideration should also be given to the possibility of reduced range of movement following stabilization, particularly in open stabilization. Rehabilitation following surgery is likely to take at least 6 months.

Elbow dislocation occurs predominantly posteriorly as a result of hyperextension of the loaded elbow, and often happens during tumbling or on the vault, but female gymnasts are also at risk on the uneven bars when falling on the outstretched arm during flight skills or changing from the low to high rail. It can be a simple dislocation, but often has an associated fracture, commonly the coronoid process or medial epicondyle apophysis, which can become incarcerated during reduction. It can be associated with both nerve and vessel injury and the distal pulse should be assessed. Once reduced, a radiograph should be taken to exclude any associated fractures. Small coronoid fractures and undisplaced radial head fractures can often be treated conservatively with a sling for comfort, but the aim of all treatment following any elbow injury should be early mobilization, as the most debilitating sequelae is stiffness, which is difficult to treat. If the elbow is unstable after reduction, due to bony or ligamentous injury, surgery should be preferred to any kind of immobilization (Athwal *et al.*, 2011).

The interphalangeal joints of the hand can dislocate, if hyperextended after falling, and can be treated with reduction, followed by radiographic assessment for fracture and subsequent protected mobilization. The thumb metacarpophalangeal joint can be injured leading to rupture of the ulnar collateral ligament if the thumb is forced into hyperabduction in activities such as landing on the parallel bars after flight moves. This will require surgical treatment.

Landing on the outstretched hand on any apparatus puts the bones and joints of the carpus at risk of scapholunate dissociation, which presents with obvious deformity of the hand, gross swelling, and requires urgent surgical treatment to restore the anatomy.

Chronic injuries

Growth-related problems

As gymnastics is a sport which is developed during skeletal maturation, and requiring long hours of repetitive training, there is a significant load placed on the growing structures which can be related to chronic problems.

Traction apophysitis

As in the lower limb, but less commonly, repetitive traction on the growing parts of the skeleton, by ligament strain and tendon pull, particularly during times of increased growth, can lead to inflammatory changes, resulting in pain. These most frequently affect the elbow, particularly the medial epicondyle, but occasionally the olecranon. As with other apophysitides, the treatment is conservative with ice, compression, anti-inflammatory medication, and activity modification, whilst addressing flexibility and strengthening as required.

Distal radius physeal stress fracture (gymnast's wrist)

This condition is mainly seen in females 12–14 years of age with a training routine exceeding 35 hours per week. The condition may be considered at three stages: stage 1 = pre-radiographic, stage 2 = radial physeal radiographic changes, and stage 3 = stage 2 with secondary ulnar positive variance (Figure 11.2).

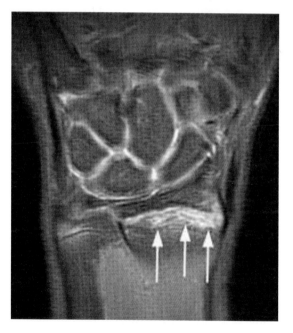

Figure 11.2 MRI scan of distal radial physeal stress fracture. Note the high signal in the physeal area (arrows).

In stage 1, diagnosis is made on clinical grounds, and gradual return to activities may be possible in 2–4 weeks. In stage 2, X-ray findings of physeal widening and cystic changes exist, and return is prolonged to 2–4 months. In stage 3, concern for ulnar abutment symptoms and subsequent symptoms apply. No correlation between MRI findings and stages of healing has been found; thus, it is not useful as a prognostic tool.

Early closure of radial physis

Experiments have shown that in a wrist with the arm in neutral rotation 80% of the load is transferred though the radius and 20% though the ulna (Albanese *et al.*, 1989). Forearm supination produces a relative negative ulnar variance, forearm pronation produces a relative positive ulnar variance. A wrist loaded with the forearm in supination produces an increase of load transmitted through the radius. Increased load through the radius may lead to excessive forces resulting in early closure of the physis of the distal radius.

Osteochondritis dissecans

Osteochondritis dissecans (OCD) of the elbow is an idiopathic, localized disorder of the subchondral bone resulting in separation and fragmentation of the articular surface and underlying bone. The first description was by König in 1887, where he thought it was caused by an inflammatory reaction of the cartilage (Edmonds & Polousky, 2013). At present no formal etiology is known, but inflammation does not play a role in the pathogenesis.

It is an increasing cause of elbow pain and dysfunction in the competitive adolescent athlete and can lead to clicking and pseudolocking. It mostly affects the young adolescent athlete involved in high-demand, repetitive overhead, or weight-bearing activities, for example, young male baseball players and female gymnasts.

It should not be confused with Panner's disease (osteonecrosis of the capitellum), which occurs in mainly male patients younger than 10 years. It may however be the same process with a different course and prognosis.

The process has best been described for throwing athletes. During the late cocking and early acceleration phases of throwing, the elbow is subjected to high valgus stress with distraction forces applied to the medial aspect of the elbow and significant compression and shear forces to the lateral radiocapitellar joint. The extreme, repetitive axial loads in young gymnasts with a frequently increased physiological valgus lead to comparative high loads in these athletes. Repeated radiocapitellar compression on the immature epiphysis from repetitive valgus strain leads to subchondral fatigue fracture. Continued compressive stress leads to ultimate breakdown and fragmentation of the overlying articular cartilage and subchondral bone.

When the subchondral fracture leads to displacement, a subsequent fracture of the overlying cartilage leads to detachment of the fragments resulting in loose bodies.

A subsequent vascular injury to the bone, with a tenuous vascular supply with one or two end vessels to the capitellum may add to the further collapse of the involved part of the capitellum.

Patients complain of pain, first during activities and subsequently during rest. Physical examination sometimes reveals a mild effusion and pain on palpation of the capitellum. Rarely, instability of the collateral ligaments is seen. When an effusion is present there is often limitation of extension.

Radiographic modalities

The classic early findings of capitellar rarefaction, radiolucency, or flattening of the articular surface can be seen on plain radiographs. The typical lesion is located on the anterolateral aspect of the capitellum. Fragmentation with demarcating sclerosis and formation of loose bodies are seen with more advanced lesions. Late findings include radial head enlargement and osteophyte formation.

While X-rays are not very sensitive, especially in determining the type of treatment advised, often MRI is added. MRI shows bone changes earlier than a plain X-ray and supplies information about the state of the articular cartilage, vascularity of the fragment (when intravenous gadolinium is used), and stability of the fragment (with the use of intraarticular gadolinium) (Figure 11.3).

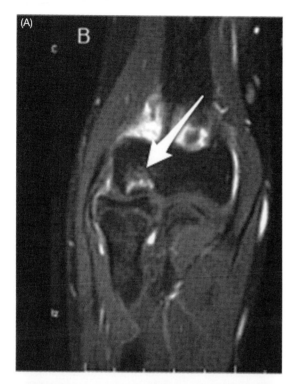

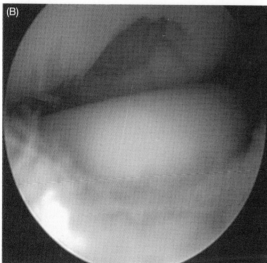

Figure 11.3 Osteochondritis dissecans (OCD) of the elbow. **(A)** MRI scan. See high signal around the capitellum (arrow). **(B)** Arthroscopy of defect after excision of loose OCD fragment.

The indications for conservative treatment are radiographic findings of subchondral flattening or radiolucency, a stable fragment as diagnosed with MRI with an open physis of the capitellum. This treatment includes immediate cessation of repetitive stress and, when the ROM is normal, exercises of the elbow. Regular X-rays and MRIs are performed at 6–12 weeks intervals. It typically takes 6 months to confirm healing.

When the fragment is unstable on MRI, or the physis is closed or a loose body is seen on the radiograph, surgery is performed. Most of the procedures can be performed arthroscopically, which enables a full inspection of the joint and leads to a faster rehabilitation. Several arthroscopic treatments are described, and there is no evidence currently for the best treatment. Generally the following guidelines can be used:

- *The fragment is still present and the overlying cartilage intact:* Either retrograde drilling, using a guide or transchondral drilling can be performed to enhance the vascularity of the bone fragment. Follow-up studies with X-ray or MRI can monitor the healing of the defect.
- *The fragment is present but unstable:* Fixation with screws, small bone pegs, or other devices can be performed.
- *If the fragment becomes detached to form a loose body:* The fragment can be removed and the lesion, either treated by drilling or curretting. It is hardly ever possible to replace the loose fragment in the defect.

Alternatively, an osteochondral graft, either from the knee or the rib can be transplanted in the defect. The prognosis of these grafts is not guaranteed and rehabilitation will take more time. Autologous chondrocyte transplantation can be considered, although little data is available on its efficacy for treatment of OCD of the elbow.

OCD of the elbow is not infrequent in young athletes with repetitive loads on the elbow. When diagnosed early and with proper conservative treatment, the athlete can usually resume their activities at the same level. Once surgery is needed, and whatever surgery is performed, the chances of regaining full activities are reduced. Newer techniques hopefully will lead to a better prognosis for the treatment of this disease (de Graaff *et al.*, 2011).

Other common injuries

Shoulder

Shoulder problems often present with pain, which often get labeled with the diagnosis of impingement. Impingement is a clinical sign, rather than a diagnosis, which is caused by irritation of the rotator cuff tendons being impinged upon by unforgiving structures in the subacromial space above (external) or the glenohumeral joint below (internal).

External impingement is divided into primary causes, which are due to outlet obstruction in the subacromial space, and secondary causes, which are due to rotator cuff dysfunction frequently found in conjunction with instability (due to cuff imbalance). Internal impingement is caused by glenohumeral joint instability, such that the cuff insertion gets trapped between the glenoid and the humeral head. This can then lead to pain inhibition compounding the problem by causing cuff imbalance. In gymnasts primary external impingement is rare, as this typically comes on as a degenerative process. Thus, gymnasts presenting with impingement need to have instability and cuff tendinopathy excluded as the underlying cause.

Rotator cuff pathology

The rotator cuff is a group of muscles deep to the deltoid, consisting of subscapularis, supraspinatus, infraspinatus, and teres minor. Together these muscles control the rotation of the shoulder and give control and stability to the glenohumeral joint, where the deltoid provides power. The rotator cuff is susceptible to problems if large loads are put on it as a result of altered biomechanics. Gymnastics is a sport that has a heavy demand of the rotator cuff and the muscles can be worked asymmetrically leading to imbalance of power, which is difficult to address with conditioning exercises. For example, many of the exercises in gymnastics require strength of internal rotation, which if not balanced by training of the external rotators can lead to the humeral head being loaded in internal rotation, which can cause both external (due to reduced subacromial space) and internal impingement (due to relative instability).

Superimposed on this impingement is the strength requirement of the disciplines and loading of the joint due to upper limb weight bearing, whilst the cuff tendons are trapped leading to damage not only from physical injury but also ischaemic injury as the blood vessels to the tendons are compressed.

If this continues, the pathology becomes chronic, which is common as the athlete continues to train "through the pain," and tendinopathy develops, which further exacerbates the imbalance.

Classically, tendinopathy presents as an insidious onset of pain, particularly with certain overhead activities and pain on strength moves of the shoulder. Plain radiographs are frequently normal, but may show some subtle abnormalities of instability, or subacromial changes, and as such are a simple screening tool. Ultrasound scans are operator dependent, and are useful for extraarticular abnormalities, but can miss deep pathology. MRI scanning shows both intra- and extraarticular abnormalities, and with contrast arthrography discovers most pathology.

Rotator cuff tears can occur acutely, after trauma or dislocation, or can develop as the end stage of the tendinopathy process. Acute tears should be picked up by examination of the affected muscle being weak after dislocation or a forced movement during muscle contraction. Chronic tears often present with insidious pain, and weakness may not be apparent as it is considered to be due to the pain. The gymnast will often maintain movement, but certain activities with the arm in abduction become difficult, until eventually they are not possible. This most frequently affects the supraspinatus muscle, but the subscapularis can also be torn, as can the infraspinatus as an extension of the supraspinatus tears.

The treatment of rotator cuff disease should ideally commence with prevention, through good conditioning, and attention to the groups of muscles, which are frequently ignored during training to maintain the balance within the rotator cuff. As the disease process develops into tendinopathy, the treatment should continue with rehabilitation to attain a stable shoulder throughout its range of movement, through stretching any tight capsule and muscle groups, and strengthening any weak groups. This treatment should be developed in conjunction with an experienced physiotherapist.

For rotator cuff tears the only solution in high-demand gymnasts is early intervention with surgical repair, to reduce the risks of propagation of the tear, and subsequent long-term disability with a view to return to pre-injury level.

Shoulder instability

Shoulder instability is a spectrum of disease ranging from recurrent dislocations, through subluxation (partial dislocation with spontaneous reduction), with a feeling of instability, to pain on certain activities typically in abduction and external rotation. The glenohumeral joint is an intrinsically unstable joint. The bony morphology is more like a golf ball set on a golf tee, than a true ball and socket joint like the hip. The humeral head maintains its position in the glenoid through a range of mechanisms both static (bony morphology, labrum, capsulolabral complex) and dynamic (rotator cuff). Both the static and dynamic stabilizers are interconnected through the proprioceptive responses generated by the movements within the shoulder. For example, as the shoulder moves into external rotation the anterior glenohumeral ligaments tighten, acting as a passive limiter ("checkrein") to further external rotation, but also send a neuronal signal to initiate contraction of the internal rotator subscapularis to stop further rotation. Without this, excessive external rotation may result in anterior translation and eventually dislocation of the humeral head.

Pathological processes, which affect any of the stabilizing mechanisms, can lead to instability of the shoulder. Instability can develop acutely as a result of dislocation (traumatic instability), or can develop in individuals who are susceptible to instability (atraumatic instability). Gymnasts require highly mobile joints, to undertake their disciplines, with a joint capsule and ligament complex that tend to be less tight than in the general population, leaving them at risk of atraumatic instability.

Traumatic dislocations tend to have more obvious underlying abnormalities, such as bony or capsulolabral defects. Those with atraumatic instability can be separated into those with and without structural abnormalities, which may be amenable to surgery. The treatment must be tailored to the individual based on pathology and symptoms.

Clinically the patient describes the shoulder dislocating or coming in and out of the joint. This is also associated with pain and apprehension doing certain activities, typically above shoulder height particularly in abduction and external rotation, although multidirectional instability may describe a feeling of looseness in many positions. Examination should reveal the direction of instability, anterior, posterior, or multidirectional, to aid further investigation. The mainstay of investigations will be through MRI or CT arthrogram, which should identify bony defects on the glenoid and humeral head, labral detachments, capsular abnormalities, and ligament injuries (Figure 11.4).

In general terms, treatment of atraumatic multidirectional instability, where no structural

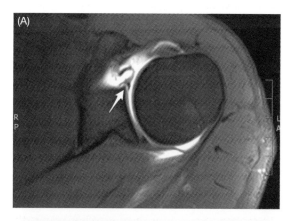

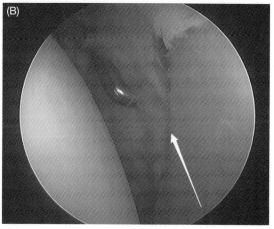

Figure 11.4 (A) Magnetic resonance arthrogram of shoulder with anterior labral tear. **(B)** Anterior labral tear as seen at arthroscopy.

abnormality has been identified, should begin with intensive physiotherapy, to develop better gleno-humeral joint control. This is achieved by improving proprioception and a course of strengthening to develop improved balance of the rotator cuff muscles, and retraining of any abnormal muscle patterning. If this is unsuccessful then there are surgical options to address generalized capsular laxity, but there is a risk of overtightening the capsule limiting the range of movement, with overall worse outcomes as compared to surgical treatment of anterior stabilization (Gaskill *et al.*, 2011).

For patients with structural abnormalities, the treatment should be to address the underlying abnormality. This is most likely to be through surgical treatment. There is debate over open or arthroscopic treatment for these conditions, and surgeon preference and experience will decide this. The benefits of arthroscopic treatment are of faster recovery and better maintenance of range of movement, but there is a slightly higher recurrence rate in certain groups such as contact sportspeople.

Long head of biceps/SLAP tears

The long head of biceps (LHB) is a tendon, which is partly intraarticular, from its origin at the superior labral complex of the glenoid, and partly extraarticular where it runs into the intertubercular groove of the humerus and develops into the biceps muscle. Its exact function is unknown, but may work as a humeral stabilizer, particularly in abduction to reduce external rotation. It can cause problems from its insertion to the superior labrum. Also, the tendon itself can become too mobile, subluxing either anteriorly or posteriorly, causing pain, and a sensation of locking, and can wear both the tendon substance or the humeral articular surface, often in association with rotator cuff pathology.

Superior labrum anterior posterior (SLAP) tears come about due to the attachment of the biceps peeling off the bony attachment along with its labral attachment (Figure 11.5). This can happen when doing a heavy lift, rotating the loaded shoulder (e.g., on the rings), or in a fall. SLAP tears often cause pain, weakness with movement into abduction and internal rotation, causing loading of the biceps anchor. There are different types of SLAP tear,

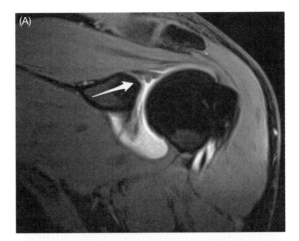

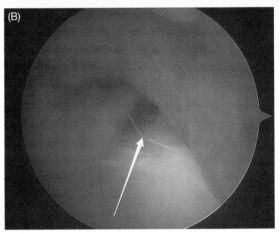

Figure 11.5 (A) Magnetic resonance arthrogram of superior labrum anterior posterior (SLAP) tear. **(B)** SLAP tear as seen at arthroscopy (arrow indicates labral tear).

and may be isolated or associated with anterior labral tears in instability. The severity ranges from fraying of the labrum, to a labral tear (stable or unstable), to a tear extending into the biceps anchor and tendon. The treatment of these conditions depends on the severity of symptoms and the underlying pathology, ranging from conservative with posterior capsular stretching, but often requires surgical repair.

Abnormalities of the LHB are commonly degenerative and develop insidiously with time. If an injury occurs, it probably exacerbates an asymptomatic problem. With time, biceps tendinopathy can eventually lead to rupture of the biceps tendon, which may alleviate the symptoms of pain, but often leads to bulging of the distal biceps muscle ("Popeye" deformity), and probably reduces the power of elbow flexion, compared to the contralateral side. The best management for biceps pathology in the shoulder is not clear. If no associated pathology such as cuff tear or labral tear is present then a period of shoulder rehabilitation should be attempted. If this fails, then surgical treatment should be considered. In isolated cases of fraying of the tendon, with no excessive mobility of the tendon, debridement may be all that is required, otherwise a tenodesis or possibly tenotomy should be undertaken.

Elbow

Tendinopathies

Lateral and medial epicondylitis (tennis and golfer's elbow, respectively) is a common condition affecting athletes and office workers alike. Symptoms arise insidiously, often after a change of activity, which requires increased/altered work of the forearm muscles. It causes pain over the epicondyles, worsened by resisted activity of the extensor (lateral) and flexor (medial) muscle groups of the forearm.

Although it has a benign natural history, refractory cases are seen and these are a therapeutic challenge: several conservative treatments have been proposed, including therapeutic ultrasound, friction massage, acupuncture, extracorporeal shock-wave therapy, corticosteroid injections, and strengthening and eccentric training. Some of these interventions are based more on tradition rather than scientific rationale, and the current evidence supporting their use is limited.

Eccentric training has demonstrated promising results for the management of lateral elbow tendinopathy, although current data is limited.

Surgical intervention is a last resort to treat this condition after failed conservative treatment, and there are multiple options, but the aim is to debride the tendinopathic tissue, and stimulate an acute inflammatory response to initiate tendon healing. The outcomes are reported as good or excellent in 80% (Solheim *et al.*, 2011).

Instability

Instability, either lateral or medial, can be caused by trauma or repetitive injury to the medial or lateral collateral ligaments of the elbow, leading to stretching or rupture.

The instability may lead to pain, and lack of confidence in the elbow when loading and rotating.

Early treatment is directed at maintaining stability and achieving a limited arc of motion while the injured structures are healing in the phase of inflammation (0–3 weeks). Protected ROM exercises are performed to prevent joint stiffness and augment healing. It is well documented that early motion nourishes the cartilage and enhances soft tissue healing.

If conservative treatment fails, which is usually only in the most severe cases, surgery can be considered. Surgery to reconstruct the ligaments is complex with uncertain outcomes, requiring a full understanding of the injury, thorough examination, and imaging to make the right decision about the surgery (Murthi *et al.*, 2011).

Posterior impingement

This condition is a result of repeated hyperextension of the elbow, which is compounded by loading the elbow (such as in tumbling). With extension, the olecranon is repeatedly impacted into the olecranon fossa, which causes synovial inflammation. As the synovium becomes inflamed it becomes swollen, and so more susceptible to impingement, and with time the bone and cartilage can become injured, eventually developing spurs, which can break and become loose bodies.

The initial treatment is physiotherapy to control the movements, and injections into the olecranon fossa of local anesthetic and corticosteroid can help alleviate the symptoms, although surgical debridement may eventually be required.

Loose bodies

Loading the elbow during gymnastic activities leads to large stresses through the joint. This can lead to the development of loose fragments of cartilage and bone, which can move through the joint. Locking of the elbow occurs if the loose bodies become stuck, until they move, unlocking the joint. Removal of these bodies can be done arthroscopically, but recovery often takes a few months.

Wrist

Overuse injuries in the wrist are quite common in gymnasts, mainly due to the severe axial and rotational load on the wrist during several exercises of the gymnasts.

There is a relationship between the exposure to a certain sport and the prevalence of injuries.

Young gymnasts, who exercise often more than 20–30 hours per week, are especially susceptible to these injuries.

Dorsal impingement syndromes

Dorsal impingement syndromes are common in all sports where repetitive dorsiflexion occurs particularly accompanied by axial loading. It is reported that more than 50% of young, beginning to midlevel gymnasts experience wrist pain (DiFiori et al., 2006).

Dorsal impingement or dorsal wrist syndrome may result from dorsal capsulitis or synovitis with resultant capsular thickening. In longstanding cases, osteophytes may occur at the dorsal rim of the distal radius or dorsal aspects of the scaphoid or lunate. Usually, plain radiographs are negative, but a CT scan may reveal the dorsal osteophytes.

Most cases resolve with splinting, rest, and nonsteroidals or injection. In refractory cases, wrist arthroscopy and debridement of synovitis, with or without osteophytes debridement, may be curative. The athlete should be counseled that return to the same activity might result in recurrence of the symptoms.

Occult dorsal ganglion may result from athletic activity and may present as a dorsal wrist syndrome. This results from injury to the scapholunate ligament with secondary degenerative changes. Diagnosis is suspected in the athlete with complaints of pain in dorsiflexion, especially with loading. Point tenderness on the scapholunate ligament is usually present. Plain radiographs are mostly negative. An MRI may reveal a small ganglion. In cases that do not respond to immobilization and rest, corticosteroid injection has been suggested, with poor results when compared to surgical excision.

Triangular fibrocartilage complex

The triangular fibrocartilage complex (TFCC) is the primary stabilizer of the distal radioulnar joint. It is divided into a central articular disc portion, which is relatively avascular, and the dorsal and palmar radioulnar ligaments, which are more vascular and are stabilizing structures of the distal radioulnar joint. The volar ulnar carpal ligaments extend from the periphery of the TFCC and ulnar styloid to the lunate and triquetrum. The ulnar extensor muscle subsheath and the ulnar collateral ligament complete the complex.

The axially loaded forearm bears about 80% of the load through the radius and 20% through the TFCC and ulna. The thickness of the TFCC varies inversely with a positive ulnar variance (relatively long ulna), and it has been shown that increased positive ulnar variance results in increased load bearing through the ulnar axis. Injuries to the TFCC are more common in the wrist with ulnar positive variance.

Traumatic tears, usually noted in young athletes, may be central or peripheral: peripheral tears may result in distal radioulnar joint instability.

Acute traumatic events involve axial load bearing with rotational stress. Gymnasts routinely load their wrists in hyperdorsiflexion and ulnar deviation (the first hand in round-offs and on the vault), and put rotational stresses through the loaded hand (on pommel horse). Acute injuries may be superimposed on chronic repetitive traumatic events.

Physical examination includes several tests with rather low sensitivity. Typically there is pain in the sulcus between the ulnar styloid and pisiform and supination lift test. There may be distal radioulnar joint instability. MRI may be useful in the diagnosis. When conservative treatment with splinting has failed, an arthroscopy can be both effective for the diagnosis as well as for the treatment of the lesion.

Arthroscopy of the radiocarpal, mid-carpal, and distal radioulnar joint may yield a diagnosis of chondral lesions of the distal radioulnar joint as well as TFCC tears and instability. Traumatic tears of the central articular disc (type 1A tears) do well with debridement. Peripheral lesions (type 1B) need a more aggressive approach with repair, with more prolonged rehabilitation.

In neutral or positive variance of the ulna a distal resection of the ulna could be considered, either with the wafer method or by an open ulnar shortening.

Other injuries

Distal radius stress fractures, scaphoid stress fractures, avascular necrosis of the lunate (Kienbock's disease), and mid-carpal instability are less frequent, but should be considered when gymnasts present with pain at the dorsum of the wrist. Gymnasts are also at risk of tendinopathies around the wrist.

Stress fracture of the scaphoid is rare, and diagnosis is made by snuffbox tenderness and MRI findings/X-ray/bone scan. Thus far in reported cases, the fracture has healed with 2–4 months of casting.

Avascular necrosis of the capitate has been reported in a gymnast and required surgical debridement and drilling. Long-term follow-up is not available.

Rehabilitation

There are few definitive studies on the most effective rehabilitation protocols for upper limb problems, but principles exist based on physiology and biomechanics:

1 *Diagnosis:* The rehabilitation can only be as good as the diagnosis, and if this is wrong it may actually lead to poor compliance and worse outcomes.
2 *Early pain relief:* Abnormal muscle patterning can be due to pain inhibition, leading the gymnast to develop abnormal positions for the arm, neck, or back. This may require a period of rest, change of routine, analgesia, and judicious use of injections.
3 *Maintenance of kinetic chain and core stability:* Whilst the upper limb is recovering from an injury, the rest of the body should not be ignored, but actively prepared for the onset of the upper limb rehabilitation through prescribed lower limb and trunk exercises.
4 *Range of movement:* Most gymnastic disciplines require a full range of movement, and conditioning and rehabilitation should aim to maintain this as soon as possible after injury, to avoid stiffness and allow muscle balance.
5 *Scapular stabilization:* The scapula is the base upon which the activity of the whole upper limb rests. In order for the arm to act to maintain its control requires the scapula to be stable, which is often jeopardized in the acute injury phase due to pain, and subclinical instability of the glenohumeral joint, in an attempt to avoid positions prone to subluxation and impingement. Closed chain exercises are the mainstay of scapula stabilization.

6 *Rotator cuff:* The rotator cuff is the key to shoulder function. It maintains the humeral head in the glenoid socket through fine motor control, allowing the larger strength muscles of the shoulder to give the shoulder power. Unfortunately, they are easily ignored and can become overpowered by these stronger muscles, giving rise to imbalance, tendinopathy, and instability. Rehabilitation requires that the cuff is addressed as a single unit, rather than as individual muscles, and is dependent on a full pain-free range of passive movement. Closed chain exercises allow the cuff to strengthen whilst avoiding shear forces on the joint, which may lead to unstable movements.
7 *Elbow:* Avoid longterm immobilization, as risk of stiffness is significant. Passive stretching of the elbow may give rise to gains in range of movement in the short term, but can lead to progressive stiffness, if the stretching results in pain. Exercises should aim at self-directed range of movement.
8 *Wrist:* Moving from stretching exercises to strengthening exercises should be undertaken, but return to training may be facilitated by judicious use of taping and bracing.
9 *Hand:* Injuries to the hand need a treatment regime that will allow early mobilization, as the risk and consequences of stiffness are significant. The aims of rehabilitation are to regain full range as quickly as possible.

Further research

Gymnastics will always be a sport that puts participants at risk of injury. More information is needed about the etiology of some of the common chronic problems associated with the sport, particularly with respect to the developing skeleton. Rehabilitation for gymnastic injuries and the best time to return to sport needs further research, as does rehabilitation for growth-related injuries, particularly the enthesopathies and the best time to return to full training. By understanding which gymnasts are at risk, at what stage of development, and doing which skills, can lead to strategies to reduce the risk of long-term problems, which will lead to inability to train, and compete.

Ideally, this could be possible through registries of participating gymnasts (within one federation or combining multiple federations) and the injuries they sustain during their training, and competition.

Summary

The upper limb is made up of complex joints, which are adapted to an upright life and to manipulate tools. Gymnastics as a sport puts an enormous strain on these joints through weight bearing, range of movement, and strength. This puts the limb at significant risk during growth and adulthood, of serious injury, which may render the sport impossible. The ideal way to avoid injury is through an understanding of the risks, adequate conditioning and training for the individual skills, and early treatment for chronic conditions as they are developing, and completion of the treatment course to avoid recurrences. This requires teamwork between the gymnast, coach, physiotherapist, and doctor, so that problems are not hidden away until they are made worse. Many conditions should successfully be treated with rehabilitation avoiding surgery, which often necessitates cessation of training for a period of time.

References

Albanese, S.A., Palmer, A.K., Kerr, D.R., Carpenter, C.W., Lisi, D., and Levinsohn, E.M. (1989) Wrist pain and distal growth plate closure of the radius in gymnasts. *Journal of Pediatric Orthopedics*, **9** (1), 23–28.

Athwal, G.S., Ramsey, M.L., Steinmann, S.P., and Wolf, J.M. (2011) Fractures and dislocations of the elbow: a return to the basics. *Instructional Course Lectures*, **60**, 199–214.

Brophy, R.H. and Marx, R.G. (2009) The treatment of traumatic anterior instability of the shoulder: nonoperative and surgical treatment. *Arthroscopy: The Journal of Arthroscopic and Related Surgery*, **25** (3), 298–304.

DiFiori, J., Caine, D., and Malina, R. (2006) Wrist pain, distal radial growth plate injury, and ulnar variance in the young gymnast. *American Journal of Sports Medicine*, **34**, 840–849.

Edmonds, E.W. and Polousky, J. (2013) A review of knowledge in osteochondritis dissecans: 123 years of minimal evolution from König to the ROCK Study Group. *Clinical Orthopaedics and Related Research*, **471** (4), 1118–1126.

Gaskill, T.R., Taylor, D.C., and Millett, P.J. (2011) Management of multidirectional instability of the shoulder. *The Journal of the American Academy of Orthopaedic Surgeons*, **19** (12), 758–767.

de Graaff, F., Krijnen, M.R., Poolman, R.W., and Willems, W.J. (2011) Arthroscopic surgery in athletes with osteochondritis dissecans of the elbow. *Arthroscopy: The Journal of Arthroscopic and Related Surgery*, **27** (7), 986–993.

Murthi, A.M., Keener, J.D., Armstrong, A.D., and Getz, C.L. (2011) The recurrent unstable elbow: diagnosis and treatment. *Instructional Course Lectures*, **60**, 215–226.

Singh, S., Smith, G.A., Fields, S.K., and McKenzie, L.B. (2008) Gymnastics-related injuries to children treated in emergency departments in the United States, 1990-2005. *Pediatrics*, **121** (4), e954–e960.

Solheim, E., Hegna, J., and Øyen, J. (2011) Extensor tendon release in tennis elbow: results and prognostic factors in 80 elbows. *Knee Surgery, Sports Traumatology, Arthroscopy*, **19** (6), 1023–1027.

Recommended reading

Dwek, J.R., Cardoso, F., and Chung, C.B. (2009) MR imaging of overuse injuries in the skeletally immature gymnast: spectrum of soft-tissue and osseous lesions in the hand and wrist. *Pediatric Radiology*, **39** (12), 1310–1316.

Kolt, G. and Caine, D. (2010) Gymnastics. In: D. Caine, P. Harmer, and M. Schiff (eds), *Epidemiology of Injury in Olympic Sports. Encyclopaedia of Sports Medicine*, vol. XVI, pp. 144–160. Wiley-Blackwell Publishers (UK) and the International Olympic Committee (IOC) Medical Commission.

McRae, R. and Esser, M. (2008) *Practical Fracture Treatment*, 5th edn. Churchill Livingstone Publishers.

Rettig, A.C. (2003) Athletic injuries of the wrist and hand. Part I: traumatic injuries of the wrist. *The American Journal of Sports Medicine*, **31** (6), 1038–1048.

Rettig, A.C. (2004) Athletic injuries of the wrist and hand: part II: overuse injuries of the wrist and traumatic injuries to the hand. *The American Journal of Sports Medicine*, **32** (1), 262–273.

Skirven, T.M., Osterman, A.L., Fedorczyk, J., and Amadio P.C. (2011) *Rehabilitation of the Hand and Upper Extremity*, 6th edn. Mosby Publishers.

Chapter 12
Treatment and rehabilitation of common lower extremity injuries

Liesbeth Lim

Sports Medical Advice Center Aalsmeer, Aalsmeer *and*
Sports Medical Advice Center Annatommie (Centers for Orthopedics and Movement), Amsterdam, The Netherlands

Introduction

The majority of Artistic Gymnastics injuries are located in the lower extremity (35.9–70.2% of injuries), with most of the literature mentioning proportions above 50%) (Kolt & Caine, 2010).

Injuries to the ankle, foot and knee are the most common, arising from high-impact loads during tumbling and acrobatic activities on the floor, vault, and balance beam, with the ankle sprain as the most common type of injury. Landings and take-offs for tumbling and vaulting or dismounts from apparatus, often from heights of more than 2.5 metres, are the high-risk moves.

Rhythmic Gymnastics (performed only by women) entails relatively low risk in terms of severe injuries (mostly strains and sprains), due to the relatively low frequency of high-impact acrobatic components in this discipline. Acute injuries are mostly sustained in the lower limbs, and certain positions in Rhythmic Gymnastics require extreme range of motion of the joints, such as the hips and the spine, so (chronic) injuries are seen frequently in the back. Choreography in this discipline is important and the injuries may be similar to those sustained by ballet dancers.

In Trampoline Gymnastics the main injuries are also located in the lower extremity and consist of ankle and knee sprains, which result from falls during incomplete and/or incorrect landings. Landings with the lower legs between the frame and the steel springs can result in cutting wounds. Compared to Artistic Gymnastics the surface properties of the trampoline serve to "cushion" the gymnast's landing, but conversely this elasticity enables the gymnast to easily rebound.

By its nature, performed on apparatus, Artistic Gymnastics predisposes to acute injuries. However, chronic injuries occur more in the higher levels, due to accumulation of microtraumas and microfractures and limited time for recovery, as training hours around 30 hours per week are "normal."

This chapter will highlight the treatment and rehabilitation of the most common lower extremity injuries incurred by gymnasts who compete in the artistic, rhythmic, and trampoline disciplines. However randomized controlled and long-term studies of treatment and rehabilitation protocols in gymnastics are lacking. Most of the available published data are case reports and arise from studies of injuries affecting (female) artistic gymnasts.

Acute injuries

Acute injuries occur from trauma (either direct or indirect) incurred during an accident on the apparatus, or a fall from the apparatus, and can also increase risk of chronic injuries if not treated adequately or rehabilitated completely.

Fractures

Fractures of the lower extremity require the same treatment strategy as for all fractures.

Gymnastics, First Edition. Edited by Dennis J. Caine, Keith Russell and Liesbeth Lim. © 2013 International Olympic Committee. Published 2013 by John Wiley & Sons, Ltd.

The general treatment management for fractures is to attain anatomical alignment and length and to prevent such as delayed union or nonunion (pseudoarthrosis), avascular necrosis and articular incongruence, which can lead to late sequelae such as osteoarthritis. The choice of therapy and the prognosis for fractures will also be determined by the type and severity of the associated soft tissue injury. Fractures should be referred to the orthopedic surgeon, preferably with interest and experience in (children's and adolescent) sports. The surgeon's choice for a therapy will also be influenced by the gymnast's level and injury history, and the gymnastics goals in consultation with the coach, and in combination with the gymnast's "competition calendar." Ideally, the choice will be made in cooperation with the responsible sports medicine professionals.

Specific fractures in children and adolescents

In children, most extraarticular fractures can be treated conservatively due to the remodeling capacity of growing bone.

The epiphysis is a vulnerable structure in the growing bones and fractures of the epiphysis can result in growth disturbances and angulation deformities, leading to altered joint mechanics and long-term disability. Epiphyseal fractures in the lower extremity usually occur around the ankle (distal tibia) and knee (proximal tibia and distal femur).

They can be classified according to the five types (I–V) of Salter and Harris (1963) or the newer Peterson classification, which added a type VI; and to the three types of Aitken. The type determines the severity of the epiphyseal fracture and thus its prognosis for developing growth disturbances (Caine *et al.*, 2006). Other factors, related to greater risks for growth disturbance are: age of the child (in a younger child), gender (on average rather in boys than in girls) or which growth plate is injured (in region of the knee).

A sprain sustained by a child or adolescent gymnast may be associated with an epiphyseal fracture and medical professionals should take this into account in their diagnosis management until proven otherwise, as initial examinations of the growth plate or ossification centers can be negative. Long-term follow-up, including X-ray examination of matching limbs at 3–6-month intervals, is necessary to monitor the child's recuperation and growth, particularly when acute epiphyseal fracture involves a joint (Caine *et al.*, 2006).

Foot and ankle fractures

In gymnastics the highest loads are incurred during landings where the impact on the foot and ankle can be several times the body weight. Due to the high energy, especially in landings on the plantarflexed foot with a forward-leaning body followed by forced dorsiflexion of the ankle, which mainly occur in the backwards tumble activities, and sometimes in combination with inversion or eversion of the ankle, different ligament or tendon injuries and fractures or dislocation of the foot and ankle can occur (see Figure 12.1).

The foot has a "complex" anatomy with several bones adjacent to each other, thus projecting over each other on plain radiographs and complicating the decision of a correct diagnosis in the acute phase. Aggravated, prolonged, or recurrent symptoms when increasing the gymnastics program need further investigation.

General treatment and rehabilitation for lower extremity injuries

The treatment strategy for the following (acute) lower extremity injuries is roughly according to the subsequent general protocol. It should be noticed, that there is lack of literature about rehabilitation programs and techniques for lower extremity injuries in gymnastics. The protocol includes recommendations from experience and is based on the guideline and general principles of Sports Medicine (see also "Recommended reading"), and has to be individualized and specified for the different gymnastics disciplines.

Acute phase

The RICE therapy for the first 3–5 days after the acute trauma may be prescribed for the relief in the acute period (reduction of swelling and pain) (Table 12.1).

Anti-inflammatory medication is prescribed for acute pain management and because of the possible side effects, the first choice is regular painkiller such as Panadol.

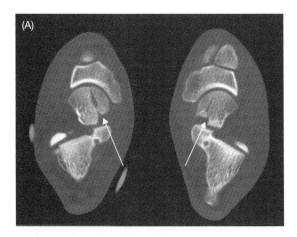

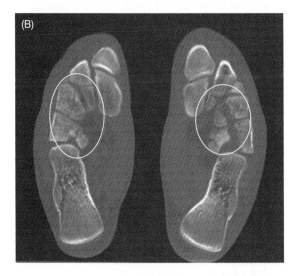

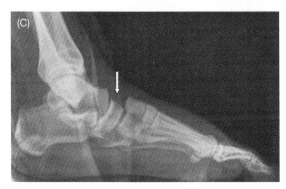

Figure 12.1 Multiple fractures in both feet. **(A)** Axial CT scan shows talar fracture in both feet (arrows); **(B)** cuboid fracture, lateral and intermediate cuneiform fracture (circles). **(C)** Plain radiograph of the lateral ankle and foot shows naviculocuneiform dislocation (arrow).

Table 12.1 RICE therapy in the acute phase after trauma.

RICE	Description of the therapy
Rest	Is recommended during the inflammatory response to the tissue damage. Controlled active dorsiflexion and plantarflexion of the ankle, or extension and flexion of the knee if possible and weight bearing are allowed within the pain threshold, otherwise shortly non-weight bearing with crutches.
Ice application	Is not proven to reduce the swelling. But intermittently application can be considered to reduce the localized pain in the short-term.
Compression	By using elastic bandage, it may have a positive effect on the decrease of swelling and pain. The relationship between a faster decrease of swelling by compression and ultimately a faster functional recovery is not proven.
Elevation	Is the most effective strategy in reducing the swelling in the short-term.

Electrotherapy, lasertherapy, and ultrasound therapy have no added value to the acute treatment.

Connective tissue massage and lymph drainage techniques are increasingly applied for reducing the swelling, but have not yet been studied in controlled trials.

During the treatment period isometric muscle strengthening can be started to prevent significant atrophy.

Recovery and rehabilitation phase

In the early recovery phase, joint mobilization and defined exercises, which can be applied at home, are important to stimulate the vascularization and neural system and to avoid joint stiffness.

Rehabilitation always consists of a well-monitored program with progressive exercises for strength (functionally or with weights), first in closed kinetic chain and later in open kinetic chain, of the pelvic/gluteal muscles, quadriceps (especially the vastus medialis) and hamstrings, and calf and foot muscles. Exercises for core stability and neuromuscular training can be started initially in the supine position.

Conditioning exercises, controlled and technical jump and landings exercises, and agility training will be finally added.

Continuing the exercise program for muscle strength and flexibility of the upper extremity, the upper body, and the back, as well as core stability regimen is a must to prevent another new injury and help ensure a faster return to gymnastics.

Treatment of any treatable predisposing factors is important to prevent recurrence or new injury.

Sports-specific phase

Proprioception and balance exercises of the injured joint must be completed before returning to basic gymnastics. Single-leg "hoptests" (particularly the "triple hoptest"), such as vertical (up–down), horizontal (forward), sideways, and "figure-of-8" hoptests are good indicators for functional recovery.

Leg activities should always be resumed on a soft surface, with (extra) mats, or on trampoline (possibly supported with spotting belt) and later on the tumbling track. Twist and "compound" landings and hard landings have to be avoided until the rehabilitation program is finished.

Finally, the gymnast can return slowly to full training when the clinical symptoms are completely resolved. Pain will be the main guideline, which can be monitored by the "visual analog scale" (VAS) score, evaluated by the gymnast ranging from 0 (no pain at all) to 10 (the most severe pain ever).

Protection by using a brace or tape for the injured ligaments during rehabilitation and when resuming (basic) gymnastics training is advisable. The preferred type of brace for the ankle is the soft brace, such as a lace-up brace or a semi-rigid brace.

To maintain the "feeling" with the apparatus during the rehabilitation phase, the gymnast is encouraged to do basic skills, without dismounts, on the "hanging" apparatus such as uneven and high bar and rings or on the "arm supportive" apparatus such as pommel horse and parallel bar.

Furthermore, this is important for female gymnasts, who do not use a dowel grip on the uneven bars, to avoid reduction of hand palm callosity.

Full muscle strength, full end range of motion, coordination, balance, and symmetric core stability should be restored before resuming competition.

Dislocation of joints

Patella

The mechanism for patellar dislocation is usually either a direct blow on the femur condyles or on the (medial) patella in a fall or a twisting injury in which the femur is internally rotated upon the fixed tibia in the flexed knee, for example, during a "stick" landing with the affected leg out of balance. This trauma mechanism is similar to that for an anterior cruciate ligament (ACL) injury, which may occur in association with this injury.

Another mechanism is a sudden burst of quadriceps activity in the landings, for example, when stepping behind with the affected leg extended for a "stick" landing (with "spread legs").

Patellar dislocation is highly predisposed in the hypermobile patellofemoral joint (in association with patella alta ("high-riding patella") and/or patellofemoral dysplasia) and is at high risk in gymnastics due to the multiple rotational landings. Muscular weakness or imbalance can be associated with, but may also be the result of, patellar dislocations. The patella dislocates laterally out of its groove onto the lateral femoral condyle and acutely spontaneous reposition often occurs, with knee extension.

An acute dislocation of the patella may be accompanied by different lesions such as a tear of the medial retinaculum and vastus medialis expansion; and avulsion fracture, osteochondral fracture or bone bruise/contusion of the medial patellar margin and/or lateral femoral epicondyle/trochlea; and chondral fractures of the patellar joint surface ("flakes").

After the primary (first-time) patellar dislocation, residual laxity of a medial retinacular injury may produce patellar instability, and this in turn may produce recurrent anterior pain and symptomatic giving-way. The anterior knee pain should be differentiated from patellofemoral pain syndrome.

Treatment of acute dislocation is repositioning of the patella, after painkiller administration or regional anesthesia, by extending the knee and putting local pressure on the patella in the medial direction.

After reduction, the initial treatment plan in cases without associated lesions is conservative with a splint in knee extension and pain management. After a week, a limited motion knee brace in 30° flexion of the knee can be prescribed, with gradually increasing knee flexion during 6 weeks, for example, with 15° every week to 45°, 60°, 75°, 90° flexion, respectively (Figure 12.2).

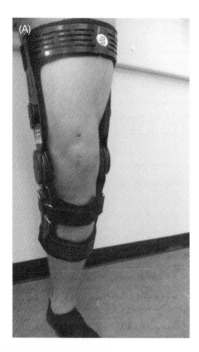

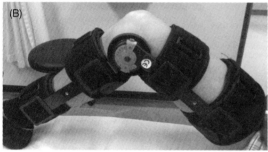

Figure 12.2 Limited motion knee braces: **(A)** in front view **(B)** in side view, with detailed hinge in degrees.

Isometric muscle strengthening can be started to prevent significant atrophy. After 6 weeks treatment, protection with a brace may be continued until full knee flexion takes place. This schedule should be individually based, dependent on the severity of pain and swelling and may be shortened or prolonged. Well-developed vastus medialis (obliquus) muscle is essential for good patellar tracking.

Arthroscopy is required in cases of osteochondral fracture or flakes of the patellar joint surface, with operative repair in cases of the medial retinaculum rupture.

The primary treatment of chronic patellar instability is the same as after the acute (first) dislocation.

But when previous symptoms and anatomic disorders are present, conservative treatment generally has a poor outcome.

Foot

The loads during landings are most essential at the tibiotalar joint and talonavicular joint (Chilvers *et al.*, 2007). As these loads are high-energetic, dislocations of the foot in gymnastics can occur in the whole foot in association with fractures, like in the tarsometarsal joints (TMT or Lisfranc's joint), the talonavicular and calcaneocuboid joints (Chopart's joint), and even in the naviculocuneiform joint (See Figure 12.1C).

Dislocation of tendons

Peroneal tendon

Dislocation of the peroneal tendon can occur in forced passive ankle dorsiflexion like in deep forward landings in gymnastics or in inversion ankle trauma with subsequent forceful contraction of the peroneus to prevent this motion. The dislocation can persist in ankle eversion and plantar flexion activities, causing recurrent ankle sprains or giving-way feeling and tenosynovitis, and this condition requires surgical treatment.

Sprains

Knee sprains

Medial collateral ligament

The medial collateral ligament (MCL) in gymnastics may be injured frequently with other intraarticular knee injuries, such as an ACL rupture and (medial) meniscal tear known as the "unhappy triad." The prognosis will depend on the most severe concomitant injury.

The injury mechanism is a (in)direct valgus stress trauma of the knee with the foot planted and slightly external rotated and the knee being forced inward, like in an off-balance landing in gymnastics. The severity of the ligament tear can be classified into grade I (mild), grade II (moderate), or grade III (complete rupture).

The treatment can be conservative for all grades with a knee brace. The more severe injuries (grade II and III) require a longer rehabilitation (about twice as long) than the mild (grade I) injuries before returning to full sports activity.

Anterior cruciate ligament

ACL ruptures in gymnastics may occur in landings with flexed (as well as extended) knees from the rotational acrobatics movements, especially in dismounts, including during the vault. A "popping sound" may be heard and usually there is swelling within few hours.

Females are more prone to ACL injuries because of the smaller ACL size and smaller intercondylar notch of the femur (Hutchinson & Ireland, 1995).

On examination, the Lachman's test and anterior drawer sign are positive and a positive Pivot shift is pathognomic for the ACL rupture. In the acute phase this is difficult to perform, since the patient cannot relax sufficiently due to the pain and swelling. The tests should be performed either in the very acute phase (within 1 hour) or in the delayed phase after 5–7 days.

History and clinical findings are most important and MRI can confirm the diagnosis and show concomitant intraarticular lesions.

Gymnastics is a "cruciate-dependent" sport. A rupture of the ACL with a positive pivot shift sign is therefore not compatible with gymnastics at elite level because of the high-demanding rotational acrobatic skills. Surgical reconstruction is then required, particularly when concomitant lesions are present.

In a skeletally immature patient, surgical treatment of an ACL rupture poses additional challenges. There are several surgical reconstructions and the goal is to recreate ACL stability without causing growth plate arrest, with leg-length discrepancy or angular deformity. The approximate degree of skeletal maturity determines the timing. Arthroscopically performed reconstruction is recommended and the choice for the graft depends on the surgeon's (and patient's) preference and experience and can be an autologous graft (the own body's tendon, with preference for hamstrings tendon in gymnasts) or allograft (cadaver's graft of a tendon). Autologous reconstruction with patellar tendon can cause patellar tendinopathy in sports with explosive and repetitive jumping activities, such as gymnastics.

A delayed reconstruction of 4–6 weeks after the injury will give better outcome as the risk for arthrofibrosis and "cyclops" formation (connective tissue mass/scar tissue nearby the entrance of the graft at the tibial plateau) is lower and the graft will better develop in a favourable intraarticular environment of the knee with slight or no swelling and a nearly normal range of motion and gait.

An intense medical and physiotherapy program should commence following the acute trauma (see Section "General treatment and rehabilitation for lower extremity injuries") for an optimal preoperative preparation.

Specifically in gymnastics, because of the nature of the sport, the rehabilitation time takes approximately 9–12 months prior to return to full gymnastics on competition level and rehabilitation management must be very well defined in time frames with written protocols. Teamwork with realistic goals is required during this period.

Initially, neuromuscular electrostimulation can be used for supporting the (muscle) exercises. And wearing a protective knee brace with hinges (e.g., CTI or Don Joy brace) is recommended, particularly in the first 6 weeks for safety.

Caution must be advised for the ingrowth of the graft tissue. In gymnasts with increased ligamentous laxity, full extension drills and mobilization techniques should be restricted.

After 6 months of post-operative period, rapid progression to functional and strength exercises specific for gymnastics can take place. Agility tests, functional tests, and isokinetic Cybex/Biodex testing can be used to evaluate the level of progression and the differences with the uninjured leg, aiming for the quadriceps strength of at least 90% of the uninjured leg and the hamstrings strength at 100%.

However, the rehabilitation schedule should be individually programmed, dependent on the function of the knee, and should be adapted based on the monitored individual symptoms and signs of the knee during and after the exercises, only allowing progress to the next step when the actual program can be performed without pain and swelling.

In reconstructions with hamstrings autologous graft, loss of full knee flexion or sometimes of full hamstrings strength may occur. A rehabilitation program similar for hamstrings muscle tear is useful.

Posterior cruciate ligament

Posterior cruciate ligament (PCL) rupture occurs more frequently in direct forced posterior trauma on the proximal tibia with the knee flexed, but in gymnastics it occurs in landings (especially on the vault apparatus) with hyperextended knees. Hyperextension trauma occurs when the gymnast does not yet expect to land, but the feet strike the ground before the leg muscles can actively absorb the landing forces on the knee.

Treatment for an isolated PCL rupture is conservative with non-weight-bearing immobilization in a brace or splint in the acute phase (for 1 week), followed by use of a knee brace for 6 weeks. Intensive strength training with stability and proprioception training show good results and returning to gymnastics to the pre-injury level is possible, despite the persisting laxity.

Surgery is indicated in the combined tears with posterolateral rotatory instability.

Meniscus

In gymnastics, acute medial as well as lateral meniscus tears can occur from rotational landings and from landings with hyperextended knees. In children and adolescents, a discoid meniscus and meniscal cyst, most frequently located on the lateral side of the knee, can mimic meniscal tear symptoms.

The treatment depends on the associated ligament tears or cartilage damage. The goal is to maintain as much of the meniscus as possible for its load absorption properties.

Minimal and stable meniscal tears (without displacement) can be treated conservatively. Persistent swelling, pain, and symptomatic locking symptoms of the knee will need arthroscopy.

Post-surgery rehabilitation will take 6 weeks, but this will not always mean full gymnastics activity or competition at the end of the 6 weeks. The rehabilitation program can take longer in cases of complicated tears or in lateral meniscal tears.

Ankle sprains

Lateral ankle ligament injuries

Ankle sprains are the most common sports injury with the anterior lateral ankle ligament being mostly injured.

The main intrinsic predisposing factors for the lateral ankle ligament injuries are the muscle strength of the lower leg, proprioception and balance characteristics, and range of motion of the ankle. Limited ankle dorsal flexion and reduced propriopception are indicative of an increased risk of sustaining lateral ankle ligament injuries, and previous ankle sprain in the past is a plausible risk factor (Kerkhoffs et al., 2012).

Extrinsic predisposing factors are for example the type of the performed sport and whether a competition is involved. Dismounts in gymnastics are always performed at the end of (complex) routines and may increase the risk of injury, as the gymnast might be fatigued with diminished levels of coordination and strength.

The diagnosis of the lateral ligament rupture after an acute ankle sprain can be made with a high degree of reliability by delayed physical examination 4–5 days after the acute trauma based on the presence of hematoma, accompanied by local pressure pain or a positive anterior drawer test or both (van Dijk et al., 1996), together with an accurate history relating to the trauma mechanism.

Functional treatment of acute ankle ligament injury is still the "gold standard" and preferred over surgical therapy.

After an acute lateral ligament injury, there is a delayed reaction time of the peroneus muscles due to the (traction) injury of the peroneal nerve and decrease of the strength of the extensor and evertor muscles, and other muscle groups around the ankle.

So the treatment management should consist of various exercises, all within the pain limits, ranging from proprioceptive training by using a wobble board as well as training on one leg with closed eyes (to turn off the optical control), muscle strength, muscle coordination, and joint mobility exercises of the whole limb. In the rehabilitation phase, the damaged ligament(s) must be protected by external support, either by tape or brace.

In an ankle sprain without rupture of the lateral ligament, the rehabilitation program is the same, but shorter in duration.

Surgical repair of ankle ligament injuries can be considered for professional and elite athletes, but on an individual basis. Even after surgery, however, it is necessary to take sufficient time for wound healing and for the rehabilitation program before returning to competitive gymnastics. So the decision to opt for surgery or for functional treatment also depends on the time of the gymnastics season and the history of chronic instability, time from trauma to diagnosis, associated ankle joint damage, and access to an experienced foot/ankle surgeon (Kerkhoffs & Tol, 2012).

Exercise therapy with proprioception, coordination and balance training, and home exercises are mostly considered as the strategy for the secondary prevention, even for longer period, up to 12 months after the first ankle ligament injury. Wearing either a brace or tape during gymnastics landing skills is useful in the prevention after a lateral ankle ligament injury. A lace-up or semi-rigid brace may be preferable to tape in the preventive strategy since for the long-term use it is better for the skin and in terms of the evaluation of cost.

Complete recovery is essential, otherwise there will be decreased performance for a prolonged time and an increased risk for a new or recurrent injury.

Medial ankle ligament injuries ("deltoid ligament")

In gymnastics, deltoid ligament rupture can occur frequently in the hyperdorsiflexion trauma mechanism with overpronation as seen in deep acrobatic landings, following initial landings on the forefoot. A rupture of the deltoid ligament can be accompanied by a (longitudinal) rupture of the tibialis posterior or the flexor hallucis longus tendon.

Rehabilitation for the deltoid ligament injury is the same as for the lateral ligament injury, but it takes twice as long before returning to full gymnastics, especially in case of calcifications in the injured deltoid ligament or a concomitant bony or chondral lesion, sometimes requiring arthroscopy.

General attention in ankle sprains

Due to the often great height of dismounts from the apparatus and incomplete rotation in the landing (increasing the impact of the landing), extreme compression in the ankle joint may lead to more severe injuries, which are not recognized at the time of the initial (clinical) presentation.

Any sprain that does not improve with adequate treatment should always be reconsidered. The possible associated injuries are: osteochondral lesions or stress fractures of the talar dome, tibial plafond, lateral talar process, posterior process of the talus (e.g., Cedell fracture, a fracture of the medial tubercle of the posterior process, however rare), and anterior calcaneal process.

Ankle impingement syndrome

Anterior soft tissue ankle impingement may develop after a ligament rupture with interposition of the torn parts of the ligament. In the bony impingement, the repetitive microtraumas in the ankle induce spur formation, such as osteophytes or ossicles, which in turn provoke the process of synovial impingement (Figure 12.3). It is not the osteophyte itself that is painful, but the compression of the inflamed soft tissue caught between the traction spurs and the osteophytes (van Dijk, 2006).

Gymnasts with anterior ankle impingement complain of limited hyperdorsiflexion when loaded with the heel on the ground, which often occurs in landings from backwards somersaults.

The treatment is initially conservative with modifications of training like decreasing the number of repetitions of acrobatic and tumbling activities with forced ankle dorsiflexion. Anti-inflammatory medication, physical therapy mobilizing techniques (translations of the talocrural joint), and taping to limit the end ranges of ankle motion may also be used.

Corticosteroid injections in case of chronic synovitis or abundant soft tissue may be indicated for the elite gymnast and if this fails, arthroscopy to remove the exostosis/spurs and osteophytes or hypertrophic synovial tissue can be performed. Arthroscopic treatment of bony impingement is more successful than treatment of soft tissue

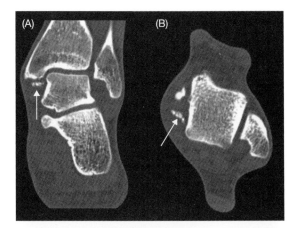

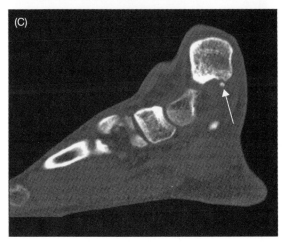

Figure 12.3 (Posterior) medial fragments in the ankle, causing impingement. CT scan of the ankle: **(A)** coronal (arrow), **(B)** axial (arrow), and **(C)** sagittal (arrow) view.

impingement, because of recurrence of scar tissue post-operatively in the latter (van Dijk, 2006).

Posterior ankle impingement may develop after an extreme plantarflexion/inversion trauma or may be caused by overuse, resulting in synovitis or tenosynovitis. Usually, a hypertrophic posterior process of the talus or a (slightly displaced) os trigonum is associated with posterior impingement, but its existence does not cause the impingement syndrome. Pathognomic is the "posterior impingement test," which elicits pain by repetitive quick passive forced hyperplantarflexion movements (in a patient sitting with the knee flexed at 90°).

Return to sport practice after arthroscopy of posterior impingement syndrome is twice as long (approximately 9 weeks) than in the anterior impingement syndrome.

Tendon ruptures

Ruptures of the achilles tendon and less frequently of the patellar tendon can occur in gymnastics in association with an uncoordinated explosive take-off or landing. The mechanism is that of a forced joint motion and a simultaneously strong contraction of the muscle (eccentric contraction) or a failure in the neuromuscular protective mechanism due to fatigue or disturbed coordination. For the elite gymnast, surgical repair is preferred for the lower rate of a rerupture or a residual lengthening of the tendon (with inability to regain the former strength).

Chronic injuries

Growth-related injuries

Physeal injuries

Young athletes are at risk for physeal injury, particularly during periods of rapid growth (Caine *et al.*, 2006).

Physeal injuries can be both acute and chronic and may both lead to growth disturbances. Stress-related physeal injuries affecting young athletes in a variety of sports, including gymnastics, are increasingly reported, including those affecting the lower extremities (Caine *et al.*, 2006).

To reduce risk of injury, training programs should be individualized and adapted to reduce the intensity and high-impact loads during periods of rapid growth. Periodic physical examination for diagnosis at an early stage and careful measurement of height at 3-month intervals to provide coaches with data to estimate growth rate, are recommended (Caine *et al.*, 2006).

Apophyseal injuries

During adolescence, apophyseal injuries are common, including in young gymnasts.

The apophyses are located at the site of attachment of major musculotendinous system to the growing bone, beyond the articulation of the joint and are subjected primarily to tensile/traction forces. They are also called "traction epiphyses" and do not contribute to longitudinal growth (Caine *et al.*, 2006).

In the immature skeleton, the apophysis is weaker than the attached musculotendinous unit or ligament, so forced incoordinated and eccentric muscle contractions or traction trauma in adolescence will cause injuries with "inflammatory" reaction ("traction apophysitis") or even an avulsion fracture with a slip and displacement, while in the adult they will cause muscle or tendon strain or rupture. Apophyseal injuries typically occur at the average ages between 8 and 15 years.

The growth rate of the apophysis is slower than that of the epiphysis of the corresponding bone, which is believed to be due to the increased number of collagen fibers in the apophysis needed to support the greater tensile forces on this structure (Peck, 1995). Subsequently, apophyseal injury may occur until late adolescence and the apophysis is most vulnerable between 12 and 16 years when the ossification center develops under hormonal influence in the rapid growth period (Lazovic *et al.*, 1996).

In girls, the fusion in the apophysis usually occurs about 2 years sooner (between 8 and 13 years) than in boys (between 10 and 15 years). In gymnastics, the incidence of apophyseal injuries among females may be high, often due to the delayed onset of skeletal maturation.

Osgood–Schlatter disease, Sinding-Larsen–Johansson syndrome

In the knee, "Osgood–Schlatter disease" at the tibial tuberosity occurs more frequently than "Sinding-Larsen–Johansson syndrome" at the inferior pole of the patella (the distal respectively proximal insertion of the patellar tendon). It is the most common apophysitis occurring at 9–15 years of age and may be associated with tight quadriceps muscle and excessive pronation of the foot.

Sever's disease

In the foot, "Sever's disease" can cause pain at the posterior calcaneus (insertion of the Achilles tendon). It may be associated with tight achilles-tendon and calf muscles and biomechanical foot abnormalities (such as tarsal coalition, hyper-pronated foot, or equinus foot). In gymnastics, increased frequency of hard landings, particularly performed on bare feet, is a common cause.

It occurs most often at the age between 7 and 10 years, until early puberty, and is the second most frequent apophyseal injury.

Pelvis

Apophyseal injuries in adolescent gymnasts may also occur frequently in the pelvis and hip as they tend to appear and fuse later (Vandervliet *et al.*, 2007).

Especially apophyseal injuries of the ischial tuberosity occur frequently in the female gymnast due to endless and explosive stretch of the hamstrings during the front split jumps and leaps and ballet sessions (flexibility exercises). The flexibility of the affected leg, measured as the straight leg raise, is significantly decreased (and often painful), whilst in gymnasts the straight leg raise can be usually extremely large (possibly around 120° or more). So an absolute limitation of the affected leg may be difficult to find, and the flexibility can be symmetric, when the unaffected leg is the "nondominant" split leg. On clinical examination both legs should always be reviewed and compared.

Hamstrings insertional tendinopathy can be associated with apophyseal injury of the ischial tuberosity (Figure 12.4).

Less frequent apophyseal injuries in gymnasts are located at the site of the iliac crest (at the abdominal muscles insertion) in imbalanced explosive muscle contractions, or at the site of the lesser trochanter (iliopsoas tendon insertion), due to the explosive side or straddle split, causing groin pain, particularly in hyperabduction and external rotation of the hip.

Use of plain radiographs is commonly difficult to distinguish apophyseal injury from an irregular apophysis, which may be caused by a normal variant of insufficient ossification or by the various ossification stages. Comparison with the other side is preferable, although apophyseal injuries may occur bilaterally as well (Figure 12.5).

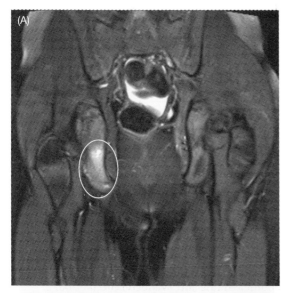

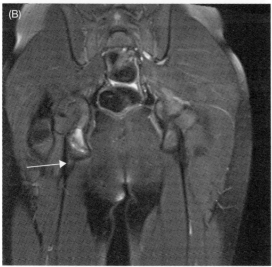

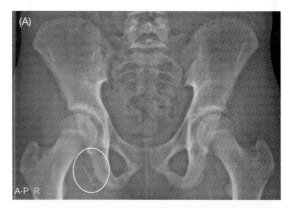

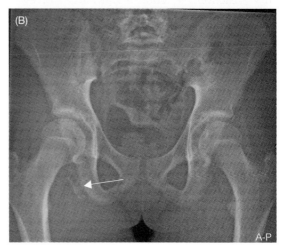

Figure 12.5 (A) Plain radiographs show irregular aspect of the ischial tuberosity on both sides, with avulsion of the apophysis on the right side and displacement of 5 mm (white circle). **(B)** After 2 months of relative rest: some callus/bone formation within the space of the avulsed apophysis (arrow).

Figure 12.4 Coronal fat suppressed T2-weighted MRI of the pelvis: apophysiolysis of the right ischial tuberosity with insertional tendinopathy of the hamstrings.
(A) High signal intensity bone marrow edema in the ischial tuberosity with widened apophysis (circle).
(B) Soft tissue edema within the thickened conjoined insertion of the hamstrings tendon (arrow). The bone marrow edema in the ischial tuberosity and the widened apophysis are also present in this view.

Usually, imaging is not necessary, unless in cases of persistent pain and to exclude other pathology. The diagnosis is based on clinical symptoms and examination. Occasionally, X-rays can show a widened or enlarged apophysis, fragmentation, irregularity, and increased density (Figure 12.5).

Ultrasound is recommended for imaging of apophyseal injuries (in the more superficial structures), while it has likely higher sensitivity in youngsters (Lazovic *et al.*, 1996). It may show the changes of the apophysis clearly, even in the absence of the ossification center or in very small centers to be seen on plain radiographs and in early phase of apophyseal injuries, where there is only soft tissue edema, appearing as hypoechogenic zone (Figure 12.6).

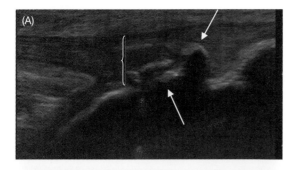

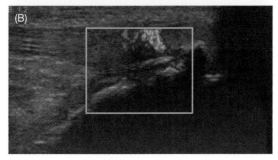

Figure 12.6 Ultrasound, sagittal view. Osgood–Schlatter's disease of the knee. **(A)** Thickened patellar tendon insertion with edema as a region with hypoechogenicity (accolade) and fragmentation of the tibal tuberosity (two arrows). **(B)** Increased flow in the thickened patellar tendon insertion (in the quadrangle): hypervascularity in the tendon (sign of inflammatory reaction), while normally there is no or few flow.

Nonoperative treatment is the first choice.

The predisposing factors, such as muscle imbalance and relatively tight muscles, and biomechanical abnormalities, if present, should be treated. Taping of the patellar tendon or heel pads and heel cups to reduce the tension of the concerning tendon can be used.

When acute pain and swelling have diminished, the gymnast can do basic apparatus training on the "hanging and arm-supporting apparatus," without dismounts.

Thereafter, the female gymnast can start with choreography on beam and floor without jumps or running and the male on floor with minimal impacts.

The rhythmic gymnast can start with choreography and basic apparatus skills, without the jumps and leaps, and without running and hopping activities.

The trampoline gymnast can resume training with a spotting belt initially, once the symptoms have diminished.

The overall prognosis is good, with complete recovery and without residual symptoms, while the condition is self-limited. Corticosteroid injections or surgery are contraindicated. Coach and gymnast need to understand the condition and modify the training activities, as symptoms may persist and recur for a long time.

The differential diagnosis for apophyseal injuries includes stress fracture, aseptic necrosis, osteochondritis dissecans, insertional tendinopathy, and bursitis. Irregularity of the apophysis on plain radiographs however may also be caused by a normal variant of insufficient ossification, which requires a different approach. A persistent apophysis after the growth may be found.

Snapping hip

The "snapping hip" is a chronic problem, seen in female gymnasts. They experience a painful snapping noise in the anterior groin during the gymnastics choreography and the flexibility exercises of the hip (in ballet or warming-up).

The "internal" snapping hip is more frequent than the "external" (which is caused by the [abductor] muscles and tendons at the lateral side of the hip), where the contracted iliopsoas tendon slides over the anterior hip capsule, femoral head, iliopectineal eminence, or lesser trochanter during active or explosive hip flexion (in abduction/external rotation of the hip) and extended legs.

The prognosis is good. Plain radiographs, MRI, and CT scan are often not necessary and are negative.

The treatment is to reassure the gymnast and explain the injury mechanism. Pelvic stability exercises, strengthening exercises, and stretching of the tight iliopsoas muscle and tendon may be helpful.

Any biomechanical disorder should be corrected or treated, for example, mobilization treatment of a blocking sacroiliac joint.

Iliopsoas bursitis or tendinopathy should be excluded as a cause of chronic groin/hip pain. In most cases, the hip only produces the "snapping" sound without pain symptoms.

Stress fractures

The direct mechanism of stress fractures consists of repetitive compressive and tensile forces, where muscular activity may play an important role, as fatigued or weak muscles have reduced capacity to absorb the forces on the underlying bone. Additionally, forceful muscle contractions can concentrate the forces across a localized area of the bone, exceeding the stress-bearing and tensile capacity of the bone.

The etiology is multifactorial; however, stress fractures are mainly due to insufficient rest periods, usually related to an increase and/or change of the training intensity and impact, volume, and frequency (e.g., in preparation for the competition period or during competition season).

Stress fractures may also be due to biomechanical imbalance, for example, excessive foot pronation (and the specific role of the tibialis posterior tendon, like in the navicular stress fractures), abnormal and altered forces (like in the tarsal coalition), or from foot and ankle injury and muscle imbalance, leading to an imbalance between bone resorption (osteoclast production) and formation (osteoblast formation). Other risk factors include nutritional and metabolic deficiencies (such as calcium and vitamin D), sleep deprivation, collagen abnormalities, and, in women, hormonal imbalances (e.g., as part of the "female athlete triad") (Boden & Osbahr, 2000).

The onset is mostly insidious with pain only in jumping activities and rapidly disappearing with rest, so allowing the gymnast to resume each time after taking some rest, which can explain the delay of the diagnosis. Eventually, it is followed by an acute onset after a poor landing or dismount.

The most common sites of stress fractures in the lower extremity are the tibial shaft and metatarsals (at the neck of the second or the third metatarsal), followed by the navicular and calcaneus stress fracture in the foot.

In determining the approach to therapy management, it is essential to assess the extent of the risks of the stress fracture regarding to its prognosis for poor healing, e.g., high-risk stress fractures tend to develop into chronic injuries with nonunion or delayed union, mainly due to their relative avascularity and therefore need more aggressive treatment (Table 12.2).

The most common sites of high-risk stress fracture in the lower extremity, also due to their morphology and anatomic site, are the middle third of the anterior cortex of the tibia (the tension side of the bone with its morphological bowing), the middle third of the navicular bone (in the relatively limited ankle dorsiflexion and excessive foot pronation), and the base of the fifth metatarsal bone.

The differential diagnosis for stress fractures is stress reaction, which can be regarded as a prefracture bone remodeling, where the bone is weakened.

Plain radiographs in the acute phase are usually negative: fewer than 10–30% demonstrate changes in the first week of the injury. Even after 2–3 weeks, plain radiographs do not show any periosteal changes until approximately 6 weeks, when early fracture healing with changes of periosteal and endosteal bone formation leading to thickening of the periosteum (the so called "callus formation"), is greatest. Occasionally, a radiolucent line can be seen (see Figure 12.7C).

Table 12.2 High-risk and low-risk sites of stress fractures (Boden & Osbahr, 2000).

Sites of high-risk stress fractures	Sites of low-risk stress fractures
Femoral neck (tension side)	Fibula
Patella	Dorsal cortex of the medial tibia
Anterior cortex of the tibia (tension side)	Calcaneus
Talus	Metatarsal bones (except fifth metatarsal)
Medial malleolus	
Navicular bone	
Fifth metatarsal bone (base)	
Hallux sesamoids	

Isotopic bone scan is often used in the acute phase to determine subtle bone pathology like stress fractures, because of the high sensitivity of the method, but it is low in specificity. Moreover this method is invasive and for children and adolescents less preferable, as nowadays MRI has become an adequate diagnostic tool for evaluating stress fractures. The T1-weighted images demonstrate diffuse hypointense area and on fat suppressed T2-weighted and short tau inversion recovery (STIR) images, an increased signal intensity confirms the diagnosis (Figure 12.7A and B).

The overall MRI can define the anatomic location and extent of injury as well as any soft tissue conditions.

In some cases of distinct stress fracture, an MRI will not add more information if CT scan is available, such as in navicular (Figure 12.8) or fifth metatarsal stress fracture.

In therapy management, all the above-mentioned risk factors have to be assessed.

Good teamwork involving a nutritionist, the coach, medical team, gymnast, and parents, is essential.

As rest periods of weeks and months are long lasting for the (elite) gymnast, depending on the period of the gymnast's season, devices such as bone growth stimulation and low-intensity ultrasound to shorten the rest period may be used (Jensen, 1998), although the effectiveness is not evidence-based. Most of the studies on these devices are animal studies and the devices are applied in the nonunion or delayed fractures, but not yet in the (sub)acute phase.

After the immobilization phase, the gymnast may start, for example, in the pool (hydrotherapy) and with light weight-bearing exercises accompanied by the physiotherapist.

High-impact loads are restricted until local pain on palpation has disappeared, using the visual analog scale (VAS), with a score 0–2 out of 10.

In general, after 3 months of rest or immobilization, there is resolution of symptoms in most athletes, but there are cases of longstanding and persistent symptoms.

In the elite gymnast, the choice for surgical intervention (in case of high-risk site) may be needed for a faster return to full gymnastics as well as to prevent recurrence (Figure 12.8D).

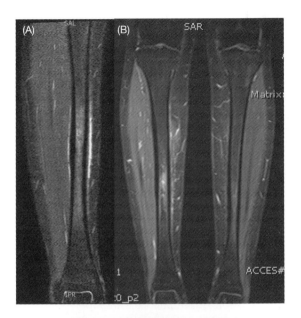

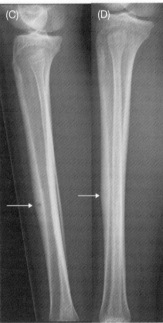

Figure 12.7 Stress fracture in the middle third of the anterior tibia in a gymnast. **(A)** Coronal fat suppressed T2-weighted MRI and **(B)** coronal T1-weighted MRI show the bone marrow edema at the left side (while the initial radiographs were negative). **(C)** The lateral radiographs show the "resorption" line and thickened cortex after 8 weeks (of totally 4 months) of immobilization (arrow) and **(D)** persistent thickened cortex after 5.5 months (arrow).

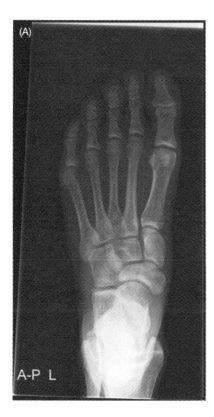

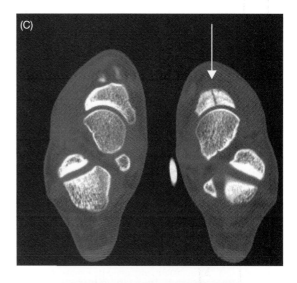

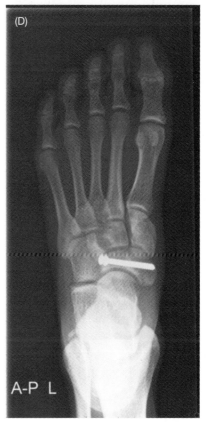

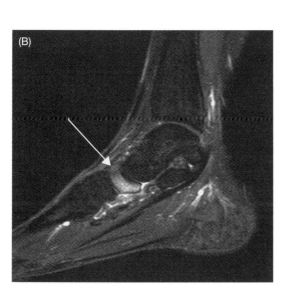

Figure 12.8 Navicular stress fracture of the left foot. **(A)** Negative plain radiograph in the subacute phase. **(B)** MRI shows bone marrow edema (arrow). **(C)** CT scan shows the fracture line classically running vertically from dorsal (arrow). **(D)** Plain radiograph after screw fixation.

Further research

There is lack of literature available on the effectiveness and the outcome of the various rehabilitation programs and techniques for the lower extremity injuries in gymnastics. Although at competition level, serious lower extremity injuries occur frequently.

Most literature on the lower extremity injuries consists of case reports and is particularly limited to Women's Artistic Gymnastics. Several suggestions for further research related to lower extremity injuries are listed below:
• Research to evaluate the long-term effects of injuries in the immature lower extremity, and prospective cohort study on the determinants of physeal injuries, are needed.
• Prospective research in each gymnastics discipline on the intrinsic and extrinsic risk factors of lower extremity injuries will help sports medicine professionals and coaches in early detection and thus appropriate training adaptations.
• Furthermore, assessment of uniform measurement methods and test protocols for the minimum required basic gymnastics physical condition are recommended as well as further research on the minimum required training hours for each age category to prevent loss of concentration, coordination, and muscle strength during long-term training.
• Studies of the effectiveness of implementation of neuromuscular training and core stability programs in the off-season and preseason period and preparticipation musculoskeletal screening are advised.
• Continuous research on the required absorbing characteristics in relation with the stiffness of the floor, mats, and springboard and on improving the spotting techniques will still be needed.

Summary

Familiarity with the specific and common gymnastics medical problems of the lower extremities and the biomechanical requirements and trauma mechanisms may prevent delayed diagnosis and long-lasting damage in the (immature) musculoskeletal system of the gymnast.

Adequate safety equipment, maintenance of balanced flexibility and strength, good (landing) technique, training modification of the number of repetitions of high-impact loads to limit pain, and proprioceptive training and taping or bracing of the ankle after ligament injury, are important tools to reduce the risk of overuse and recurrent injuries of the lower extremities.

Further research on the outcome of the various rehabilitation programs and techniques of the lower extremity injuries is recommended to ultimately develop uniform and effective rehabilitation programs and protocols and training procedures.

Acknowledgments

With thanks to The Medical Library of St Lucas Andreas Hospital, Amsterdam, for supplying the articles and Mrs M.A.Th.P. Wienk, MD, and Mr M.C. de Jonge, MD, Radiologists (St Lucas Andreas Hospital, Amsterdam and Zuwe Hofpoort Hospital, Woerden, The Netherlands) for their support in supplying the specific images.

References

Boden, B.P. and Osbahr, D.C. (2000) High-risk stress fractures: evaluation and treatment. *Journal of the American Academy of Orthopaedic Surgeons*, **8** (6), 344–353.

Caine, D., DiFiori, J., and Maffulli, N. (2006) Physeal injuries in children's and youth sports: reasons for concern? *British Journal of Sports Medicine*, **40** (9) 749–760.

Chilvers, M., Donahue, M., Nassar, L., and Manoli, A. (2007) Foot and ankle injuries in elite female gymnasts. *Foot & Ankle International*, **28** (2), 214–218.

Hutchinson, M.R. and Ireland, M.L. (1995) Knee injuries in female athletes. *Sports Medicine*, **19** (4), 288–302.

Jensen, J.E. (1998). Stress fracture in the world class athlete: a case study. *Medicine and Science in Sports and Exercise*, **30** (6), 783–787.

Kerkhoffs, G.M. and Tol, J.L. (2012) A twist on the athlete's ankle twist: some ankles are more equal than others. *British Journal of Sports Medicine*, **46** (12), 835–836.

Kerkhoffs, G.M., van den Bekerom, M., Elders, L.A., van Beek, P.A., Hullegie, W.A., Bloemers,

G.M., de Heus, E.M., Loogman, M.C., Rosenbrand, K.C., Kuipers, T., Hoogstraten, J.W., Dekker, R., Ten Duis, H.J., van Dijk, C.N., van Tulder, M.W., van der Wees, P.J., and de Bie, R.A. (2012) Diagnosis, treatment and prevention of ankle sprains: an evidence-based clinical guideline. *British Journal of Sports Medicine*, **46** (12), 854–860.

Kolt, G.S. and Caine, D.J. (2010) Gymnastics. In: D.J. Caine and P.A. Harmer (eds), *Epidemiology of Injury in Olympic Sports*, pp. 144–158. Wiley-Blackwell, Chichester.

Lazovic, D., Wegner, U., Peters, G., and Gosse, F. (1996) Ultrasound for diagnosis of apophyseal injuries. *Knee Surgery, Sports Traumatology, Arthroscopy*, **3** (4), 234–237.

Peck, D.M. (1995) Apophyseal injuries in the young athlete. *American Family Physician*, **51** (8), 1891–1898.

Salter, R.B. and Harris, W.R. (1963) Injuries involving the epiphyseal plate. *Journal of Bone and Joint Surgery [American]*, **45**, 587–622.

van Dijk, C.N. (2006) Anterior and posterior ankle impingement. *Foot and Ankle Clinics*, **11** (3), 663–683.

van Dijk, C.N., Mol, B.W., Lim, L.S., Marti, R.K., and Bossuyt, P.M. (1996) Diagnosis of ligament rupture of the ankle joint. Physical examination, arthrography, stress radiography and sonography compared in 160 patients after inversion trauma. *Acta Orthopaedica Scandinavica*, **67** (6), 566–570.

Vandervliet, E.J., Vanhoenacker, F.M., Snoeckx, A., Gielen, J.L., Van, D.P., and Parizel, P.M. (2007). Sports-related acute and chronic avulsion injuries in children and adolescents with special emphasis on tennis. *British Journal of Sports Medicine*, **41** (11), 827–831.

Recommended reading

Blatnik, T.R. and Briskin, S. (2013) Bilateral knee pain in a high-level gymnast. *Clinical Journal of Sport Medicine*, **23** (1), 77–79.

Brukner, P. and Khan, K. (2012) *Clinical Sports Medicine*, 4th ed. Sydney: McGraw-Hill.

Caine, D.J. and Nassar, L. (2005) Gymnastics injuries. *Medicine and Sport Science*, **48**, 18–58.

Caine, D.J. and Golightly, Y.M. (2011) Osteoarthritis as an outcome of paediatric sport: an epidemiological perspective. *British Journal of Sports Medicine*, **45** (4), 298–303.

Guideline for "the acute inversiontrauma of the ankle". Dutch Society for Sports Physicians (VSG).

Harringe, M.L., Renstrom, P., and Werner, S. (2007) Injury incidence, mechanism and diagnosis in top-level team-gym: a prospective study conducted over one season. *Scandinavian Journal of Medicine and Science in Sports*, **17** (2), 115–119.

Kerkhoffs, G.M., Versteegh, V.E., Sierevelt, I.N., Kloen, P., and van Dijk, C.N. (2012) Treatment of proximal metatarsal V fractures in athletes and non-athletes. *British Journal of Sports Medicine*, **46** (9), 644–648.

Kirialanis, P., Malliou, P., Beneka, A., and Giannakopoulos, K. (2003) Occurrence of acute lower limb injuries in artistic gymnasts in relation to event and exercise phase. *British Journal of Sports Medicine*, **37** (2), 137–139.

Marshall, S.W., Covassin, T., Dick, R., Nassar, L.G., and Agel, J. (2007) Descriptive epidemiology of collegiate women's gymnastics injuries: National Collegiate Athletic Association Injury Surveillance System, 1988–1989 through 2003–2004. *Journal of Athletic Training*, **42** (2), 234–240.

Chapter 13
Treatment and rehabilitation of common spine/trunk/head injuries

Larry Nassar

College of Osteopathic Medicine, Michigan State University, East Lansing, MI, USA

Introduction

Spinal and head trauma is common in the variety of sports included under the umbrella term known as gymnastics. Unfortunately, the epidemiology of gymnastics injuries has been sparse over the last decade. Harringe *et al.* (2007) performed the most recent prospective study over one gymnastics season in Scandinavia and reported no head injuries; however, 24.4% and 31.3% of all injuries involved the spine in female and male teamgym gymnasts, respectively. A study by O'Kane *et al.* (2011), which is the most recent article on club-level gymnastics injuries, was a retrospective study performed in the Seattle, Washington, USA area. It included five gymnastics clubs and 96 gymnasts. They reported that 15–30% of the gymnasts had a concussion depending on how they defined concussion. There were 5 acute back injuries reported (8.8% of all acute injuries) and 14 overuse back injuries (18.4% of all overuse injuries). Further research is needed to better understand the epidemiology of club-level gymnastics.

Concussion management constantly changes as more information about the etiologies and treatments emerge from the medical community. An overview of concussion management in the gymnast is reviewed. Controversy also exists in

Gymnastics, First Edition. Edited by Dennis J. Caine, Keith Russell and Liesbeth Lim. © 2013 International Olympic Committee. Published 2013 by John Wiley & Sons, Ltd.

some of the treatments regarding spinal injuries. The purpose of this chapter is to review treatment and rehabilitation of common spine/trunk/head injuries affecting gymnasts. This chapter will also review several spinal conditions and recommend therapeutic interventions that may be best applied to the injured gymnast to enhance their recovery.

Concussions

Concussions are the most common type of traumatic brain injury that the gymnast sustains. A concussion is a milder form of traumatic brain injury. It is defined as a complex pathophysiological process affecting the brain, induced by traumatic biomechanical forces secondary to direct or indirect forces to the head (McCrory *et al.*, 2009). Direct contact with the safety mats and the apparatus is frequently the cause of this injury. Direct impact with cervical flexion and extension may result in concussion and is the most common type of mechanism of injury. Rotational forces of the head and neck are not as common but may lead to more severe symptoms. Gymnasts may land hard on their buttocks and sustain a concussion through impulsive forces transmitted up the trunk and spinal column to the brain.

Neck strength is important (Daneshvar *et al.*, 2011). The neck muscles are able to assist in absorbing the traumatic forces thereby decreasing brain pathology. Neck muscles are able to support the head and absorb the forces with flexion/extension motion patterns better than in a rotational pattern. Forceful cervical rotation may create greater brain pathology than experienced with cervical flexion and extension. Commonly, males will have stronger neck muscles and proportionally smaller heads than female gymnasts. The male gymnast may sustain greater forces and yet have a milder concussion if their neck musculature is able to absorb the forces well.

Most concussions are a disturbance of the brain related to neurometabolic dysfunction rather than structural brain injury and are therefore associated with normal CT scans and MRIs of the brain. Concussion may or may not involve a loss of consciousness or loss of memory. These forms of brain injury result in a complex mixture of physical, cognitive, emotional, and sleep-related symptoms. Recovery may take from several minutes to days, weeks, months, or even longer in more significant injuries. Fortunately, most typical concussions have a rapid onset of short-lived neurologic dysfunction that resolves spontaneously. Evaluation and grading of concussion is an ongoing debate in the medical community (Guskiewicz & McLeod, 2011).

The treatment for concussions is focused on physical and cognitive rest until the gymnast is asymptomatic. It is not uncommon to find that it takes 7–10 days for all the symptoms of a concussion to resolve. Similar to resting an injured joint to allow for healing to take place, the brain needs rest after it is concussed. During the initial rest phase it is beneficial for the gymnast to avoid reading, texting, keyboarding, video/computer games, watching television, loud music, bright lights, and of course physical activity in and out of the gymnastics venue. This may require the school-aged gymnast to stay home from school to rest the brain. Once the gymnast is asymptomatic then the brain may be challenged again just as you would add back exercises to an injured joint.

The gymnast should start with adding back stimuli outside of the gym to the brain including all activities of daily living: reading, texting, keyboarding, and a return to school work. Next, the gymnast should add back light aerobic activity to increase their heart rate to a maximum of 70% of their predicted maximum heart rate. The next step is in adding gymnastics-sport-specific exercises.

The most basic of this type of activity would be leaps and jumps in the gym. The next step would be to add back skills requiring inversion of the body like handstands and walkovers. Basic flipping and twisting acrobatic skills are added next followed by the more advanced skills of the gymnast that require multiple flips and twists and advanced skills on the variety of apparatus.

Cervical spine injury

The cervical spine has the overall greatest range of motion when compared to the rest of the spine. Normally, there is a lordotic curvature of the cervical spine. When there is injury, the cervical muscles tend to spasm to splint the spine. This tends to create a straightening of the cervical lordosis and may create a reversal of the lordotic curve. A key point in cervical injuries is to have a high suspicion of pathology after a gymnast lands on their head. Initially there may be no signs of radiculopathy or myopathy and no point tenderness with palpation. However, if significant muscle spasm is present, imaging studies need to be performed to insure that a vertebral, disc, or spinal cord injury did not occur.

Vertical compression injuries occur with axial loading of the head with forces transmitted to the cervical spine. A Jefferson's fracture of the anterior and posterior arches of C1 and burst fractures of the lower cervical spine may occur. In addition, an acute herniated disc may occur with vertical compression injuries.

Hyperflexion injuries to the cervical spine create an anterior translation of the vertebra. Significant ligament disruption, facet subluxation, veterbra dislocation, and vertebra teardrop fracture may occur. These injuries are unstable and require surgical intervention. The clay-shoveler's fracture (a stable fracture of the spinous process of the lower cervical vertebra) and simple wedge fractures are usually stable injures. Acute disc herniation may also be the result of a hyperflexion cervical trauma.

Hyperextension injuries to the cervical spine create a posterior translation of the vertebra. Avulsion fractures of the anterior arch of the atlas and teardrop fractures occur in the anterior vertebral column. Fractures of the posterior arch of the atlas and extension teardrop fractures occur in the posterior column. More significant pathology occurs when the hyperextension injury creates damage in multiple vertebrae at the same time. Hangman's fracture (an unstable fracture of both pedicles or pars interarticularis of the C2 vertebra), vertebra dislocations, and vertebra subluxations are examples of these more severe injuries.

Treatment and rehabilitation of cervical injuries are dependent on the severity of the pathology. It is beyond the scope of this chapter to enter into the details of the severe traumas. However, for the strains and sprains of the cervical spine, physical therapy (PT) is recommended to decrease the inflammation, decrease the pain, and return to full musculosketal function.

Overuse injuries

Gymnastics require the athlete to combine amazing strength and flexibility of the spinal structures. If a musculoskeletal imbalance develops, back pain often follows. These imbalances may lead to strains, sprains, facet syndromes, and even stress fractures if they are not attended to in a timely fashion. When a gymnast presents with gradual onset, nonacute back pain, the most important aspect of the treatment is to first determine the cause. Knowledge of the cause of the back pain allows the medical specialist and coach to best prepare a treatment plan. By addressing the cause a better long-term resolution of the gymnast's symptoms may be developed. Rest from the aggravating activity is often not all that is required. After the rest period is completed and the gymnast returns to the activity, the pain may well return. By taking the same gymnast with the same body mechanics and returning them to the same activity, the same pathology may eventually return. The gymnast's body or the gymnast's activity may need to be changed. In many cases, both the gymnast's body and the activity need to be changed.

In order to change the gymnast's body the first step is to identify the risk factors that the gymnast's body may possess that place him or her at higher risk for back pain. This requires a detailed biomechanical analysis of the gymnast's body. Gymnasts may have well-defined muscle structure. However, superficial appearance of muscle structure may be deceiving. It is not always how the gymnast looks. More importantly, it is how the gymnast functions that is the vital key in understanding the cause of the mechanical back pain. The gymnast needs to be evaluated to see what muscles test as strong and what muscles test as weak. They need to be evaluated to test their flexibility. Kinesthetics and proprioception are additional factors that need to be assessed (Table 13.1). This may require a team effort involving the medical professional and the coach.

The assessment of these muscle imbalances of tight and weak muscles needs to be analyzed to ascertain if in fact the weak muscles are actually weak or just inhibited in their action. Research has demonstrated that certain groupings of tight muscles can directly affect the function of other muscles by neurologically inhibiting their ability to appropriately contract (Jull & Janda, 1987). The medical practitioner/coach may test this by stretching the tight muscles and then immediately retesting the strength of the weak muscles. If the weak muscles test strong, then there is an underlying neuromuscular inhibition of the weak muscle by the tight muscle.

Evaluation of how the upper and lower extremities affect the core needs to be performed. For example, does the gymnast experience increased back pain when performing trunk active range of motion with the arms raised up over head when compared to arms next to the side. This may indicate that a restriction involving the shoulder complex may be contributing to the back pain. This information is valuable in the construction of the rehabilitation program for the injured gymnast.

It is one thing to isolate specific muscles and test their function of strength and flexibility and it is another thing to functionally test these muscle groups. Just like an injured gymnast with a sprained ankle needs to regain the ability to balance on the injured extremity by performing static and dynamic proprioceptive drills, the gymnast with back pain needs to be able to restore proper static and dynamic proprioception and kinesthetic awareness. They need to be able to restore their ability to coordinate the function of the muscles to

Table 13.1 Overview of muscle and joint tightness (restrictions), weakness (inhibition), and kinesthetic/proprioception.

Muscles prone to tightness	Muscles prone to weakness	Muscle and joint kinesthetics/ proprioception
Gastocnemious/ soleus	Peroneals	Control of the core in a static neutral position
Hip adductors	Anterior tibialis	Control of the core in a static flexed position (posterior pelvic tilt)
Hamstrings	Vastus medialis and lateralis	Control of the core in a static extended position (anterior pelvic tilt)
Rectus femoris/ illiopsoas	Gluteal muscle group	Dynamic control of the core as it moves through flexed, neutral, and extended motion patterns
Tensor fascia latae	Rectus abdominus	Coordinated control of the core with dynamic motions of the upper quadrants
Piriformis	Transverse abdominus	Coordinated control of the core with dynamic motions of the lower quadrants
Erector spinae	Serratus anterior	Coordinated control of the core with dynamic motions of the upper and lower quadrants
Quadratus lumborum	Rhomboids	
Pectoralis major	Lower trapezious	
Upper trapezius		
Levator scapulae		
Sternocleidomastoid		
Scalenes		
Lattisimus dorsi		

adequately control the spine with static positional holds and through dynamic core motions. The gymnast should able to "sense" and to "feel" that the appropriate muscles are working when performing the movement and know where their extremities are in positional relationship to their core. The gymnast may think they are positioning their core in proper alignment with their drill/skill.

However, they may actually be in a piked or arched position in their core with a posterior or anterior tilted pelvis. The medical professional can have the gymnast perform specific clinical exercises to assess their body alignment awareness. In addition, the coach may have the gymnast perform some basic skills and analyze the gymnast's body position with these movements too. There needs to be crossover from the medical clinic to the gym. Enhancement of the function of the gymnast's skills with pain resolution is the ultimate goal.

Rapid growth during adolescence is another area to investigate when an adolescent gymnast presents with gradual onset of low back pain. With lengthening of the limbs and trunk, a loss of coordination and imbalance may occur. With this same lengthening a gymnast's strength-to-length ratio may be altered and they become relatively weaker. The gymnast may also experience a relative tightness in muscles that were more flexible prior to the rapid change in growth. Female gymnasts experience a change in their pelvic shape during adolescence. This may alter their core dynamics.

During adolescence, congenital issues of the spine may be brought to light. The gymnast may have a structural anomaly that was asymptomatic prior to the alteration in body size. This anomaly may then become symptomatic. With gradual onset of low back pain during adolescence, the medical professional should consider the possibility that the gymnast has a transitional lumbosacral vertebra, hemisacralization of the fifth lumbar vertebra, or partial lumbarization of the first sacral vertebra (Figure 13.1). These anomalies may create facet inflammation or sacralillitis due to the altered mechanics. Thoracic spine pain may be a result of the development of Scheuermann's disease. Scoliosis may become more significant. The medical professional needs to be aware of these issues and include them in the differential diagnosis. Further discussion on these topics will occur elsewhere in this chapter.

Rehabilitation of overuse injuries requires more than just rest. Rest is a relative term for a gymnast. In more significant and severe cases, complete rest from all gymnastics activity is required. However, in most mild to moderate cases, the gymnast requires relative rest. Relative rest is described as resting the gymnast from the aggravating skills and allowing

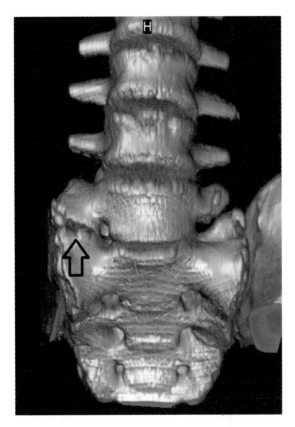

Figure 13.1 3D CT scan showing a L5 vertebra with right-sided hemisacralization. (With courtesy of Lawrence Nassar.)

that muscle for up to an hour and coaches generally avoid this type of activity (Marek *et al.*, 2005). However, with rehabilitation, the understanding of muscle inhibition needs to be first addressed. Therefore, it is important to start the rehabilitation session with muscle flexibility before the strengthening portion. By stretching the tight muscles first and then adding the strengthening drills, the gymnast's muscle inhibition may be reduced and the inhibited muscle may respond better to the exercises. If this inhibition is not reversed, then the gymnast may actually reinforce the pathological pattern of muscle compensation. The use of foam rollers, massage sticks, and massage balls are beneficial for use to assist in the flexibility of muscles. The medical professional may perform myofascial release techniques: teach the gymnast special tri-plane myofascial unwinding exercises (Figure 13.2) and specific stretches to perform as part of a routine that initiates each rehabilitation session. Shoulder flexibility (Figure 13.3) and upper thoracic mobility assist with creating lower lumbar stability. The gymnast should be able to lift upwards through their arms pressing the upper thoracic spine caudad and anterior as they arch/extend their back creating a lengthening affect to the spine. They should be advised against shortening their spine by collapsing down and hinging at the lower lumbar spine.

him/her to continue participation in those skills that do not negatively influence the injury. The coach may be asked to participate in analyzing the skills that aggravate the gymnast's spine to see if there is a flaw in the gymnast's technique that needs to be addressed. The coach may assist in the recovery of the injured gymnast by breaking down the skill into its basic components and having the gymnast "relearn" the skill with improved form and technique. This may lend itself to less stress on the gymnast's spine. These skills should not only include acrobatic skills but also dance skills.

The rehabilitation from a therapeutic exercise standpoint should be centered on the biomechanical evaluation of the gymnast. The tight muscle groups should first be addressed. Rehabilitation is different than conditioning. With conditioning, over-stretching of a muscle at the start of a practice may negatively impact the power generating capacity of

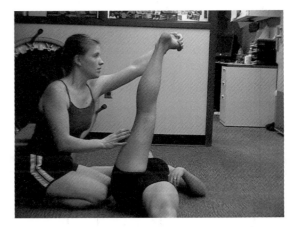

Figure 13.2 Tri-plane myofascial unwinding of the lower extremity with hip flexion, hip adduction, and hip internal rotation combined with ankle inversion and ankle dorsiflexion. This can be done with a partner or with the use of a stretch cord. (With courtesy of Lawrence Nassar.)

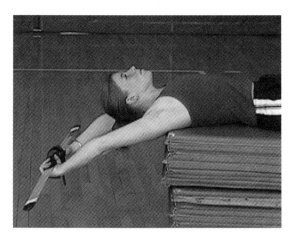

Figure 13.3 Shoulder flexibility may be performed with the gymnast lying on a panel mat. The gymnast holds onto a light weight to assist with the stretch. They should keep their ribs flat, hips flat, and legs adductor together. The stretch should not cause them to arch their back and they should not allow their ribs to flare out. This helps to isolate the stretch to the shoulder complex. (With courtesy of Lawrence Nassar.)

During the flexibility phase of the rehabilitation session, the gymnast may benefit from slow deep breathing. It may be beneficial to have the gymnast hold the stretch for a certain number of deep slow breaths (i.e., 5–10 deep slow breaths) instead of having them focus on holding a stretch for a certain time period. They need to allow their bodies to relax to best respond to the flexibility activities. It may be important for the gymnast to perform short periods of stretching several times a day to improve their flexibility, that is, maybe 10–15 minutes of stretching per session, three to five sessions a day.

The strengthening of weak and inhibited muscles requires the gymnast to think. They need to be engaged mentally to ensure that the actual muscle/muscle groups are activating with the exercise. If the gymnast is distracted and not focused on the exercises, they may allow for further compensation to occur thus reinforcing the pathologic muscle patterning that created the back pain. If the gymnast is given a number of repetitions to do in a set, they should focus on proper technique with each repetition. If their form breaks down, they need to stop even if they have not completed the required number of repetitions. They need to build their strength with proper form first and then increase the number of repetitions. These types of details are important for a rehabilitation program to best accomplish its goals.

Strengthening exercises can be performed in a variety of ways. Static positional holds such as a side and prone planks are important to perform as part of the basic foundation of the rehabilitation program. Advancing to core exercises in which the gymnast is performing the exercises on a softer or wobbly surface may enhance the difficulty of the drills. The medical professional may incorporate the use of a Swiss ball, Bosu ball, wobble discs, and other such devices for this purpose. These devices may assist in not only strengthening the spine but also in enhancing the proprioception and kinesthetic awareness of the spine.

It is important to progress beyond static exercises. Dynamic exercises in which the spine is moved through a controlled range of motion, are beneficial to assist in the gymnast's strength and kinesthetic awareness. The pelvic clock in which the gymnast learns to tilt their pelvis in a variety of directions using the face of a clock as a means to direct their motion is a basic dynamic core exercise. Side planks with arm and leg movements, twisting side planks, and rotational trunk motions while seated on a Swiss ball, are all examples of more advanced dynamic core exercises. In addition, core stability performed with the gymnast in a pike handstand and handstand position is beneficial to incorporate stability through the upper quadrant. For example, performing pike handstands on a wobble disc with the gymnast pressing through their shoulders to create clockwise and counterclockwise circles while maintaining a stable core position is a challenging core exercise (Figure 13.4).

Manual medicine techniques for realignment of the spine and the extremities may be performed during the rehabilitation. These realignment techniques may allow the gymnast to improve the function and kinesthetic awareness of the spine. This may prove beneficial with assisting the gymnast's recovery.

Therapeutic modalities involving a variety of means to heat and cool the injured tissue, augmented soft tissue mobilization techniques, acupuncture, vacuum cupping, laser light therapy, electrical stimulation, and therapeutic ultrasound

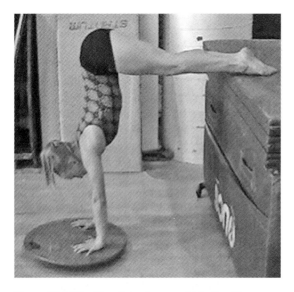

Figure 13.4 Piked handstand on a wobble disc. The gymnast presses through their shoulders to create clockwise and counterclockwise circles while maintaining a stable core position. (With courtesy of Lawrence Nassar.)

are some of the commonly administered treatments as part of a comprehensive PT plan. The uses of rigid, semi-rigid, and soft elastic compression lumbar braces are frequently employed to alleviate more painful conditions. Adhesive strapping has been used for many decades; most recently Kinesio Taping techniques have been applied to the injured gymnast to assist with the treatment of spinal pain. The use of these therapeutic modalities requires further investigation since their evidence-based effectiveness has not been fully established.

Rehabilitation programs may become overwhelming for a gymnast if they are told to do many exercises without a plan as to how to incorporate the exercises into their daily routine. The medical professional and coach should work together on implementing such a plan of action. First the number of strengthening exercises may be divided into four groups. If each group holds 3–4 core exercises, the gymnast is easily able to perform 12–16 different core exercises effectively in a week without overwhelming the gymnast by doing too many at one time. Each group can have a balance between static and dynamic exercises, incorporate a good variety of exercises so as not to overemphasize one motion pattern in a single group, and avoid quickly fatiguing a specific muscle group. This helps to prevent the gymnast from going into a pathological compensatory muscle firing pattern while performing their rehabilitation exercises. The gymnast may perform one of the exercise groups at the beginning of each practice and one of the exercise groups at the end of each practice on Monday, Wednesday, and Friday. Repeat this template with the other two exercise groups for Tuesday, Thursday, and Saturday. In addition, the flexibility/mobility of the restricted muscles and body regions needs to be incorporated into the schedule as well. Finding time to stretch/foam roll three to five times a day may be a difficult task if it is not planned out in advance for the gymnast. Please see Table 13.2 below for an overview of a weekly plan for a spinal rehabilitation program.

Table 13.2 Chart overview of a weekly spinal rehabilitation program. Flexibility refers to the use of stretches, foam roller, myo stick, myo ball, and so on, to enhance motion of a restricted/tight muscle or body region. Group A, Group B, Group C, and Group D refer to the four different exercise groups to enhance core strength and core proprioception/kinesthetic awareness.

	Monday	Tuesday	Wednesday	Thursday	Friday	Saturday	Sunday
Morning	Flexibility	Flexibility	Flexibility	Flexibility	Flexibility	Flexibility	Flexibility
Beginning of practice	Flexibility Group A	Flexibility Group C	Flexibility Group A	Flexibility Group C	Flexibility Group A	Flexibility Group C	
Mid-practice	Flexibility	Flexibility	Flexibility	Flexibility	Flexibility	Flexibility	Flexibility
End of practice	Flexibility Group B	Flexibility Group D	Flexibility Group B	Flexibility Group D	Flexibility Group B	Flexibility Group D	
Before bedtime	Flexibility	Flexibility	Flexibility	Flexibility	Flexibility	Flexibility	Flexibility

Spondylolysis and spondylolisthesis

Stress fractures to the spine most commonly occur in the lower lumbar posterior column. Spondylolysis is the term used for these types of fractures. Spondylolysis is defined as a fatigue fracture of the vertebral arch usually occurring at the pars interarticularis. Spondylolysis may also occur through the pedicle portion of the posterior vertebra, but this is far rarer. This is a stress overuse injury that is created by repetitive hyperextension and rotation of the spine (Standaert & Herring, 2000). An acute traumatic event creating a microfracturing of the bone may be an initial insult. The fracture is then completed by the repetition of extension and rotation forces. The fifth and fourth lumbar vertebrae are the most common location of these fractures. Spondylolysis that occurs above L4 may take longer to heal then those that are at L4 or L5. Unilateral spondylolysis, either on the right side or left side of the vertebra (Figure 13.5), has an easier course of recovery, in general, than a bilateral spondylolysis in which both sides are damaged.

Spondylolithesis is a condition in the spine in which there is a translation of one vertebra on another vertebra. The superior vertebra generally moves anterior to the inferior vertebrae. Spondylolisthesis is commonly grouped into two main types: isthmic and degenerative (Wiltse *et al.*, 1975). Degenerative spondylolithesis results from degeneration of the intervertebral disc. The degenerative type of spondylolisthesis may result in anterior or posterior translation. Anterior translation is called anterolisthesis and posterior translation is called retrolisthesis. Isthmic spondylolisthesis is the most common type of spondylolithesis seen in gymnastics. Isthmic spondylolisthesis is categorized into grades based upon how far the superior vertebra translates anterior to the inferior vertebra (Meyerding, 1932). Grade 1 spondylolisthesis is a translation of the superior vertebra up to 25% of the distance of the vertebral body of the inferior vertebra. Grade 2 is a translation from 25 to 50%. Grade 3 is a translation from 50 to 75%. Grade 4 is a translation from 75 to 100% and grade 5 is when the superior vertebra has translated past the inferior vertebrae and an angle is created between the two vertebrae (Figure 13.6). Progression of low-grade (grades 1 and 2) spondylolithesis is very low. Only about 4–5% of adolescents will show progression (Lonstein, 1999). Many gymnasts with grade 1–2 isthmic spondylolisthesis are asymptomatic.

The use of a bone stimulation unit is controversial but may be of benefit to use to enhance bone healing. If the gymnast does not have pain with normal

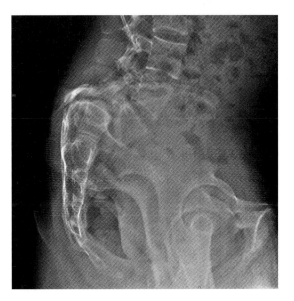

Figure 13.6 Grade 5 spondylolisthesis. 17-year-old female athlete walked into the medical clinic with concerns about how her back looked and denied any significant pain with her dance or acrobatics.

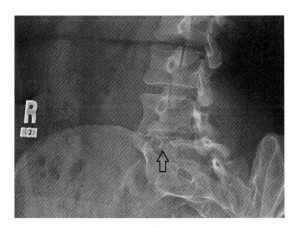

Figure 13.5 Spondylolysis is demonstrated on the right side of the L5 at the pars articularis.

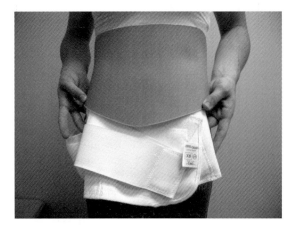

Figure 13.7 A "warm and form" lumbar support is a type of brace that is an elastic soft lumbar support with a pocket in the back. The orthotist warms a plastic insert and molds it to the gymnast's back and inserts it into the pocket.

life (activities of daily living outside of the gym) then do not place them in a brace for their back. If the gymnast has pain with normal life, then place them in a Criss Cross warm and form type of back brace (see Figure 13.7). They may need to wear the brace 23 hours a day, removed only to shower/bathe. The goal is to relieve them from pain with normal life activities, including sleeping. This then allows the injury to heal quicker since the gymnast is not irritating the pathological site. It also helps prevent muscle spasms. Most gymnasts do not want to be in the brace, but after they use it to sit in school and they notice that they can sit much better with less pain, then they are more compliant with wearing the brace. If after 1–2 weeks in the warm and form back brace they still have pain with normal life, then place them in a customized thoracolumbosacral orthosis (TLSO). This is a more rigid and motion restricting brace (see Figure 13.8). They need to wear the brace 23 hours a day. They may remove it to shower and do therapeutic exercises. Once in the TLSO, they remain in that brace until they can arch without pain. Then, they may remove the TLSO and return to the smaller more flexible warm and form brace if needed. Bracing for spondylolysis and spondylolisthesis is controversial. The medical literature is mixed with some articles recommending bracing and others finding it to be of no help and others have found bracing causes increased stress to the

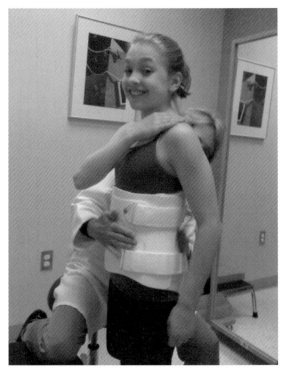

Figure 13.8 A thoracolumbosacral orthosis is a customized rigid brace. (With courtesy of Lawrence Nassar.)

pars (Standaert, 2005). See Figure 13.9 for an overview of the use of a brace presented here.

In general, after 4 weeks reassess the gymnast. If their exam is significantly better and they have full pain-free range of motion, then they may be placed on the fast track and they wear the warm and form brace only 12 hours a day for the next 2 weeks. At 6 weeks recheck them and if they are doing well, the brace is then only used in the gym. At 8 weeks the hard plastic is removed from the back pouch of the warm and form brace and then by 10–12 weeks they progress to full gymnastics. The soft brace is completely removed once they have been able to return to full gymnastics. The benefit of the soft brace is a reminder to the gymnast and the coach to continue doing the rehabilitation exercises and progress with caution. It is also a proprioceptive reminder to control the core better.

After 4 weeks if their exam is improved but they still have pain with trunk extension then they are on the standard track. They then use the back brace

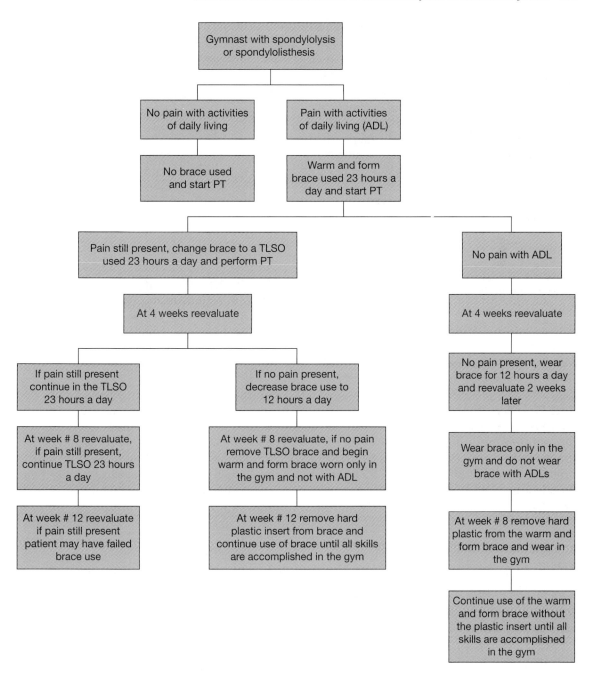

Figure 13.9 Overview of the use of a brace for the treatment of spondylolysis and spondylolisthesis. ADL, activities of daily living; PT, physical therapy; TLSO, thoracolumbosacral orthosis.

for 12 hours per day for the next 4 weeks and they may not need to be rechecked again until week 8. If they are then able to arch fully pain-free then they wear the brace only while in the gym. If at 8 weeks they still have pain with full extension then they stay in the brace 12 hours a day and recheck them again at 12 weeks. If they are able to arch pain-free then they only wear the brace in the gym and remove the hard plastic back out of the warm and form brace. Continue the brace without the plastic insert until they are back to full gymnastics, then they remove the brace completely. By wearing the warm and form brace without the hard plastic insert, the soft elastic corset helps to remind the gymnast to keep their core muscles engaged. Some medical professionals will place all symptomatic gymnasts into a TLSO for 12 weeks without reevaluation until week number 12. If pain is still present after 12 weeks of TLSO brace use, then either consider further brace use or begin evaluation for possible fusion of the fracture (Cavalier *et al.*, 2006).

As soon as the gymnast is diagnosed with spondylolysis or spondylolisthesis it is recommended that the gymnast starts PT to correct any muscle imbalances found and improve their overall core stability and function. In addition to flexibility of the extremities, for the first 4 weeks they work with neutral trunk-to-trunk flexion bias. If they are on the fast track then by week 6 they start working into trunk extension in PT. If they are on the standard track, they start working trunk extension somewhere between 8 and 12 weeks. If they are placed into the TLSO then in general they are not able to start extension work until about 12 weeks. They must be pain-free with normal life before starting to work into extension in PT. They gradually increase their trunk strength in extension. It may be easier to start to challenge the spine in extension by working the hips into extension first, then add trunk extension, and finally add trunk and hip extension combined at the same time. They must be able to arch first in PT with their exercises before they are allowed to do arching skills in the gym.

The key generic points in PT to be addressed:
• Shoulder flexibility and upper thoracic mobility restrictions need to be addressed.
• Iliopsoas/quadriceps/iliotibial band/erector spinae flexibility.
• Normal muscle firing patterns need to be restored.
• Gluteus medious strength, gluteus maximus inferior fibers strength, and lower abdominal strength need to be enhanced.
• Just like other joints in the body, kinesthetic awareness and proprioception of the spine needs to be restored.

• Overall, the therapist needs to correct all the musculoskeletal imbalances that are risk factors for low back pain to prevent reoccurrence of the injury.

Lumbar facet syndrome

The facet joints are synovial joints reinforced by fibrous capsule that connect the inferior vertebral arch of one vertebral to the superior vertebral arch of another vertebra. Facet syndrome of the spine was defined in 1933 as lumbosacral pain, with or without sciatica, which was likely to occur after a sudden rotation trauma to the lumbosacral spine (Ghormley, 1933). Further investigations showed that not only compression of the facet joints but also repetitive distraction forces of the facet joints from lateral trunk bending and forward trunk flexion frequently create pathology (Cohen & Raja, 2007). The nature of activities involved with gymnastics places them at risk for trauma to their facet joints. It is not uncommon to find the gymnast with significant low back pain who has no sign of fracture on imaging studies, to have a facet syndrome. The gymnast with facet pain may experience more discomfort than a gymnast with spondylolysis when the gymnast is asked to move into trunk flexion, moving from a trunk flexed position to an extended position, and with lateral side bending. Forceful landings with the trunk flexed places great strain on the lumbar facet capsules.

Treatment of a gymnast with lumbar facet syndrome should begin with rest from the aggravating activity. The medical professional should perform a physical examination to investigate for biomechanical/neuromuscular patterns that may be underlying risk factors. Therapeutic intervention should be conservative to start with. PT to treat the physical examination findings needs to be employed. If pain persists, then invasive procedures, that is, facet blocks, may need to be performed. The role of facet blocks for facet syndromes still remains controversial and more medical research in this area needs to be conducted (Cohen & Raja, 2007). Furthermore, lumbar facet syndrome, as a whole, is a controversial topic in the medical literature. The pathological cause, evaluation, and treatment procedures all need further investigation to better understand this syndrome.

Other spine and back conditions

Scheuermann's disease and endplate fractures

Scheuermann's disease is described as three or more consecutive thoracic vertebrae with irregularity of the endplates creating a wedging of the vertebra body of at least 5°, Schmorl's nodes, and loss of disc space height that creates a hyperkyphosis of greater than 40° (Sorensen, 1964). The cause of Scheuermann's disease is unknown. However, it has been documented in the medical literature that Scheuermann's disease may be caused by repeated or acute trauma to the immature spine (Tribus, 1998). The endplates (vertebral body growth plates) of a gymnast are at risk to damage from the stress of the sport especially with hyperflexion injuries. In general, however, the presentation of Scheuermann's disease is a nontraumatic gradual onset of thoracic spine pain with loss of thoracic spine mobility. Atypical Scheuermann's disease is the type of vertebral body wedging with endplate irregularity that does not possess the hyperkyphosis. This pathology may occur at the thoracolumbar junction or in the lumbar spine alone. In general, this condition is self-limited and the pain associated with the condition resolves with endplate closure as the gymnast progresses through adolescence. Pain associated with this condition seems to be increased with the atypical form (Figure 13.10).

Treatment of Scheuermann's disease is mainly symptomatic and includes rest from aggravating activities, PT, occasional use of bracing to relieve more moderate to severe levels of pain, and rarely surgical correction of the hyperkyphosis.

Endplate fractures from acute or repetitive stress involved with gymnastics may give a similar appearance as Scheuermann's disease but this would be rare to occur at three consecutive levels. Schmorl's nodes may or may not be present. Frequently, disc space narrowing may be present since the trauma

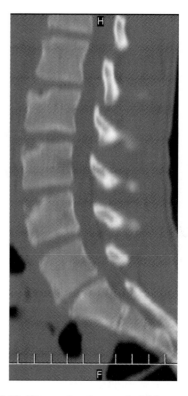

Figure 13.10 CT scan showing atypical Scheuermann's disease of the lumbar spine.

that created the endplate fracture may also cause insult to the disc. Endplate fractures may be difficult to diagnose when the endplates are not readily seen on radiographs. This occurs when the endplates are very immature. However, as the spine matures, the vertebra may develop with a wedge shape due to the damage. The endplate fracture may look like a chip off the anterior superior or anterior inferior edge of the vertebra. Less commonly the posterior portion of the vertebral endplate is involved. It is not uncommon for endplate fractures to occur between T10 and L2 at the thoracolumbar junction (Figure 13.11) and the L4, L5, and S1 levels at the lumbosacral junction (Katz & Scerpella, 2003). Endplate fractures are also referred to as anterior limbus fracture and avulsion of the ring apophysis.

Treatment of endplate fractures is similar to treatment of spondylolysis. Bracing is used, if needed, to help reduce pain. Rest from all activity that creates pain is important. PT similar to that described with spondylolysis may prove to be beneficial.

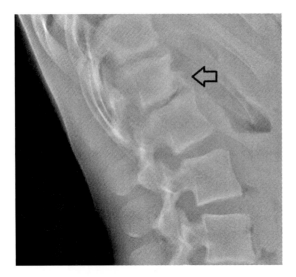

Figure 13.11 L1 endplate fracture.

Scoliosis

Idiopathic scoliosis is not uncommon in gymnasts. It has been reported in the medical literature that rhythmic gymnasts have a high occurrence of idiopathic scoliosis. It has been hypothesized that ligamentous/joint laxity combined with delay in menarche and asymmetrical repetitive loading of the spine from favoring or dominance of one side of the trunk more than the other in rhythmic routines may explain this finding in the Rhythmic Gymnastics population (Tanchev *et al.*, 2000). Frequently, idiopathic scoliosis is asymptomatic. Historically, in the early medical literature written at the beginning of the 1900s, "gymnastics" was the mainstay of nonsurgical treatment for scoliosis. Unless there is significant pain, rest from gymnastics is not required. The strength training and inherent core stability needed to be successful in the sport of gymnastics works as an advantage. It may be of benefit for the coach to review the gymnast's skills and try to incorporate a balance in their skill set so as not to overuse one side of the spine in their routines. Formal PT to improve the strength of the lengthened/weakened muscles on the convexity side of the curve coupled with stretching of the tight/shortened muscles on the concavity side of the curve form the basics of the therapeutic exercises. Bracing may be required depending on the

maturity of the gymnast, rate of change of the curvature, and degree of curvature. Surgical correction is recommended if the curvature of the spine creates compromise to the cardiovascular/pulmonary function of the gymnast.

Discogenic back pain

Disc pathology has been classified as disc bulges, disc herniations, disc protrusions, disc extrusions, and disc degeneration. The medical literature has identified that up to one-third of the normal population may have disc bulges and yet are asymptomatic (Boden *et al.*, 1990). The finding of a disc bulge on a gymnast with a painful back condition may not necessarily be the cause of their pain. It is recommended to search for other causes of the back pain that may be of greater influence to the pain the gymnast perceives. Disc herniation, protrusions, and extrusions may be more symptomatic depending on their influence on the spinal cord and the spinal nerves. Disc degeneration has a high correlation with the complaints of back pain.

The disc may be damaged by an acute traumatic event or by chronic mechanical loading of the disc. Gymnasts with significant disc pathology find it difficult to sit for prolonged periods of time. Sitting with an unsupported back may actually decrease the stress on the facets and increase the load on the disc when compared to standing. Disc degeneration places more stress on the facet joints and may create facet pathology compared to disc herniation.

The mainstay of treatment for discogenic pain is PT. Manual medicine to improve the alignment is of benefit too. If pain persists with conservative care, then invasive use of steroids with epidurals may be of value for disc herniations/protrusions/extrusions. The tertiary care would be a form of disectomy surgery. Fortunately, most gymnasts respond well to the conservative care with the therapeutic interventions.

Pelvic floor dysfunction

The impact forces that the female gymnast sustains during acrobatic and trampoline skills place significant stress on her pelvic floor. Published studies (Nygaard *et al.*, 1994; Eliasson *et al.*, 2002) have demonstrated that 80% of elite female trampoline gymnasts and as high as 67% of female artistic gymnasts report involuntary urinary leakage during training. Compared to other sports including basketball, tennis, field hockey, track, swimming, volleyball, softball, and golf, the female gymnast has the highest occurrence of urinary incontinence. The intraabdominal forces with gymnastics may become so intense and the female urethra is so short that the pelvic floor is frequently unable to prevent urinary leakage. Medical research has demonstrated the importance of the pelvic floor in the facilitation of stability in lumbopelvic stability. Fatigue of the pelvic floor muscles creates increased urinary leakage as demonstrated by medical research with increased leakage occurring near the end of a gymnastics training session (Eliasson *et al.*, 2002). Male gymnasts also sustain high-impact forces, however, due to the increased length of the male urethra, urinary leakage has not been reported. Instead of stress-induced incontinence, the male gymnast sustains symptoms of lumbopelvic pain.

The pelvic floor muscles are required to quickly and forcefully respond to the impact forces to withstand the deceleration forces of the abdominal viscera. Gymnasts, unfortunately, have shown increased laxity of noncontractile elements (reduction in their tissue collagen concentration). This may be related to the increased prevalence of hypermobile joints found in the gymnast. The combination of the forces applied to the pelvic floor and the reduction of tissue collagen concentration may well lead to the stress urinary incontinence demonstrated (Kruger *et al.*, 2007).

Musculoskeletal ultrasonography of the pelvic floor musculature of gymnasts compared to ballet dancers, and others has shown that gymnasts actually have adapted to the impact forces of their sport. Compared to the other sports studied, gymnasts demonstrated increased mean diameter of their pubovisceral muscles and greater bladder neck descent with a valsalva activity (Bo, 2004).

The use of the pelvic floor musculature to assist in lumbopelvic stability has been well known in the dance art of ballet as the dancer learns from an early age to "lift" through their floor. Some professional ballet companies utilize musculoskeletal ultrasonography to allow the ballerina to see her pelvic floor muscles contract. This is a useful tool that can be incorporated into therapeutic exercise programs to improve lumbopelvic stability, which may not only assist with the reduction of stress urinary incontinence but also reduce lumbopelvic mechanical pain.

It is recommended that gymnasts learn to perform Kegels exercises as part of their therapeutic intervention for low back pain. A simple way of incorporation of this into their program is to have the gymnast learn to co-contract the pelvic floor with the transverse abdominal muscle to start each spinal stability exercise. Once these muscles have been contracted, then the gluteal and other abdominal muscles are contracted and the exercise is then performed. By incorporation of this extra step, urinary incontinence may be decreased, spinal stabilization may be enhanced, and back pain may be reduced.

Further research

There is a need for continued research in the understanding of the biomechanics of the gymnastics skills. The forces applied to the human body by the various gymnastics skills continue to increase as the difficulty of the skills continue to progress with each change of the Code of Points by the International Federation of Gymnastics (FIG). It is important to continue investigation on how high these forces are and how they affect the anatomical structures of the immature and mature gymnasts' musculoskeletal systems.

The equipment used in gymnastics evolves over time and it is vital to have an in-depth understanding of how the equipment influences the gymnasts' skills, the forces applied to their bodies, and the forces absorbed from their bodies. Further research in this area is beneficial to help minimize the stress the gymnast sustains and yet, maximize their performance.

A continued investigation into the benefits of therapeutic modalities, core exercises, and strapping/taping/bracing of the spine is of high importance to enhance the recovery of the gymnast's spinal injuries.

Further understanding of the pathophysiology of a concussion, functional and structural evaluation of this injury, and therapeutic intervention for treatment of a concussion is of vital need for all athletes and nonathletes alike.

Summary

Spinal and head injuries are complex in nature and the understanding of these injuries continue to develop over time as medical technology improves and evidence-based medicine sheds light on these acute and chronic injuries. It is important for the coach and medical professional to keep current their understanding of the mechanics of the sport of gymnastics and how the forces of the skills affect the gymnasts' bodies. Therapeutic interventions for the treatment of spinal and head trauma continue to evolve. This chapter has provided sample treatment protocols that may prove beneficial for the coach and medical professional to utilize with their injured gymnast.

References

Bo, K. (2004) Urinary incontinence, pelvic floor dysfunction in exercise and sport. *Sports Medicine,* **34** (7), 451–464.

Boden, S., Davis, D., and Dina, T. (1990) Abnormal magnetic resonance scans of the lumbar spine in asymptomatic subjects; a prospective investigation. *Journal of Bone and Joint Surgery, America,* **72**, 403–408.

Cavalier, R., Herman, M., Cheung, E., and Pizzutillo, P. (2006) Spondylolysis and spondylolisthesis in children and adolescents: diagnosis, natural history, and nonsurgical management. *Journal of the American Academy of Orthopedic Surgeons,* **14** (7), 417–424.

Cohen, S. and Raja, S. (2007) Pathogenesis, diagnosis, and treatment of lumbar zygapophysial (facet) joint pain. *Anesthesiology,* **106** (3), 591–614.

Daneshvar, D., Nowinski, C., McKee, A., and Cantu, R. (2011) The epidemiology of sport-related concussion. *Clinics in Sports Medicine,* **30** (1), 1–17.

Eliasson, K., Larsson, T., and Mattsson, E. (2002) Prevalence of stress incontinence in nulliparous elite trampolinists. *Scandinavian Journal of Medicine and Science in Sports,* **12** (2), 106–110.

Ghormley, R. (1933) Low back pain with special reference to the articular facets, with presentation of an operative procedure. *Journal of the American Medical Association,* **101**, 1773–1777.

Guskiewicz, K. and McLeod, T. (2011) Pediatric sports-related concussion. *Physical Medicine and Rehabilitation,* **3**, 353–364.

Harringe, M., Renstrom, P., and Werber, S. (2007) Injury incidence, mechanism and diagnosis in top-level team gymnastics: a prospective study conducted over one season. *Scandinavian Journal of Medicine and Science in Sports,* **17**, 115–119.

Jull, G. and Janda, V. (1987) Muscles and motor control in low back pain. In: L.T. Twomey and J.R. Taylor (eds), *Physical Therapy for the Low Back: Clinics in Physical Therapy,* pp. 253–278. Churchill Livingstone, New York.

Katz, D. and Scerpella, T. (2003) Anterior and middle column thoracolumbar spine injuries in young female gymnasts. Report of seven cases and review of literature. *The American Journal of Sports Medicine,* **31**, 611–616.

Kruger, J., Dietz, H., and Murphy, B. (2007) Pelvic floor function in elite nulliparous athletes. *Ultrasound in Obstetrics & Gynecology,* **30**, 81–85.

Lonstein, J. (1999) Spondylolisthesis in children: cause, natural history, and management. *Spine,* **24**, 2640–2648.

Marek, S., Cramer, J., Fincher, A., Massey, L., Dangelmaier, S., Purkayastha, S., Fitz, K., and Culbertson, J. (2005) Acute effects of static and proprioceptive neuromuscular facilitation stretching on muscle strength and power output. *Journal of Athletic Training,* **40** (2), 94–103.

McCrory, P., Meeuwisse, W., Johnston, K., Dvorak, J., Aubry, M., Molloy, M., and Cantu, R. (2009) 2008 consensus statement on concussion in sport – the 3rd International Conference on concussion in sport held in Zurich. *South African Journal of Sports Medicine,* **21** (2), 36–46.

Meyerding, H. (1932) Spondylolisthesis. *Surgery, Gynecology & Obstetrics,* **54**, 371–377.

Nygaard, I., Thompson, F., Svengalis, S., and Albright, J. (1994) Urinary incontinence in elite nulliparous altheles. *Obstetrics & Gynecology,* **84**, 183–187.

O'Kane, J., Levy, M., Pietila, K., Caine, D., and Schiff, M. (2011) Survey of injuries in Seattle area levels 4 to 10 female club gymnasts. *ClinicalJournal ofSport Medicine,* **21**, 486–492.

Sorensen, K. (1964) *Scheuermann's Juvenile Kyphosis: Clinical Appearances, Radiography, Aetiology, and Prognosis.* Munksgaard, Copenhagen.

Standaert, C. (2005) The diagnosis and management of lumbar spondylolysis. *Operative Techniques in Sports Medicine,* **13**, 101–107.

Standaert, C. and Herring, S. (2000) Spondyloysis: a critical review. *British Journal of Sports Medicine,* **34**, 415–422.

Tanchev, P., Dzherov, A., Parushev, A., Dikov, D., and Todorov, M. (2000) Scoliosis in rhythmic gymnasts. *Spine,* **25**, 1367–1372.

Tribus, C. (1998) Scheuermann's kyphosis in adolescents and adults: diagnosis and management. *Journal of the American Academy of Orthopedic Surgeons*, **6**, 36–43.

Wiltse, L., Widell, E., and Jackson, D. (1975) Fatigue fracture: the basic lesion isthmic spondylolisthesis. *Journal of Bone and Joint Surgery*, **57**, 17–22.

Recommended reading

Akuthota, V., Ferreiro, A., Moore, T., and Fredericson M. (2008) Core stability exercise principles. *Current Sports Medicine Reports*, **7** (1), 39–44.

Bennett, D., Nassar, L., and Delano, M. (2006) Lumbar spine MRI in the elite-level female gymnast with low back pain. *Skeletal Radiology*, **35** (7), 503–509.

Caine, D. and Nassar, L. (2005) Gymnastics injuries. In: D.J. Caine and N. Maffulli (eds), *Epidemiology of Pediatric Sports Injuries; Individual Sports*, vol. 48, pp. 18–58., Karger, Basel.

Faulkner, K. (2010) The female pelvic floor in women's artistic gymnastics. *Sport Health*, **28** (2), 32–33.

Kokkonen, J. and Lauritzen, S. (1995) Isotonic strength and endurance gains through PNF stretching. *Medicine and Science in Sports and Exercise*, **27** (Suppl.), S22.

Kruse, D. and Lemmen, B. (2009) Spine Injuries in the sport of gymnastics. *Current Sports Medicine Reports*, **8** (1), 20–28.

Marshall, S., Covassin, S., Dick, R., Nassar, L., and Agel, J. (2007) Descriptive epidemiology of collegiate women's gymnastics injuries: National Collegiate Athletic Association Injury Surveillance System, 1988–1989 through 2003–2004. *Journal of Athletic Training*, **42** (2), 234–240.

McNeal, J. and Sands, W. (2001) Static stretching reduces power production in gymnasts. *Technique*, **21** (10), 5–6.

Chapter 14
Gymnastics injury prevention

Marita L. Harringe[1], Dennis J. Caine[2]

[1]Stockholm Sports Trauma Research Center *and* Care Sciences and Society, Karolinska Institutet, Stockholm, Sweden
[2]College of Education and Human Development, University of North Dakota, Grand Forks, ND, USA

Introduction

Avoiding injury is essential if one is to reach top-level gymnastics. Although it is impossible to eliminate all injuries, attempts to reduce them are obviously warranted. Prevention strategies deal with intrinsic factors such as physical and mental preparation and extrinsic factors such as the environment, safety equipment, and rules and regulations surrounding the gymnastics discipline. The preparation of a gymnast is to achieve goals for success, but to be successful the gymnast must be correctly prepared and, as far as possible, remain injury-free. This chapter is based on the scientific evidence regarding different aspects of injury prevention. To find the correct injury preventive strategy is not easily accomplished and the process is time consuming.

Sports injury prevention research involves a "sequence of prevention" (van Mechelen *et al.*, 1992). First, research establishes the extent of injury. Second, research explores its etiology (i.e., the causes and implications of injury). Third, research creates a prevention strategy to reduce the injury burden. Last, research evaluates the effectiveness of the implemented prevention strategy by reexamining the extent of injury (Figure 14.1, also described in Chapter 10). From a research perspective, it is preferable to evaluate the effect of preventive measures by means of a randomized

control trial (RCT) (Meeuwisse & Bahr, 2009). RCTs and quasi-experimental studies regularly compare new interventions to routine training protocols. Those studies typically cluster random participants by team or school in order to avoid cross-contamination among teammates. Unfortunately, it is not easy to set up an RCT in an ongoing high-level sport such as gymnastics, which is continuously changing with respect to skill level, technique, equipment, apparatus, and the FIG (Fédération International de Gymnastique) Code of Points.

There are only a few studies that have scientifically tested preventive measures in gymnastics. Additionally, to date, no studies have examined factors that impact the likelihood of a prevention strategy being adopted by the gymnastics community (i.e., translational research). However, studies in other sports have shown that it is difficult to implement injury prevention programs unless the extra practice also adds a quality or improved performance to the sport itself. The fact that the prevention programs may reduce the amount of injuries does not seem to be enough. One reason may be that prevention programs are time consuming, and to be effective should be implemented before injury—when it actually does not seem to be needed. A change in behavior must therefore be achieved. If the prevention programs are considered ordinary training and not extra training, this may be accomplished. With respect to what is known about learning and behavior we believe that prevention programs should be implemented from a young age. The prevention programs should be regarded as recovery and reactivation of

Gymnastics, First Edition. Edited by Dennis J. Caine, Keith Russell and Liesbeth Lim. © 2013 International Olympic Committee. Published 2013 by John Wiley & Sons, Ltd.

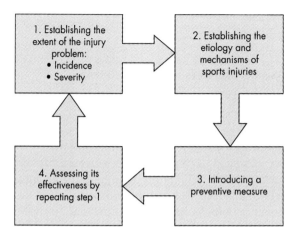

Figure 14.1 Four-step sequence of injury prevention research. (Source: Van Mechelen W., Hlobil H., Kemper J.C.G. (1992) Springer Healthcare © Adis Data Information BV 2012. All rights reserved.)

the neuromuscular system and the body control, essential for the performance, not as extra practice. Since there are few studies regarding prevention of injury in gymnastics, recommendations in this chapter are in some cases drawn and presented from studies carried out in other sports.

Intrinsic strategies

Specific balance and agility training, joint stability and neuromuscular exercises, plyometric strength training as well as general strength, and stretching exercises are included in successful prevention programs in sports such as soccer and European team handball (Schiff *et al.*, 2010). These preventive measures are also included in ordinary gymnastics training, and several of the exercises, used in prevention programs, originate from gymnastics. The neuromuscular control has to be working properly in order to avoid injury and since gymnasts spend a tremendous amount of time in practice, fatigue leading to decreased neuromuscular control may be a problem. Consequently, effective recovery of the neuromuscular control system would be one means of prevention. This may be achieved by rest, proper nutrition, and neuromuscular control exercises such as joint stability training and basic balance and agility training.

Joint stability

The stability of a joint depends on active as well as passive structures such as the joint capsule, ligaments, and deep stabilizing muscles. These structures provide joint stiffness while large force-producing muscles enable movements. The demands on each and every structure are high in gymnastics, especially since gymnasts are strong and at the same time flexible. Gymnasts practice to perfection, which means that they spend several hours repeating and practicing a skill. Although it may seem as if the muscles and the neuromuscular control system work properly there is a risk of fatigue in the deep stabilizing system. Decreased neuromuscular control of the deep stabilizing muscles may finally lead to functional joint instability, delayed muscle onset, pain, and severe injury. The importance of a well-working muscle system is obvious for a gymnast and stabilizing muscles of the joints do not seem to recover without specific activation. Therefore, a program including low-intensity specific exercises may help the recovery and prevent more severe injuries to occur. Since warm-up is part of the preparation of a gymnast, these exercises would preferably be implemented in the warm-up and target one or more joints. Balance boards, elastic bands, and gym balls as well as ordinary gymnastics equipment may be fun and helpful tools in this practice. There are several books and scientific articles presenting specific exercises for strengthening the core and joints such as the knee, ankle, and shoulder. A few exercises to provide stiffness of the lower back are presented later in this chapter.

Muscles contributing to lumbar stiffness

Muscles such as the transversus abdominis, obliquus internus, diaphragm, iliocostalis, multifidus, and quadratus lumborum have been suggested to be active in protecting and stabilizing the lumbar spine. Of the local muscles, the transversus abdominis and the lumbar multifidus are the most discussed and studied muscles to especially contribute to lumbar stiffness. However, since the transversus abdominis muscle works closely with, and sometimes fuses with, the obliquus internus, the obliquus internus may also be considered an important contributor to the stiffness of the lumbar spine. The transversus abdominis is the abdominal muscle most closely associated with control of intraabdominal pressure and it also influences stiffness and intersegmental motion of the lumbar spine through its connection to the thoracolumbar fascia. Furthermore, this muscle preactivates during a movement of the upper or lower extremity, even before the primary movers of the actual extremity. This activation is delayed in patients with low back pain. The multifidus muscles are best developed in the lumbar region of the spine and their contribution to lumbar stiffness has been shown in a variety of studies. These muscles are impaired in patients with low back pain and recovery of the multifidus muscles does not appear to be automatic after resolution of an acute, first-episode of low back pain.

Prevention of nonspecific low back pain

Injury involving the low back is not uncommon among gymnasts and low back pain is a common complaint. Specific segmental exercises of the lumbar muscles have shown promising results regarding treatment and prevention of low back pain in young teamgym gymnasts (Harringe *et al.*, 2007). The idea is to add specific, low-intensity exercises to the lower back, as a complement to the ordinary strength and preparation training for gymnasts. The exercises should be implemented in the regular training, for example, in the warm-up, and be continuously performed. This type of training has also been used with success in the treatment of more severe injuries such as disc herniations and spondylolysis (O'Sullivan *et al.*, 1997). However, it is important to remember that the exercises do not replace ordinary trunk muscle training. A study on collegiate gymnasts performing a 15-minutes general trunk muscle training program, twice a week, 10 weeks preseason, also appeared to reduce episodes of low back pain (Durall *et al.*, 2009). As long as there is no fatigue or injury the core muscles work properly and co-activate without specific exercises. However, once there is disturbed activity such as fatigue or injury the deep stabilizing muscles do not work properly. To ensure well-functioning core muscles, the specific

exercises should be introduced as a complement to ordinary trunk muscle training.

Specific exercises for lumbar stiffness

In the early 1990s, Richardson and Jull (1995) presented specific muscle exercises to control the lumbar spine. The specific exercises were suggested to reactivate the local muscles of the lumbar spine and to control pain in patients with low back pain. The base for this training is the draw-in action, also called abdominal hollowing. It is an isometric muscle contraction to not only activate the transversus abdominis and/or obliquus internus but also enhance co-activation with the lumbar multifidus muscles. The abdominal hollowing is performed by gently drawing in the abdominal wall, especially of the lower abdominal area. It is an isometric contraction and the time length for which the exercise is held, as well as to maintain a normal rate of breathing, is important. A pressure bio-feedback unit (Chattanooga group, Inc., USA) (Figure 14.2) may be used to control for correct muscle contraction.

The device is helpful, in particular during the learning phase, for guidance of performing the muscle contraction correctly. The specific training

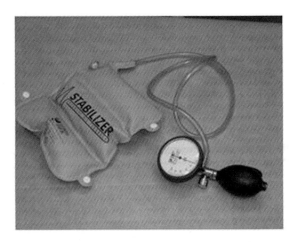

Figure 14.2 A pressure bio-feedback unit. The unit is inflated to 70 mmHg pressure and placed under the lower abdomen while the subject is lying in prone position. When the correct contraction is performed, pressure decreases by approximately 6–8 mmHg.

is commenced in the four point kneeling and prone positions, of which the four point kneeling position may be the easiest to start with (Figure 14.3). In this position the rectus abdominis muscle is difficult to activate and thus helpful since the aim of the training is to activate the deeper part of the abdominal wall. Once the gymnast knows how to perform the exercise, the positions should become more sport-specific. The gymnast may, for example, perform the abdominal hollowing in a static position such as a handstand or in a dynamic situation walking on the hands or in a tumble or a vault (see Weeks 5–8 in Section "Eight-weeks introduction program"). However, it is important to keep one or two of the basic exercises to ensure correct performance and to ensure a reactivation of potentially fatigued muscles. The bio-pressure feedback unit is fun to use and, when used correctly, provides accurate feedback.

Eight-weeks introduction program

Hereunder an introduction program to the specific muscle control exercises is presented (Harringe *et al.*, 2007). The idea is to introduce an exercise to reactivate fatigued or injured deep stabilizing muscles of the lower back. It should be implemented during ordinary training. Once the gymnasts master the abdominal hollowing it may be an exercise to use in the warm-up, just to make sure that the muscles work properly, or in different training modalities for core stability. There are several books on core stability or core training and these may give ideas on how to progress with the training. However, the key to success is to keep it simple in the learning phase to be sure to target the deep muscles. Remember that these exercises complement heavy load training and it is important to ensure correct technique in the exercises.

Weeks 1–2: Introduce the abdominal hollowing in prone and four-point kneeling positions (Figure 14.3). Use the pressure bio-feedback unit (Figure 14.2) to control for correct execution in prone position. Each exercise should be repeated 10×10 seconds and included in the warm-up.

Weeks 3–4: Keep the basic exercise in the four-point kneeling position. Add diagonally elevation of the arm and leg in the prone position. Repeat each exercise 10×10 seconds. Also add abdominal hollowing in an upright position on a balance board. Position the body on both feet, with slightly flexed knees while moving the arms up and down in front of the body. The exercise is easy to perform, although it increases the demands on the deep stabilizers of the lumbar spine. The exercise should be performed for 5 minutes at each training session. To increase the difficulty the gymnast may add some weight, for example, light dumbbells in the hands, while moving the arms up and down. However, it is important to keep the control of the abdominal hollowing during the exercise.

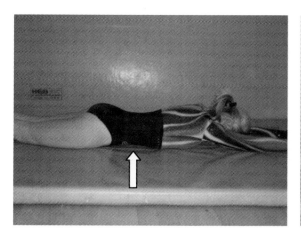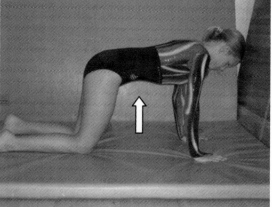

Figure 14.3 Abdominal hollowing in a prone and a four point kneeling position. (Source: Harringe *et al.* (2007) with kind permission from Springer Science and Business Media.)

Weeks 5–8: Continue with the exercises from previous weeks. Add sports-specific positions with the instruction to keep emphasis on the abdominal hollowing. In the study on teamgym gymnasts by Harringe *et al.* (2007), 12 basic trampette skills were added. Unstable surfaces such as balance boards, trampolines, and trampettes have shown to activate stabilizing muscles of the lumbar spine and thus improve core stability. The sports specificity of the exercises should be chosen to fit the different disciplines.

Prevention of lower extremity injuries

The lower extremity is the most commonly injured body region in Artistic Gymnastics. Injuries involving the knee and ankle, in particular, occur frequently in Artistic Gymnastics (see Chapter 10). There is little gymnastics-based evidence on how to prevent these injuries, although some studies, in other sports, suggest that general strength training, neuromuscular control exercises, and plyometric strength training may reduce injuries to the lower extremity (Schiff *et al.*, 2010). Unpublished data on recreational gymnasts suggest that plyometric training may improve the gymnasts' performance and reduce the frequency of knee injuries and a limited study on young artistic female gymnasts showed reduced pain with neuromuscular control exercises (Marini *et al.*, 2008).

In studies on soccer and European team handball different control and balance exercises combined with plyometric training have reduced the incidence of anterior cruciate ligament injuries (Schiff *et al.*, 2010). Exercises including cutting and landing have been used and may also be useful in gymnastics since many injuries occur due to poor landing technique, and specific focus on landing has been proposed in the prevention of gymnastics injuries. Plyometric strength training engages the muscle-tendon stretch-shortening cycle and studies have shown rapid effects on strength gain with this type of technique. A newly published study set up in a biomechanics laboratory concluded that only one training session (six sets of three repetitions) using a countermovement jump may improve performance through neural modulation (Hirayama *et al.*, 2012). This could possibly mean

that this technique may help the gymnasts to regain neural control after intensive gymnastics training. However, the plyometric training is intensive and should not be performed when the gymnast is tired. Most studies implement the prevention exercises in the warm-up and the most successful prevention programs have been carried out during the entire season, linked to education of coaches and athletes. Further studies are needed in order to establish its role in gymnastics injury prevention.

Prevention of upper extremity injuries

Injuries to the upper extremity (e.g., shoulder or wrist) are more common in male gymnasts compared to female counterparts (in whom ankle and lower back injuries predominate) possibly due to the different types of apparatus used in men's gymnastics. However, wrist pain, as well as more severe wrist injury, is common in the young growing gymnast. Most scientific work in this field consists of case reports and some studies suggest possible, though not tested, preventive strategies (DiFiori *et al.*, 2006). Strength training and stabilizing exercises as well as taping or bandaging are frequently used in ordinary training. Biomechanical and clinical studies indicate that protective wrist bracing may prevent acute wrist injury; however, this preventive measure has not been tested in a controlled trial on gymnasts. Another approach would be to reduce the impact by alternating between different skills such as swinging and support-type movements during practice. An optimal gymnastics technique and recovery can most probably minimize the high impact on the body structures.

Muscle and joint symmetry

A decreased joint or muscle range of motion may result in bad timing and asymmetric force transformation through the body. Using the take-off going into a tumble or vault as an example, the forces are transformed from the ankle through the body into the gymnastics skill. The timing has to be exact in order to perform the perfect skill. If there is an asymmetry in muscle or joint range of motion the forces may be unevenly transformed and possibly result in poor technique and increased risk of injury. This is of course even more important in advanced skills since the forces are greater and consequently the impact on the gymnast higher. A slight mistake may be devastating. Equal attention to the right and left side is necessary and may prevent injuries.

Mental preparation

It is not necessarily the most difficult skills that cause acute injury. It has been shown that gymnasts are often injured in skills they know well. Since gymnastics is a very demanding sport and focus and control are qualities needed, mental preparation should be included in the prevention of injury. It would seem important to put emphasis on quality of workouts rather than repetitiveness at all times. Imagery techniques that cause no physical impact may allow a gymnast to train more hours without increased injury risk. However, the role of mental practice in reducing injuries has not been investigated in gymnastics.

An interesting but underresearched area of injury risk in gymnastics is the role played by psychosocial factors. A relation between extent of negative life stress and the frequency and severity of injury has been reported in several studies. It would seem important that gymnasts be encouraged to share with their coach, medical personnel, and parents any concerns they might have, including difficulty of skills practiced or pain experienced. "No pain— no gain" is inappropriate in gymnastics.

Extrinsic strategies

Safety equipment and gymnastics apparatus

Safety equipment such as foam pits, trampolines, bungee straps, and spotting belts are frequently used in daily practice sessions. This equipment is helpful not only in reaching new levels of performance but also in reducing the impact and risks for injuries to occur. The apparatus and landing mats have changed over time due to the continuous development of the sport, not only with respect to level of performance but also due to the protection of the gymnasts. During the last 10 years, new landing material to reduce the ground reaction forces has been introduced. These mats seem to put more strain on the forefoot, but less total ground reaction force. The construction and model/form of the vaulting apparatus (the new Pegasus) to lower the incidence of head and neck injuries, and the coverage around the trampolines and springboards are also examples on what has been done to prevent and reduce the incidence of injuries in gymnastics. However, the effectiveness of these preventive measures has not been investigated.

Health support system

Regular medical check-ups are important and necessary in prevention of injury. However, medical monitoring of gymnasts is rare in gymnastics settings below the college level. We recommend a preparticipation physical examination (PPE) for each gymnast prior to entry in competitive gymnastics, before any change in competitive level, and before returning to practice following injury. The medical history and physical examination can identify underlying conditions that require special attention or that predispose the gymnast to injury unless appropriate preventive measures are followed.

Gymnasts are generally young and growth should be monitored closely, especially since the injury risk may increase during periods of rapid growth. Research has shown that physeal strength is decreased during pubescence. Furthermore, bone mineralization may lag behind bone linear growth during the growth spurt, leading to an increased risk for injury. It is important and may be injury preventive to individualize training and skill development to accommodate possible size, physique, strength, performance, and maturity differences among chronological age peers. Thorough medical check-ups should be carried out to keep track of growth and maturation as well as nutrition, recovery, and overload. If risk behavior or pain can be captured early in time, injuries may be avoided or at least the severity of the injuries reduced.

We also recommend that gymnastics clubs include within their cost structure sufficient funds to hire an athletic trainer, physical therapist and/ or a physician with interest/expertise in sports injuries, at least on a part-time basis. This health professional should be available to provide immediate care of injuries and to supervise rehabilitation as well as to oversee special rehabilitation programs for injured or injury-prone gymnasts prior to returning to practice and competition. Early recognition of injury is important, and is improved by the presence of competent medical personnel. If the availability of a trainer or therapist is limited, their time is perhaps best focused on advanced-level gymnasts who appear at greatest risk of injury.

Gymnastics is a very demanding sport as well as an aesthetic sport. This may lead to body fixation and an increased risk for developing sports anorexia. Low levels of nutrition may lead to decreased performance and injury. A recent study reported low levels of vitamin D in elite female gymnasts (Lovell, 2008). Other studies have shown low total energy intake as well as low levels of micronutrients such as iron, zinc, and calcium (Caine *et al.*, 2001).

If possible, a multidisciplinary team including coaches, medicine support staff, nutritionists, and psychologists should be working together regarding the strategies for prevention of injury.

Training diary and periodic planning

A training diary may be useful in detecting and preventing the gymnast from injury. A diary should be easy to fill out and may contain preprinted questions. It should include training parameters such as skill level, training volume, training intensity, and training quality. The diary should also include other important factors for optimal performance such as how the gymnast feels today—alert or tired, and other outside gymnastics events that may interfere with gymnastics and rest and sleeping quality. Furthermore, a diary is helpful in planning the practice and in the transition from skill training to routine training. This transition takes time and should be well planned.

Full routines put another type of strain and demand on the gymnast. An emphasis on quality of workouts rather than repetition may be injury preventive. It is important to slowly increase the intensity and carry over from regular preparation and practice to full routine performance and competition. A perfect technique is necessary to decrease the risk for injury and therefore the gymnast has to be well prepared and only perform skills and routines he or she feels secure with during competition.

Education

Education is important and may provide coaches, gymnasts, and parents with knowledge important for the right decisions to be made regarding injury prevention. Through education the coaches should keep themselves updated with respect to changes in gymnastics including equipment and apparatus, skill techniques and levels of difficulty. In addition, education should include knowledge about growth and maturation of children and adolescents as well as an understanding that an injury, especially if insufficiently rehabilitated, may predispose the gymnast to another injury or recurrence of the same injury. A coach has to have adequate and demonstrated gymnastics competence for the level of gymnastics he or she is teaching. We recommend that in order to be hired as a gymnastics coach he or she should meet a minimum level of qualification as determined by the national gymnastics federation. With the USA Women's Artistic Gymnastics program, for example, one may achieve four progressive certification options: (1) Instructor, (2) Jr. Olympic Development Coach, (3) Jr. Olympic Team Coach, and (4) National Coach. Each certification offers a unique set of courses to equip coaches with the knowledge required to achieve excellence and better ensure the safety of gymnasts.

The first line of protection from injury belongs with the gymnast. A well-educated and thoroughly trained gymnast may detect and avoid potentially injurious situations. Furthermore, the gymnast has to be educated from an early age to distinguish between different types of pain and to listen to the signals from his or her body. Pain may signal possible or actual injury, or the achievement of optimum workload to produce a physical conditioning effect. Studies have shown that young gymnasts are capable of distinguishing between soreness from exertion and acute pain owing to injury. This is important knowledge, and may help the gymnast and those surrounding him or her to make better decisions about pain management and continued practice.

Further research

There is no doubt that gymnastics participation brings with it a wealth of personal and health-related benefits. Physical activity reduces the risk of premature mortality in general, and of coronary heart disease, hypertension, colon cancer, obesity, and diabetes mellitus in particular. However, gymnastics participation may also give rise to injury, which may undermine the many benefits of being physically active and contribute to long-term disability. Establishing sound epidemiologic research to determine the rate and severity of gymnastics-related injury and then using these data as basis for systematically identifying risk factors and developing effective prevention interventions is imperative.

Gymnastics lacks good-quality descriptive data, the fundamental building blocks of epidemiology, and which provides a basis for conducting meaningful analytical studies. This is reflected in the generally sparse listing of intrinsic and extrinsic risk factors and the extreme paucity of epidemiologic studies on preventive measures (see Chapter 10). Furthermore, most of the epidemiological research on injury in gymnastics was published prior to 2000, a major concern given the ever-changing nature of skills practiced and performed in this sport. This finding is especially disturbing given the young age of many gymnastics athletes and the relatively high incidence and severity of gymnastics injury reported in the literature.

There is a pressing need for studies designed to test risk factors and to identify and determine the effect of injury-prevention measures on reducing the rate of injury among gymnasts. Injury-prevention measures of particular interest include neuromuscular training programs, preseason conditioning, programs to enhance landing and skill mechanics, and use of taping and bracing to prevent ankle and wrist injuries. It is imperative that gymnastics organizations, including artistic, rhythmic, and trampoline, sponsor ongoing injury surveillance systems to provide an accurate picture of the incidence and severity of gymnastics-related injury and to serve as a basis for identifying and testing risk factors and preventive measures. Descriptive epidemiological studies inform us that injuries and conditions such as ankle sprains, heel pain, wrist pain, and low back pain occur frequently in gymnastics and require special attention. Increased frequency of injury following periods of competitive routine preparation, as well as per unit time during competition, also signal increased attention.

Summary

Prevention of injuries is highly important and has to be central for the team surrounding a gymnast. Few studies have investigated prevention programs and therefore little epidemiological evidence is available on how to actually prevent injuries in gymnastics. However, this chapter provides the reader with a summary of what we know today and can understand from previous epidemiology studies and health care professionals' experience. The basics of prevention must be to understand the sport, implement correct technique, and be sure to obtain adequate and complete recovery. Further research, including injury surveillance systems, is definitely needed to prevent gymnastics injuries and establish guidelines for gymnasts and coaches in the future.

References

Caine, D., Lewis, R., O'Connor, P., Howe, W., and Bass S. (2001) Does gymnastics training inhibit growth of females? *Clinical Journal of Sports Medicine*, **11**, 260–270.

DiFiori, J., Caine, D., and Malina, R. (2006). Wrist pain, distal radial growth plate injury, and ulnar variance in the young gymnast. *American Journal of Sports Medicine*, **34**, 840–849.

Durall, C.J., Udermann, B.E., Johansen, D.R., Gibson, B., Reineke, D.M., and Reuteman, P. (2009) The effects of preseason trunk muscle training on low back pain occurrence in women collegiate gymnasts. *Journal of Strength and Conditioning Research*, **23**, 86–92.

Harringe, M.L., Nordgren, J.S., Arvidsson, I., and Werner, S. (2007) Low back pain in young female gymnasts and the effect of specific segmental muscle control exercises of the lumbar spine: a prospective controlled intervention study. *Knee Surgery, Sports Traumatology, Athroscopy*, **15**, 1264–1271.

Hirayama, K., Yanai, T., Kanehisa, H., Fukunaga, T., and Kawakami, Y. (2012) Neural modulation of muscle-tendon control strategy after a single practice session. *Medicine and Science in Sports and Exercise*, doi: 10.1249/MSS.0b013e3182535da5.

Lovell, G. (2008) Vitamin D status of females in an elite gymnastics program. *Cinical Journal of Medicine*, **18**, 159–161.

Meeuwisse, W. and Bahr, R. (2009) A systematic approach to sports injury prevention, Chapter 2. In: R. Bahr and L. Engebretsen (eds), *Handbook of Sports Medicine and Science. Sports Injury Prevention, An IOC Medical Commission Publication*. Wiley-Blackwell Publishers, West Sussex.

Marini, M., Sgambati, E., Barni, E., Piazza, M., and Monaci, M. (2008) Pain syndromes in competitive elite female artistic gymnasts. Role of specific preventive-compensative activity. *International Journal of Anatomy and Embryology*, **113**, 1–8.

O'Sullivan, P.B., Twomey, L.T., and Allison, G.T. (1997) Evaluation of specific stabilizing exercise in the treatment of chronic low back pain with radiologic diagnosis of spondylolysis or spondylolisthesis. *Spine*, **22**, 2959–2967.

Richardson, C.A. and Jull, G.A. (1995) Motor control – pain control. What exercises would you prescribe?. *Manual Therapy*, **1**, 2–10.

Schiff, M., Caine, D., and O'Halleron, R. (2010) Injury prevention in sports. *American Journal of Lifestyle Medicine*, **4**, 42–64.

Van Mechelen, W., Hlobil, H., and Kemper, C.G. (1992) Incidence, severity, aetiology and prevention of sports injuries. A review of concepts. *Sports Medicine*, **14**, 82–99.

Recommended reading

Bahr, R. and Engebretsen L. (eds) (2009) *Handbook of Sports Medicine and Science. Sports Injury Prevention. An IOC Medical Commission Publication*. Wiley-Blackwell Publishers, West Sussex.

Bahr, R. (2003) Preventing sports injuries. In: R. Bahr and S. Maehlum (eds), *Clinical Guide to Sports Injuries*, pp. 41–53. Human Kinetics, Champaign, IL.

Hootman, J.M., Dick, R., and Agel, J. (2007) Epidemiology of collegiate injuries for 15 sports: summary and recommendations for injury prevention. *Journal of Athletic Training*, **42** (2), 311–319.

Jemmett, R. (2003) *Spinal Stabilization, The New Science of Back Pain*. 2nd edn. Novant Health Publishing, Halifax, NS.

Kolt, G. and Caine, D. (2010) Gymnastics. In: D. Caine, P. Harmer and M. Schiff (eds), *Epidemiology of Injury in Olympic Sports. Encyclopaedia of Sports Medicine*, vol. XVI, pp. 144–160. Wiley Blackwell Publishers (UK) and the IOC Medical Commission.

Schiff, M. and O'Halleron, R. (2010) Injury prevention in sports. In: D. Caine, P. Harmer, and M. Schiff (eds), *Epidemiology of Injury in Olympic Sports. Encyclopaedia of Sports Medicine*, vol. XVI, pp. 491–499. Wiley Blackwell Publishers (UK) and the IOC Medical Commission.

USA Gymnastics (2009) *Safety Course Handbook: Gymnastics Risk Management*. USA Gymnastics, Inc. Indianapolis, IN.

Weaver, J., Moore, C., and Howe, W. (1996) Injury prevention. In: D Caine, C. Caine, and K. Lindner (eds), *Epidemiology of Sports Injuries*, pp. 439–447. Human Kinetics Publishers, Champaign, IL.

Index

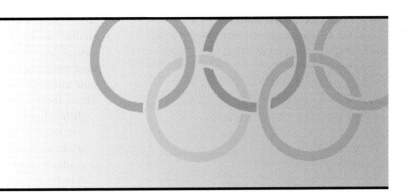

Gymnastics, First Edition. Edited by Dennis J. Caine, Keith Russell and Liesbeth Lim. © 2013 International Olympic Committee.
Published 2013 by John Wiley & Sons, Ltd.